I0875936

The Use of Nutritional Supplements and Antioxidants in Women's Infertility Treatment

In recent years, nutritional supplements and antioxidants have been increasingly considered as adjuncts in the management of female infertility. However, the scientific evidence supporting their use remains heterogeneous, and clinical decision-making in this area often lacks clear, evidence-informed guidance. This edited volume aims to provide a clinically oriented overview of the use of nutritional supplements and antioxidants in the treatment of women's infertility.

Clinicians, reproductive health specialists, and researchers who are involved in the care of women with infertility will welcome this structured, evidence-based overview of nutritional and antioxidant interventions within a clinical framework.

The Use of Nutritional Supplements and Antioxidants in Women's Infertility Treatment

A Clinical Guide

Edited by
Maryam Azizi-Kutenaei, MD, PhD
Fertility and Infertility Research Center
Hormozgan University of Medical Sciences
Bandar Abbas, Iran

Farzaneh Fesahat, PhD
Reproductive Immunology Research Center
Shahid Sadoughi University of Medical Sciences
Yazd, Iran

CRC Press
Taylor & Francis Group
Boca Raton London New York

CRC Press is an imprint of the
Taylor & Francis Group, an **informa** business

Designed cover image: Editors

First edition published 2027
by CRC Press
2385 NW Executive Center Drive, Suite 320, Boca Raton FL 33431

and by CRC Press
4 Park Square, Milton Park, Abingdon, Oxon, OX14 4RN

CRC Press is an imprint of Taylor & Francis Group, LLC

ISBN: 978-1-041-24362-5 (hbk)
ISBN: 978-1-041-23552-1 (pbk)
ISBN: 978-1-003-74154-1 (ebk)

DOI: 10.1201/9781003741541

Typeset in Palatino
by Apex CoVantage, LLC

Contents

Preface

Infertility is a complex clinical condition influenced by multiple biological, environmental, and lifestyle-related factors. In recent years, nutritional supplements and antioxidants have been increasingly considered as adjuncts in the management of female infertility. However, the scientific evidence supporting their use remains heterogeneous, and clinical decision-making in this area often lacks clear, evidence-informed guidance.

This edited volume aims to provide a clinically oriented overview of the use of nutritional supplements and antioxidants in the treatment of women's infertility. The chapters are written as narrative reviews by contributors with relevant clinical and research experience, each addressing a specific category of supplements, underlying mechanisms, or clinical contexts. The first chapter introduces the biological rationale and clinical background for supplement use in infertility, while the final chapter synthesizes the main findings and discusses their implications for clinical practice. Rather than promoting supplementation as a universal or definitive solution, this book seeks to critically examine existing evidence; highlight areas of consensus and uncertainty; and support clinicians in making informed, patient-centered decisions. Particular attention is paid to clinical applicability, safety considerations, and the limitations of current research.

This book is intended for clinicians, reproductive health specialists, and researchers who are involved in the care of women with infertility and who require a structured, evidence-based overview of nutritional and antioxidant interventions within a clinical framework.

Contributors

Ali Afrasiabi
Reproductive Immunology Research Center
Shahid Sadoughi University of Medical Science
Yazd, Iran

Somaye Dehghani-Sanij
Department of Medical Library and Information Science
School of Health Management and Information Sciences
Iran University of Medical Sciences
Tehran, Iran

Samaneh Harimi
Reproductive Immunology Research Center
Shahid Sadoughi University of Medical Sciences
Yazd, Iran

Amir Masoud Firouzabadi
Department of Biology
Ashk. C., Islamic Azad University
Ashkezar, Yazd, Iran

Mohammadjavad Mohammadifard
Reproductive Immunology Research Center
Shahid Sadoughi University of Medical Sciences
Yazd, Iran

Negar Nouri
Department of Genetics and Molecular Biology
Faculty of Medicine
Isfahan University of Medical Sciences
Isfahan, Iran

Abolfazl Taghinejad
Reproductive Immunology Research Center
Shahid Sadoughi University of Medical Sciences
Yazd, Iran

Minoo Vahedi Raad
Fertility and Infertility Research Center
Hormozgan University of Medical Sciences
Bandar Abbas, Iran

Erfan Zaker
Skin Diseases and Leishmaniasis Research Center
Department of Dermatology
Isfahan University of Medical Sciences
Isfahan, Iran

Hadi Zare-Zardini
Department of Biomedical Engineering
Meybod University
Meybod, Iran

1 Introduction

Hadi Zare-Zardini, Somaye Dehghani-Sanij, Maryam Azizi-Kutenaei, and Farzaneh Fesahat

1.1 BACKGROUND ON FEMALE INFERTILITY

1.1.1 Definition and Epidemiology

Infertility is a complex and multifactorial condition defined by the World Health Organization (WHO) as the failure to achieve a clinical pregnancy after 12 months or more of regular, unprotected sexual intercourse. This definition is widely accepted in both clinical practice and research. Infertility can be classified as primary (when a woman has never conceived) or secondary (when a woman has previously conceived but is unable to do so again) (1).

Globally, infertility affects an estimated 8–12% of couples of reproductive ages, translating to approximately 48–186 million individuals worldwide. The prevalence varies by region, with higher rates reported in certain parts of South Asia, sub-Saharan Africa, and the Middle East, often due to higher rates of untreated reproductive tract infections and limited access to healthcare (Table 1.1). In developed countries, lifestyle factors and delayed childbearing are increasingly significant contributors (2, 3).

1.1.2 Female Factor Infertility: An Overview

Female factor infertility is a significant component of reproductive challenges and is estimated to be responsible for approximately 40–50% of infertility cases, either as the sole cause or in combination with male factors. Infertility is therefore best understood as a shared issue between partners rather than a problem attributable to one sex alone. The causes of female infertility can be broadly categorized into several major groups. One of the most common is ovulatory disorders, which account for about 25–30% of female infertility (4). These disorders involve irregular, infrequent, or absent ovulation and include conditions such as polycystic ovary syndrome (PCOS); hypothalamic amenorrhea related to stress, weight changes, or excessive exercise; hyperprolactinemia caused by elevated prolactin levels; and premature ovarian insufficiency, in which ovarian function declines before the age of 40 (5). Another major category is tubal factor infertility, which results from damage to or blockage of the fallopian tubes. When the tubes are compromised, the sperm and oocyte cannot meet, preventing fertilization. Common causes of tubal damage include pelvic inflammatory disease, often secondary to sexually transmitted infections; endometriosis involving the tubes; and scarring or adhesions following previous pelvic or abdominal surgeries. Endometriosis itself is a chronic inflammatory condition characterized by the presence of endometrial-like tissue outside the uterine cavity, such as on the ovaries, peritoneum, or other pelvic structures. It affects an estimated 6–10% of women of reproductive age and is identified in up to 50% of women who present with infertility (6). Endometriosis can impair fertility through distortion of pelvic anatomy, formation of adhesions, altered immune and inflammatory responses, and negative effects on oocyte and embryo quality. Uterine and cervical factors also play a role in female infertility. Structural abnormalities of the uterus, such as fibroids (particularly submucosal fibroids that project into the uterine cavity), endometrial polyps, and congenital malformations like septate or bicornuate uterus, can interfere with implantation or increase the risk of miscarriage (7, 8). Cervical issues, including cervical stenosis or abnormalities of cervical mucus, may hinder the transport of sperm from the vagina into the uterine cavity and onward to the fallopian tubes (9). Another important cause is diminished ovarian reserve, which refers to a reduction in both the quantity and quality of available oocytes. While this decline is strongly associated with advancing maternal age, especially after the mid-30s, it can also occur earlier due to genetic predispositions; autoimmune conditions that target ovarian tissue; or iatrogenic factors such as chemotherapy, pelvic radiotherapy, or ovarian surgery. Diminished ovarian reserve reduces the likelihood of successful conception and is a key consideration in fertility evaluation and treatment planning (10, 11). Overall, understanding these categories of female factor infertility is essential for accurate diagnosis, individualized management, and timely intervention (Figure 1.2).

DOI: 10.1201/9781003741541-1

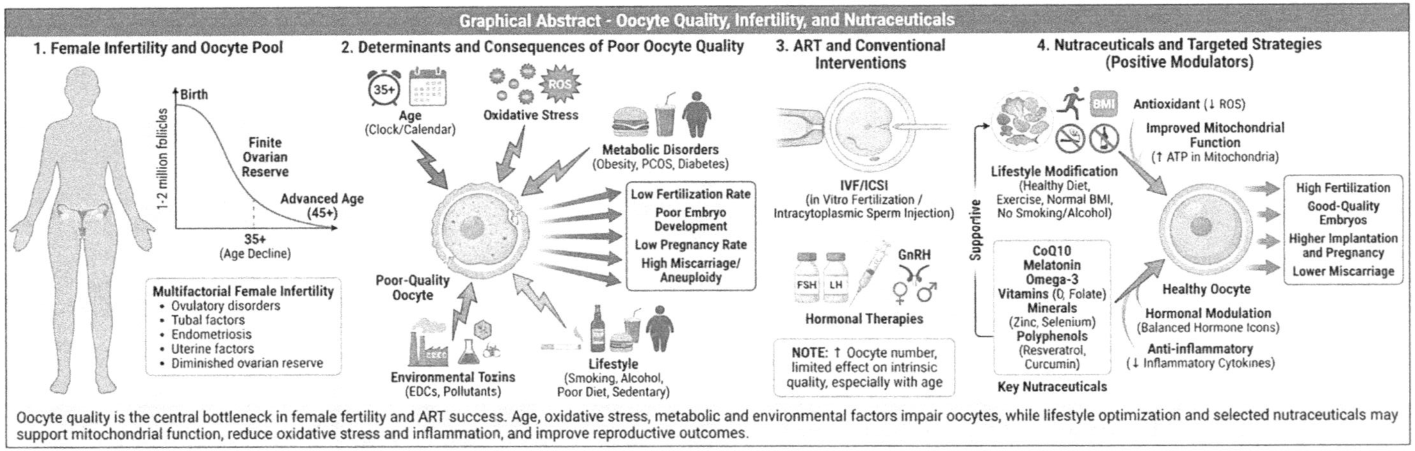

Figure 1.1 Graphical abstract. (Original figure created by the authors.)

Table 1.1: Prevalence of Infertility by Region

Region	Estimated Prevalence (%)
North America	10–15
Europe	8–12
Sub-Saharan Africa	15–30
South Asia	12–18
Middle East	10–20

Source: WHO, 2023; Adapted from (1), Licensed under CC BY 4.0.

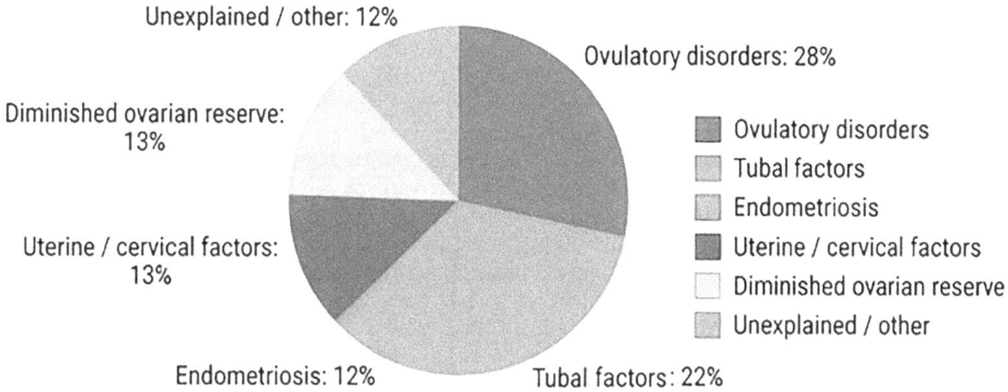

Figure 1.2 Major causes of female infertility. (Adapted from (10, 11), licensed under CC BY 4.0.)

1.1.3 The Role of Oocyte Quality and Quantity

The human female is born with a finite number of oocytes, estimated at approximately 1–2 million at birth. This number declines significantly by the time of puberty, leaving about 300,000–400,000 oocytes in the ovaries. Over the course of a woman's entire reproductive lifespan, only about 400–500 of these oocytes will actually be ovulated (12). Both the quantity, often referred to as the ovarian reserve, and the quality, meaning the ability of the oocyte to be successfully fertilized and develop into a healthy embryo, are critical determinants of overall fertility. Oocyte quality is influenced by several key factors. Age is the most important, as there is a marked decline in both the number and the functional capacity of oocytes after the age of 35, which leads to reduced fertility and increased risk of adverse reproductive outcomes (Table 1.2) (13, 14). Genetic and chromosomal integrity is also crucial, because errors during meiosis can result in aneuploidy, a condition in which the oocyte has an abnormal number of chromosomes. Aneuploidy is a major cause of miscarriage and congenital abnormalities. Another important element is mitochondrial function. Mitochondria are responsible for producing the energy required for oocyte maturation, fertilization, and early embryonic development, so any compromise in mitochondrial performance can negatively affect developmental potential. In addition, proper cytoplasmic maturation of the oocyte is essential. This involves the accurate accumulation and organization of mRNA, proteins, and cellular organelles within the oocyte cytoplasm, which together support normal fertilization and early embryogenesis. Disruptions in any of these factors can impair oocyte competence and therefore reduce the chances of a successful pregnancy (15).

1.1.4 Risk Factors and Contributing Elements

Risk factors and contributing elements play an important role in the development of female infertility, either by directly damaging the reproductive organs or by disrupting the hormonal and metabolic pathways necessary for normal reproductive function. Several lifestyle factors have been clearly associated with reduced fertility (16). Cigarette smoking accelerates the loss of ovarian follicles, increases the risk of ectopic pregnancy and miscarriage, and is linked to earlier

Table 1.2: Age-Related Changes in Ovarian Reserve and Oocyte Quality

Age (years)	Average Ovarian Reserve	Oocyte Quality	Risk of Aneuploidy (%)
<30	High	High	<20
30–34	Moderate	Moderate	20–30
35–39	Low	Decreasing	30–50
≥40	Very Low	Poor	>50

menopause. Excessive alcohol consumption can interfere with ovulation, hormone balance, and implantation. Obesity is associated with insulin resistance, chronic inflammation, and hormonal imbalance, all of which can contribute to anovulation and poorer outcomes in fertility treatments. Conversely, being underweight or having poor nutrition can impair hormone production and disrupt normal menstrual cycles (17). Environmental exposures are another important contributor. Contact with endocrine-disrupting chemicals, including certain pesticides, phthalates found in plastics and personal care products, and bisphenol A (BPA) used in some food and drink containers, can alter hormonal signaling and impair ovarian function, potentially reducing oocyte quality and affecting menstrual regularity. Several medical conditions also negatively impact fertility. Poorly controlled diabetes can disrupt hormonal regulation and increase the risk of miscarriage (18). Thyroid disorders, both hypothyroidism and hyperthyroidism, can cause menstrual irregularities and ovulatory problems. Autoimmune diseases may directly target ovarian tissue or create a chronic inflammatory state that interferes with implantation and pregnancy maintenance. Sexually transmitted infections, such as chlamydia and gonorrhea, can lead to pelvic inflammatory disease, resulting in scarring and blockage of the fallopian tubes. Iatrogenic causes – those resulting from medical treatments – can significantly affect reproductive potential as well (19). Chemotherapy and pelvic radiation used in cancer treatment can damage ovarian follicles, leading to diminished ovarian reserve or premature ovarian insufficiency. Pelvic or uterine surgeries, including those for fibroids, endometriosis, or other gynecologic conditions, may cause adhesions or structural changes in the uterus, tubes, or ovaries that impair fertility. Psychological stress is another contributing element (20). Chronic stress can disrupt the hypothalamic–pituitary–gonadal (HPG) axis, altering the release of gonadotropin-releasing hormone (GnRH) and subsequently luteinizing hormone (LH) and follicle-stimulating hormone (FSH). This disruption can lead to irregular cycles, anovulation, or hypothalamic amenorrhea. Together, these factors illustrate that female infertility is often multifactorial, arising from the interaction of lifestyle, environmental, medical, and psychological influences on reproductive health (21) (Figure 1.3).

1.1.5 Pathophysiology of Female Infertility

The pathophysiology of female infertility is complex and often multifactorial, involving disruptions at hormonal, cellular, immune, and structural levels. A central mechanism is hormonal imbalance, particularly in the secretion or regulation of gonadotropins such as follicle-stimulating hormone and luteinizing hormone, as well as prolactin and thyroid hormones (22). Altered FSH and LH secretion can impair normal folliculogenesis, prevent appropriate maturation of the dominant follicle, and disrupt the LH surge required for ovulation. Elevated prolactin levels can inhibit gonadotropin-releasing hormone and lead to anovulation, while both hypo- and hyperthyroidism can disturb menstrual regularity and ovulatory function. Inflammation and immune dysfunction also play a major role in the development of infertility (23). Chronic inflammatory states, such as those seen in endometriosis or autoimmune diseases, can damage the ovaries, fallopian tubes, or endometrium; create a hostile pelvic environment; and interfere with fertilization, embryo transport, and implantation. Abnormal immune responses may target reproductive tissues or embryos, impairing implantation and increasing the risk of early pregnancy loss. Oxidative stress is another important contributing mechanism (24). Excessive production of reactive oxygen species (ROS), beyond the capacity of the body's antioxidant defenses, can damage the DNA, lipids, and proteins of oocytes, sperm, and endometrial cells. This reduces oocyte quality, impairs fertilization, affects embryo development, and can compromise endometrial receptivity. Structural abnormalities of the reproductive tract further contribute to infertility by physically obstructing or altering the pathways required for conception and implantation (25). Congenital malformations of the uterus, such as septate or bicornuate uterus, and acquired conditions such as fibroids, intrauterine adhesions, or polyps, can distort the uterine

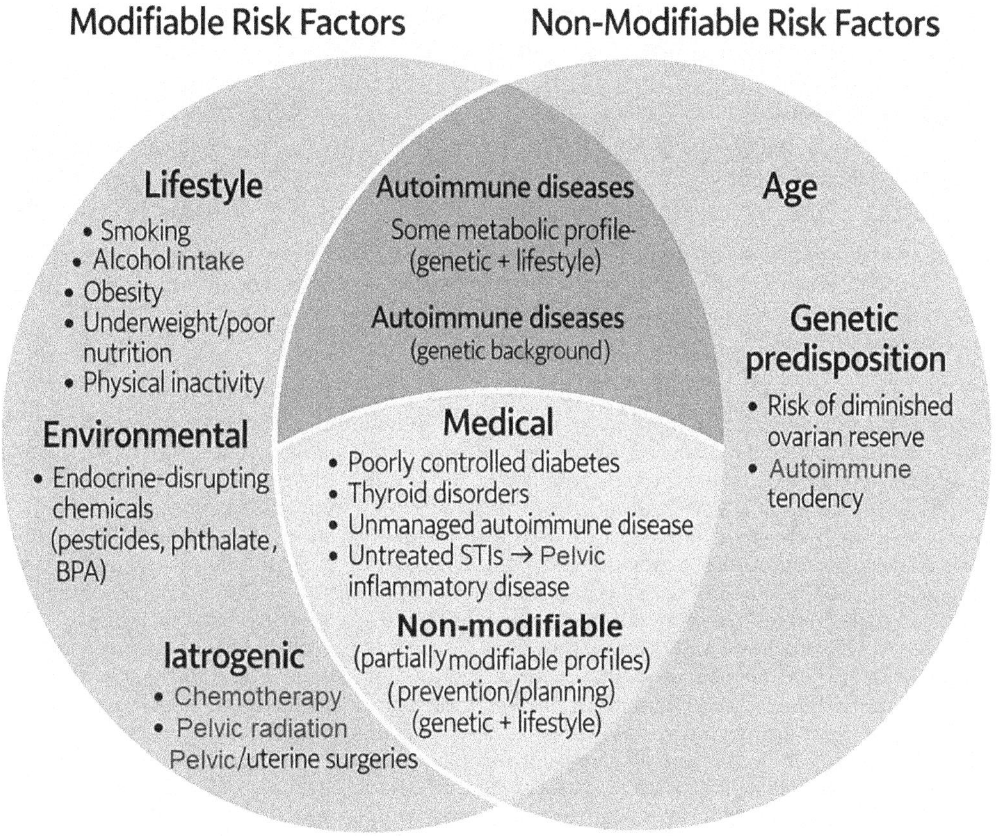

Figure 1.3 Modifiable and non-modifiable risk factors for female infertility. (Original figure created by the authors. Description concept based on data from (21). Licensed under CC BY 4.0.)

cavity and interfere with implantation or increase the risk of miscarriage. Damage or blockage of the fallopian tubes – whether from infection, surgery, or endometriosis – prevents the meeting of sperm and oocyte or the normal transport of the embryo to the uterus. Cervical abnormalities, including stenosis or scarring, can hinder sperm passage into the uterine cavity. Together, these mechanisms illustrate that female infertility usually arises from the interaction of multiple pathophysiological processes rather than a single isolated cause (26).

1.1.6 Psychological Impact

Infertility is not only a medical condition but also a profound social and psychological challenge that can affect nearly every aspect of an individual's life (Table 1.3). In many cultures, parenthood is closely tied to personal identity, social status, and marital stability, so the inability to conceive may lead to stigma, feelings of inadequacy, and social isolation. Women, in particular, may face blame or pressure from families and communities, even when infertility is due to male or combined factors. These social expectations can strain relationships and contribute to marital discord, with conflicts arising over treatment decisions, financial burdens, and differing coping styles between partners. Psychologically, infertility is associated with increased rates of stress, anxiety, depression, and a reduced overall quality of life (27). Many individuals experience grief, loss of control, and cycles of hope and disappointment with each failed attempt to conceive or each unsuccessful treatment cycle. The emotional burden is often intensified by the financial costs of investigations and assisted reproductive technologies, which may be only partially covered – or not covered at all – by insurance. The uncertainty surrounding treatment outcomes, the physical demands of medications and procedures, and the time-consuming nature of treatment further

Table 1.3: Psychological Effects of Infertility on Women

Psychological Effect	Prevalence (%)
Anxiety	30–60
Depression	20–50
Social Isolation	15–40
Marital Stress	25–50

contribute to emotional exhaustion. Together, these factors highlight that managing infertility requires not only medical interventions but also psychosocial support, including counseling, support groups, and open communication within relationships to mitigate its societal and psychological impact (28).

1.1.7 Historical Perspective and Advances in Diagnosis

Historically, infertility was frequently and unjustly attributed solely to women, often resulting in social ostracism, blame, and a lack of effective treatment options. This gender-biased perspective persisted for centuries, despite the fact that male factors account for a substantial proportion of infertility cases. Over the past century, however, advances in reproductive medicine have transformed the understanding, diagnosis, and management of infertility, reframing it as a shared medical condition rather than a moral or social failing. One of the major breakthroughs has been the development of hormonal assays, which allow for precise measurement of key reproductive hormones, including follicle-stimulating hormone, luteinizing hormone, estradiol, anti-Müllerian hormone (AMH), prolactin, and thyroid hormones. These assays have made it possible to more accurately assess ovarian reserve, evaluate ovulatory function, diagnose endocrine disorders, and guide individualized treatment strategies. Imaging techniques have also played a central role in advancing infertility diagnosis. Transvaginal ultrasound has become an essential tool for monitoring follicular development, assessing ovarian morphology, detecting uterine abnormalities such as fibroids or polyps, and evaluating endometrial thickness and pattern (29). Hysterosalpingography, an X-ray procedure using contrast dye, has enabled visualization of the uterine cavity and fallopian tubes, allowing clinicians to detect tubal blockages, structural anomalies, and intrauterine defects that may interfere with conception or implantation. The advent and evolution of assisted reproductive technologies (ART) represent another pivotal milestone. The introduction of in vitro fertilization (IVF) made it possible to retrieve oocytes from the ovaries, fertilize them with sperm outside the body, and transfer resulting embryos into the uterus, offering a chance of pregnancy to couples with severe tubal damage, male factor infertility, or unexplained infertility (30). The development of intracytoplasmic sperm injection (ICSI), in which a single sperm is injected directly into an oocyte, further expanded treatment options for those with severe male factor infertility or previous fertilization failure. More recently, preimplantation genetic testing (PGT) has allowed for the genetic analysis of embryos before transfer, enabling the selection of embryos that are chromosomally normal or free of specific inherited genetic disorders, thereby improving implantation rates and reducing the risk of miscarriage and genetic disease in selected cases (31). Despite these substantial advances, the success rates of ART remain limited and are strongly influenced by female age and oocyte quality. Women of advanced maternal age or those with significantly diminished ovarian reserve often face lower chances of live birth, higher rates of cycle cancellation, and increased risk of pregnancy loss, even with the use of sophisticated technologies. These limitations underscore the biological constraints of human reproduction and highlight the continuing need for research into oocyte biology, embryo development, and strategies to optimize reproductive outcomes (32).

1.1.8 Current Trends and Future Directions

Current trends in female infertility reflect broader social, environmental, and medical changes and are reshaping both the prevalence and the nature of reproductive challenges. One important trend is delayed childbearing, as more women choose to postpone pregnancy for educational, career, or personal reasons. While this shift has many social and economic benefits, it has also led to a higher prevalence of age-related infertility, given the natural decline in both the quality and quantity of oocytes with advancing maternal age. At the same time, there is a rising prevalence of obesity and metabolic disorders such as insulin resistance and type 2 diabetes. These conditions are closely linked to ovulatory dysfunction, poorer oocyte and embryo quality, and reduced success rates in both natural conception and assisted reproductive technologies. Environmental and occupational exposures are also playing a growing role. Urbanization and industrialization have increased contact with reproductive toxins and endocrine-disrupting chemicals in air, water, food, and workplaces, which may impair ovarian function, alter hormone balance, and affect implantation and pregnancy outcomes. Against this backdrop, the field is moving toward personalized medicine. Advances in genomics, proteomics, and molecular biology are enabling more individualized approaches to infertility diagnosis and treatment, allowing clinicians to tailor interventions based on a woman's specific genetic profile, hormonal milieu, and ovarian reserve status rather than relying solely on generalized protocols. Looking ahead, future research is heavily focused on elucidating the molecular mechanisms underlying oocyte aging, including mitochondrial dysfunction, DNA damage, and changes in epigenetic regulation. Scientists are working to identify novel, more sensitive biomarkers of ovarian reserve and oocyte competence that go beyond traditional measures like FSH and AMH. There is also growing interest in exploring new therapeutic strategies, including targeted nutraceuticals with antioxidant or anti-inflammatory properties, as well as regenerative medicine approaches such as stem cell–based therapies, ovarian tissue engineering, and techniques to preserve or restore fertility in women at risk of premature ovarian failure. Together, these developments are shaping a more nuanced, biology-driven, and individualized future for the management of female infertility.

1.2 THE ROLE OF OOCYTE QUALITY IN FEMALE FERTILITY

1.2.1 Definition and Significance of Oocyte Quality

Oocyte quality is a critical determinant of female fertility and reproductive success. It refers to the intrinsic ability of an egg (oocyte) to undergo successful fertilization, support normal embryonic development, and ultimately result in the birth of a healthy child. Unlike oocyte quantity, which is the number of eggs available in the ovaries, oocyte quality encompasses a range of cellular and molecular characteristics that influence the developmental competence of the egg (33).

High-quality oocytes are essential for successful fertilization by sperm, proper chromosomal segregation during meiosis, normal embryonic cleavage and development, implantation in the uterine lining, and sustaining a healthy pregnancy (34).

1.2.2 Cellular and Molecular Features of Oocyte Quality

The competence of an oocyte is determined by several key features:

- *Chromosomal Integrity*: The oocyte must have the correct number of chromosomes and be free from genetic abnormalities. Errors in chromosomal segregation during meiosis can lead to aneuploidy, which is a leading cause of implantation failure, miscarriage, and congenital disorders such as Down syndrome.
- *Cytoplasmic Maturation*: The cytoplasm of the oocyte must accumulate sufficient mRNA, proteins, and organelles to support early embryonic development. Proper cytoplasmic maturation is essential for the activation of the embryonic genome and the transition from oocyte to embryo.
- *Mitochondrial Function*: Mitochondria are the energy-producing organelles in the cell. Oocytes require a high level of ATP to support maturation, fertilization, and early embryonic divisions. Mitochondrial dysfunction is associated with reduced oocyte quality and poor reproductive outcomes.
- *Epigenetic Regulation*: Epigenetic modifications, such as DNA methylation and histone acetylation, play a crucial role in gene expression during oocyte maturation and early embryogenesis (35, 36).

1.2.3 Consequences of Poor Oocyte Quality

Poor oocyte quality is a major limiting factor in female fertility and directly affects the success of both natural conception and assisted reproductive technologies. When oocyte quality is compromised, fertilization may fail to occur, even with advanced techniques such as in vitro fertilization or intracytoplasmic sperm injection, because the oocyte may lack the structural or molecular integrity necessary to support normal fertilization. Even if fertilization does take place, poor-quality oocytes often give rise to embryos with limited developmental potential, leading to arrested embryonic development or embryos of poor morphological and genetic quality. This, in turn, reduces the likelihood of successful implantation in the uterine lining and contributes to higher rates of implantation failure in both natural and assisted cycles. Another critical consequence of poor oocyte quality is an increased risk of miscarriage, largely due to chromosomal abnormalities (aneuploidy) arising from errors in meiotic division within the oocyte. Embryos derived from such oocytes are more likely to have genetic imbalances that are incompatible with ongoing pregnancy, resulting in early pregnancy loss. Collectively, these factors significantly reduce the overall probability of achieving a live birth (37–39). As summarized in Table 1.4, high-quality oocytes are generally associated with high fertilization rates, optimal embryo development, higher clinical pregnancy rates, and lower miscarriage rates, whereas low-quality oocytes are linked to poor fertilization, suboptimal or arrested embryo development, reduced pregnancy rates, and a higher likelihood of miscarriage.

1.2.4 Factors Affecting Oocyte Quality

Oocyte quality is shaped by a complex interplay of genetic, metabolic, environmental, lifestyle, and age-related influences, all of which can affect the ability of an oocyte to be fertilized and develop into a healthy embryo (Figure 1.4). Among these, maternal age is the most significant determinant. As women age – especially after 35 years – oocyte quality declines due to a higher incidence of chromosomal abnormalities resulting from meiotic errors, as well as progressive mitochondrial dysfunction that impairs the energy supply required for maturation and early embryonic development. Genetic factors also play a critical role; inherited mutations, chromosomal rearrangements, or subtle genetic variations can compromise the structural and functional integrity of oocytes, reducing their developmental competence. Oxidative stress is another key contributor. Excessive production of reactive oxygen species overwhelms antioxidant defenses and damages DNA, proteins, and lipids within the oocyte, leading to impaired maturation, abnormal fertilization, and poor embryo formation. Metabolic disorders, including obesity, diabetes, and polycystic ovary syndrome (PCOS), create an altered hormonal and metabolic milieu characterized by insulin resistance, hyperandrogenism, and chronic low-grade inflammation. These changes disrupt folliculogenesis, impair nuclear and cytoplasmic maturation, and are associated with reduced oocyte quality and lower success rates in assisted reproduction. Environmental toxins add an additional layer of risk. Exposure to endocrine-disrupting chemicals such as pesticides, phthalates, and bisphenol A, as well as heavy metals and industrial pollutants, can interfere with hormone signaling and directly impair oocyte development, increasing the likelihood of infertility and adverse reproductive outcomes. Lifestyle factors further modulate oocyte quality. Cigarette smoking accelerates follicular depletion, increases oxidative stress, and is linked to higher rates of aneuploidy. Excessive alcohol intake can disrupt hormonal balance and follicular development. Poor diet, particularly those high in processed foods and low in antioxidants, together with physical inactivity, contributes to metabolic dysfunction and oxidative damage. Collectively, these factors interact to determine the overall competence of oocytes, highlighting the importance of both intrinsic biological factors and modifiable external influences in female reproductive potential (40, 41).

1.2.5 Age and Oocyte Quality: A Closer Look

The decline in oocyte quality with age is one of the most well-documented phenomena in reproductive biology. Women are born with a finite pool of oocytes, and these cells age in parallel with the individual, undergoing cumulative cellular and molecular changes over time. As women grow older, several age-related alterations occur within oocytes that compromise their developmental competence. A key change is the increased incidence of chromosomal segregation errors during meiosis, which leads to a higher rate of aneuploidy and is closely linked to implantation failure, miscarriage, and chromosomal disorders in offspring. In addition, there is a progressive accumulation of mitochondrial DNA mutations and a decline in mitochondrial function, reducing the energy supply required for proper oocyte maturation, fertilization, and

Table 1.4: Impact of Oocyte Quality on Reproductive Outcomes

Oocyte Quality	Fertilization Rate	Embryo Development	Pregnancy Rate	Miscarriage Rate
High	High	Optimal	High	Low
Low	Low	Poor	Low	High

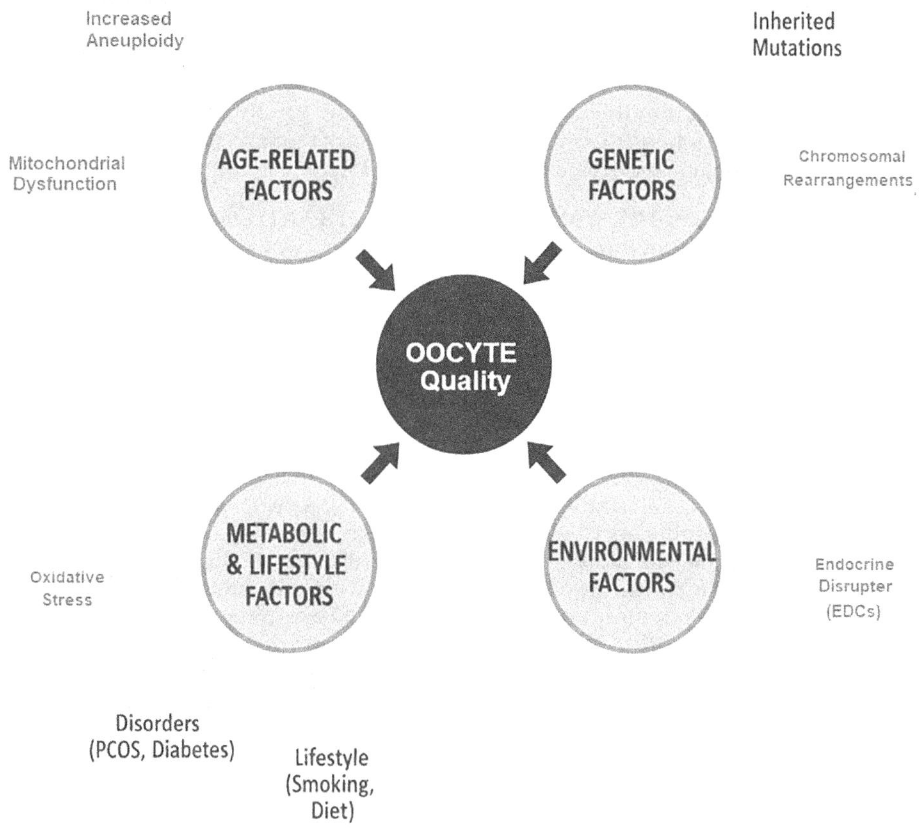

Figure 1.4 Factors affecting oocyte quality. (Original figure; created by the authors.)

early embryonic development. The aging oocyte also exhibits a diminished capacity to detect and repair DNA damage, allowing genetic lesions to persist and be transmitted to the embryo. Furthermore, the epigenetic landscape of the oocyte becomes altered with age, affecting patterns of DNA methylation and histone modification that regulate gene expression during early development. Together, these changes substantially lower the chances of successful fertilization, normal embryo development, and ongoing pregnancy, while simultaneously increasing the risk of miscarriage and chromosomal abnormalities in the resulting offspring (42, 43).

1.2.6 Clinical Implications

Understanding the role of oocyte quality in female fertility has several important clinical implications that directly influence counseling, diagnostic strategies, and therapeutic approaches. First, it emphasizes the importance of early fertility assessment and timely counseling, particularly for women who are considering delaying childbearing for educational, professional, or personal reasons. Awareness of the age-related decline in oocyte quantity and quality allows clinicians to discuss options such as earlier attempts at conception or fertility preservation strategies, including oocyte or embryo cryopreservation. Second, the central role of oocyte quality highlights the need for interventions aimed at preserving or improving oocyte competence. These include evidence-based lifestyle modifications – such as smoking cessation, weight optimization, balanced nutrition, regular physical activity, and moderation of alcohol intake – as well as the potential use of antioxidant supplementation and emerging therapies like targeted nutraceuticals designed to reduce oxidative stress and support mitochondrial function. Although many of these approaches are still under investigation, they represent promising adjuncts to conventional fertility treatments. Third, a focus on oocyte quality drives the development and refinement of diagnostic tools and biomarkers to assess oocyte competence in clinical practice. Beyond traditional measures like age, antral follicle count, and serum anti-Müllerian hormone, research is directed toward identifying molecular, genetic, and metabolic indicators that more accurately reflect oocyte health and developmental potential. Such biomarkers could improve prognostic counseling, guide individualized treatment planning, optimize stimulation protocols in assisted reproductive technologies, and ultimately enhance reproductive outcomes by tailoring interventions to each woman's specific oocyte profile (44, 45).

1.3 CHALLENGES IN THE TREATMENT OF FEMALE INFERTILITY

The management of female infertility has evolved significantly over the past few decades, with the advent of assisted reproductive technologies such as in vitro fertilization and intracytoplasmic sperm injection. Despite these technological advances, the overall success rates of infertility treatments remain suboptimal, especially for women with compromised oocyte quality or advanced maternal age. Several persistent challenges continue to limit the effectiveness of current therapeutic approaches (46).

1.3.1 Age-Related Decline in Ovarian Reserve and Oocyte Quality

One of the most significant challenges in female infertility treatment is the natural, age-related decline in both the quantity and quality of oocytes (Table 1.5). As women age, the ovarian reserve diminishes, and the remaining oocytes are more likely to have chromosomal abnormalities, mitochondrial dysfunction, and reduced developmental competence. This decline becomes particularly pronounced after the age of 35, resulting in lower fertilization rates, poor embryo quality, increased miscarriage rates, and reduced live birth rates, even with ART (47).

1.3.2 Limited Effectiveness of Current Pharmacological Interventions

Current pharmacological interventions, such as ovulation induction agents (e.g., clomiphene citrate, letrozole) and gonadotropin stimulation, are effective for certain causes of infertility, particularly ovulatory disorders. However, these treatments have limited efficacy in improving oocyte quality, especially in women with diminished ovarian reserve or advanced age. Additionally, repeated cycles of ovarian stimulation can be physically and emotionally taxing, with diminishing returns over time (48).

1.3.3 High Emotional and Financial Burden on Patients

Infertility and its treatment can impose a significant emotional and psychological toll on individuals and couples. The stress of repeated treatment failures, uncertainty about outcomes, and the invasive nature of many procedures can lead to anxiety, depression, and relationship strain. Furthermore, the financial burden of infertility treatments is substantial, as ART procedures are often expensive and not always covered by insurance. Many couples face difficult decisions about how many cycles to pursue, given the high costs and uncertain success rates (Figure 1.5) (49).

1.3.4 Potential Side Effects and Risks Associated with ART Procedures

Although assisted reproductive technologies have made it possible for many couples to achieve pregnancy, these procedures are associated with a range of potential side effects and risks that must be carefully considered in clinical practice. One of the most significant complications is ovarian hyperstimulation syndrome (OHSS), which can occur in response to the medications

Table 1.5: ART Success Rates by Age Group

Age Group (years)	IVF Live Birth Rate (%)
<35	40–45
35–37	30–35
38–40	20–25
41–42	10–15
>42	<5

Source: Society for Assisted Reproductive Technology (SART), 2023; adapted from (47); licensed under CC BY 4.0.

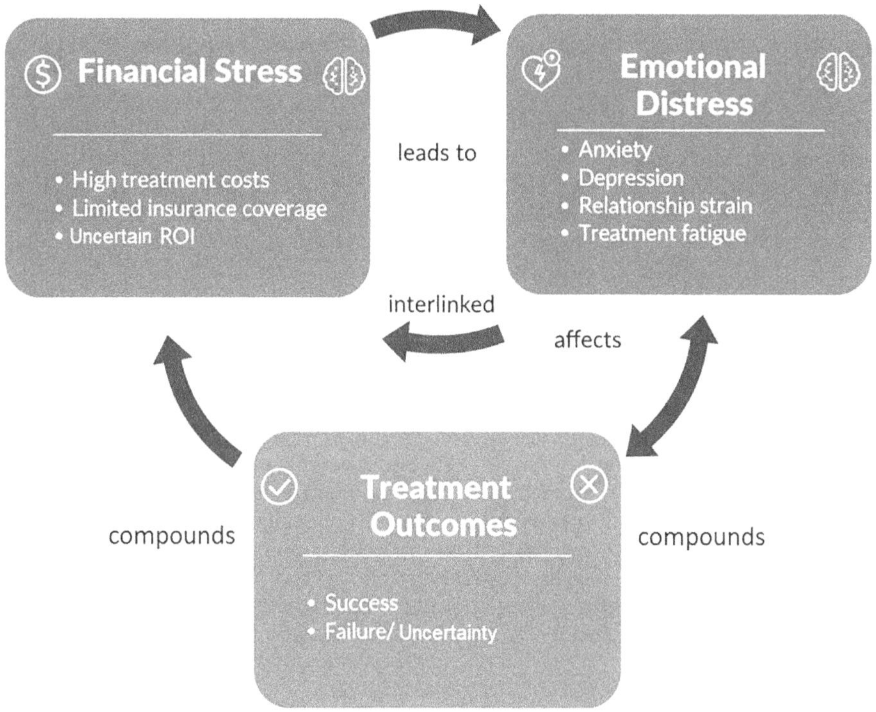

Figure 1.5 The emotional and financial impact of infertility treatment. (Original figure created by the authors based on data from (49). Licensed under CC BY 4.0.)

used to stimulate the ovaries. OHSS is characterized by enlarged, painful ovaries and fluid accumulation in the abdomen or chest, and in severe cases it can lead to thromboembolic events, kidney dysfunction, or respiratory compromise, requiring intensive monitoring and treatment. ART also increases the likelihood of multiple pregnancies, particularly when more than one embryo is transferred. Twin or higher-order multiple gestations are associated with higher rates of preterm birth, low birth weight, pregnancy-induced hypertension, gestational diabetes, and neonatal complications, as well as greater maternal morbidity. Procedure-related risks are another important consideration. Egg retrieval, which is typically performed under transvaginal ultrasound guidance and light anesthesia, carries small but real risks, including bleeding, infection, injury to pelvic organs, and complications related to sedation or anesthesia. Embryo transfer is generally low risk but may occasionally cause cramping, spotting, or, very rarely, infection. In addition to these immediate concerns, there are ongoing questions about the long-term health effects of repeated ovarian stimulation and ART cycles. Some studies have explored potential associations with ovarian tumors or other health issues, but current evidence is inconclusive and does not establish a clear causal relationship. Nevertheless, these uncertainties underscore the need for careful patient selection, individualized stimulation protocols, ongoing surveillance, and informed consent that fully addresses both the benefits and the possible risks of ART (50).

1.3.5 Lack of Personalized Treatment Approaches

Another major challenge is the lack of truly personalized or individualized treatment strategies. Most current protocols are based on population averages rather than tailored to the unique genetic, metabolic, and environmental profiles of individual patients. This "one-size-fits-all" approach may not be optimal for all women, particularly those with complex or unexplained infertility. There is a growing recognition of the need for precision medicine approaches that incorporate genetic, epigenetic, and lifestyle factors to optimize treatment outcomes (51).

1.3.6 The Need for Novel Strategies

The need for novel strategies to address poor oocyte quality is increasingly evident in light of the biological constraints of aging, the limited success rates of current ART in women with diminished oocyte competence, and the potential risks and costs associated with repeated treatment cycles. To overcome these challenges, research is progressively shifting toward more precise, mechanism-based approaches aimed at enhancing oocyte quality and improving reproductive outcomes. One major area of focus is the identification of reliable biomarkers of oocyte competence, including molecular, genetic, metabolic, and epigenetic signatures that can more accurately predict which oocytes and embryos have the highest developmental potential. Such biomarkers would allow for better prognostic counseling, more refined patient selection, and individualized stimulation and embryo transfer strategies. In parallel, efforts are underway to develop targeted therapies that address specific causes of poor oocyte quality, such as mitochondrial dysfunction, oxidative stress, and age-related chromosomal instability. These may include agents designed to support mitochondrial activity, reduce DNA damage, or modulate key signaling pathways involved in oocyte maturation. There is also growing interest in the role of lifestyle interventions, antioxidants, and nutraceuticals as adjuncts to conventional fertility treatments. Optimizing diet, physical activity, and body weight, along with the judicious use of antioxidant and micronutrient supplementation, may help mitigate oxidative stress and improve the metabolic environment of the oocyte, although robust clinical evidence is still evolving. Finally, advances in technologies for oocyte preservation and rejuvenation – such as improved vitrification techniques, ovarian tissue cryopreservation and transplantation, and emerging regenerative approaches aimed at restoring or enhancing ovarian function – hold promise for extending reproductive options and improving outcomes for women at risk of diminished ovarian reserve. Together, these lines of investigation reflect a shift toward more personalized, preventive, and biology-driven strategies in reproductive medicine (52).

1.4 THE IMPORTANCE OF OOCYTE QUALITY IN INFERTILITY TREATMENT

1.4.1 Oocyte Quality as a Central Factor in ART Success

Oocyte quality is widely recognized as one of the most critical determinants of success in assisted reproductive technologies, including in vitro fertilization and intracytoplasmic sperm injection. While both male and female factors contribute to infertility, research consistently demonstrates that the quality of the oocyte plays a more decisive role in determining the outcome of ART cycles. High-quality oocytes are essential for successful fertilization, normal embryo development, implantation, and the achievement of a healthy pregnancy (53).

1.4.2 Evidence from Clinical Studies

Numerous clinical studies have shown that the majority of failed IVF cycles are attributable to poor oocyte and embryo quality, rather than issues with sperm function or uterine receptivity. For example, even when high-quality sperm and optimal endometrial conditions are present, poor oocyte quality can result in failed fertilization, abnormal embryo development, and early pregnancy loss. Conversely, when oocyte quality is high, the chances of successful fertilization, embryo viability, and live birth are significantly increased (54).

1.4.3 Impact on Key ART Outcomes

Oocyte quality has a direct and pervasive impact on several key outcomes in assisted reproductive technologies. First, it strongly influences the fertilization rate: high-quality oocytes, with intact chromosomal and cytoplasmic structures, are more likely to be successfully fertilized by sperm and to form normal, healthy zygotes, even when ART techniques such as IVF or ICSI are used. Second, embryo development is heavily dependent on the intrinsic competence of the oocyte. Oocytes with optimal nuclear and cytoplasmic maturation provide the necessary organelles, mRNA, proteins, and energy reserves to support orderly embryonic cleavage, blastocyst formation, and overall embryo viability. This increases the chances of obtaining embryos of sufficient quality for transfer or cryopreservation. Third, pregnancy rates are closely tied to oocyte quality, because embryos derived from competent oocytes are more likely to implant successfully in the endometrium and progress to a clinical pregnancy and ongoing gestation. Finally, poor oocyte quality is a major contributor to chromosomal abnormalities (aneuploidy) in embryos, which significantly raises the risk of early pregnancy loss and miscarriage. Thus, reduced oocyte competence not only lowers fertilization and implantation rates but also increases the likelihood that pregnancies, once achieved, will not continue to term (55, 56).

1.4.4 Mechanisms Linking Oocyte Quality to ART Outcomes

The ways in which oocyte quality affects ART outcomes are multifactorial and operate at genetic, metabolic, and cellular levels. One key mechanism is genetic integrity. High-quality oocytes maintain intact chromosomal structures and proper meiotic division, which minimizes the risk of aneuploidy and reduces the likelihood of genetic disorders in the resulting embryos. This directly improves fertilization success, embryo viability, implantation, and the chances of an ongoing pregnancy.

Mitochondrial function is another crucial factor. Mitochondria in the oocyte supply the ATP required for processes such as spindle formation, chromosome segregation, fertilization, and early embryonic cleavage. Adequate mitochondrial number and function support normal development to the blastocyst stage, whereas mitochondrial dysfunction is associated with poor fertilization, embryo arrest, and lower implantation rates.

Epigenetic regulation also plays a central role. During oogenesis, the oocyte establishes specific epigenetic marks – such as DNA methylation and histone modifications – that control gene expression during early embryogenesis. Properly set epigenetic patterns are essential for normal development, imprinting, and placental function; disturbances in these marks can lead to abnormal gene expression, impaired embryo development, and adverse pregnancy outcomes.

Finally, cytoplasmic maturation is critical for oocyte competence. Beyond nuclear maturation, a high-quality oocyte must accumulate and correctly organize mRNA, proteins, organelles, and signaling molecules within its cytoplasm. This cytoplasmic preparedness provides the early embryo with the molecular toolkit it needs before its own genome becomes fully active. Inadequate cytoplasmic maturation results in embryos with reduced developmental potential, lower quality at the cleavage and blastocyst stages, and poorer ART outcomes overall (57).

1.4.5 Clinical Implications and the Need for Targeted Interventions

Clinical implications and the need for targeted interventions are closely tied to the central role of oocyte quality in determining the success of assisted reproductive technologies. Because the competence of the oocyte underpins fertilization, embryo development, implantation, and the likelihood of an ongoing pregnancy, interventions specifically aimed at supporting and enhancing oocyte health are of paramount importance in clinical practice. One major area of focus is lifestyle modification, including the promotion of a balanced, nutrient-rich diet, regular physical activity, weight optimization, and the avoidance of harmful substances such as tobacco, excessive alcohol, and recreational drugs. These changes can help reduce oxidative stress, improve metabolic and hormonal balance, and create a more favorable environment for folliculogenesis and oocyte maturation. In addition, antioxidant and nutraceutical supplementation is being explored as a means to mitigate oxidative damage and support cellular function within the oocyte and surrounding follicular environment. Agents such as vitamins C and E, coenzyme Q10, melatonin, omega-3 fatty acids, and other targeted micronutrients may help enhance mitochondrial performance and reduce reactive oxygen species, although robust clinical evidence and standardized protocols are still under development. Another key strategy involves the optimization of ovarian stimulation protocols. By tailoring the type, dose, and timing of gonadotropins and adjunct medications to each patient's age, ovarian reserve, and previous response, clinicians aim to maximize both oocyte yield and quality while minimizing the risk of complications such as ovarian hyperstimulation syndrome. Individualized protocols may improve the proportion of mature, competent oocytes retrieved in each cycle, thereby increasing the chances of generating high-quality embryos. Looking to the future, emerging therapies are being actively investigated to further enhance oocyte competence. These include experimental approaches such as mitochondrial transfer to improve the energetic capacity of aging oocytes, the use of specific growth factors or cytokines to support follicular development, and regenerative medicine strategies – such as stem cell–based interventions or ovarian tissue engineering – designed to restore or augment ovarian function. While many of these approaches remain in the research phase, they highlight a growing shift toward biologically targeted, mechanism-based treatments. By prioritizing interventions that improve oocyte quality, clinicians can meaningfully increase the likelihood of successful ART outcomes, reduce the number of treatment cycles required, lessen the emotional and financial burden on patients, and ultimately enhance the chances of achieving a healthy, term pregnancy (58, 59).

1.4.6 Current Approaches to Improving Oocyte Quality

The quality of oocytes is a pivotal factor in determining the success of infertility treatments. As such, a variety of strategies have been developed and investigated to enhance oocyte quality, particularly in women undergoing assisted reproductive technologies. These approaches range from lifestyle interventions to advanced pharmacological and adjunctive therapies, as well as emerging and experimental techniques (60).

1.4.6.1 Lifestyle Modifications

Lifestyle factors play a significant role in reproductive health and oocyte quality, and many modifiable behaviors and environmental exposures can either support or impair ovarian function. A healthy diet is fundamental: a balanced eating pattern rich in fruits, vegetables, whole grains, lean proteins, and healthy fats supplies essential vitamins, minerals, and antioxidants that help protect cells from oxidative damage and support optimal follicular development. In contrast, diets high in processed foods, trans fats, and refined sugars have been associated with insulin resistance, systemic inflammation, and poorer reproductive outcomes. Regular exercise is also important. Moderate physical activity helps maintain a healthy body weight, improves insulin sensitivity, and reduces inflammation, all of which are beneficial for oocyte quality and overall reproductive function. However, very intense or excessive exercise, especially when accompanied by low caloric intake, can disrupt the hypothalamic–pituitary–ovarian axis, leading to menstrual irregularities and impaired ovulation. Avoidance of smoking and excessive alcohol consumption is strongly recommended. Smoking increases oxidative stress, causes DNA damage, accelerates ovarian follicle depletion, and is linked to earlier menopause and reduced success with assisted reproductive technologies. Excessive alcohol intake can disturb hormonal balance, impair follicular development, and negatively affect implantation and pregnancy outcomes. Weight management is another key component. Both obesity and being underweight are associated with hormonal imbalances, anovulation, altered levels of insulin and sex steroids, and reduced oocyte quality. Obesity, in particular, is linked to chronic low-grade inflammation and poorer responses to ovarian stimulation. Achieving and maintaining a healthy body mass index (BMI) through balanced nutrition and appropriate physical activity is therefore recommended to optimize oocyte competence and reproductive potential (61, 62).

1.4.6.2 Antioxidant Supplementation

Oxidative stress is a major contributor to oocyte aging and dysfunction. Reactive oxygen species can damage DNA, proteins, and lipids within the oocyte, thereby compromising its structural integrity and developmental competence. Antioxidant supplementation is intended to neutralize excess ROS and protect oocytes from this cumulative damage. Among the most studied antioxidants are vitamins C and E, which act as potent free radical scavengers and help reduce oxidative injury within follicular and reproductive tissues. Coenzyme Q10 (CoQ10), a key component of the mitochondrial electron transport chain, supports ATP production and has been shown in experimental and some clinical studies to improve mitochondrial function in oocytes, potentially enhancing their quality, especially in older women or those with diminished ovarian reserve. Melatonin, best known for its role in regulating circadian rhythms, is also a powerful antioxidant that accumulates in ovarian follicles, where it can reduce oxidative stress, support oocyte maturation, and may improve embryo quality and implantation potential (63, 64).

Although early clinical data on antioxidant use in infertility and ART are promising in certain subgroups, important questions remain. The optimal types of antioxidants, their dosages, timing, and duration of use, as well as the most effective combinations, have not yet been firmly established. Furthermore, excessively high doses or inappropriate combinations may be counterproductive, potentially disrupting normal redox signaling. As a result, antioxidant supplementation should be considered as a supportive, adjunctive strategy, ideally guided by emerging evidence and individualized patient assessment, rather than a stand-alone cure for poor oocyte quality (65).

1.4.6.3 Hormonal Therapies

Hormonal therapies are central components of most assisted reproductive technology protocols and are primarily designed to optimize ovarian stimulation, control cycle timing, and promote follicular development. Exogenous gonadotropins, including follicle-stimulating hormone with or without luteinizing hormone, are administered to stimulate the simultaneous growth and maturation of multiple follicles, thereby increasing the number of oocytes available for retrieval in in vitro fertilization cycles. To prevent a spontaneous LH surge and premature ovulation, gonadotropin-releasing hormone agonists or antagonists are used to suppress or modulate pituitary function, allowing clinicians to precisely control the timing of final oocyte maturation and egg retrieval and to better synchronize follicular development. In women with ovulatory disorders, such as polycystic ovary syndrome or hypothalamic dysfunction, other hormonal agents like clomiphene citrate or letrozole may be employed to induce or regulate ovulation in a more targeted manner, either alone or in preparation for ART.

While these hormonal therapies are highly effective at increasing the number of follicles recruited and oocytes retrieved, their direct impact on intrinsic oocyte quality is less clear, particularly in women with diminished ovarian reserve or advanced maternal age. In such cases, stimulation can maximize the yield of available oocytes but cannot fully overcome age-related declines in genetic integrity, mitochondrial function, or other intrinsic cellular factors that determine oocyte competence. This limitation underscores the importance of combining optimized hormonal protocols with strategies aimed at preserving or enhancing oocyte quality, as well as providing realistic counseling regarding prognosis and expected ART outcomes in different patient populations (66, 67).

1.4.6.4 Adjunctive Therapies

Adjunctive therapies are increasingly being investigated as potential tools to enhance oocyte quality, especially in women with poor ovarian response, diminished ovarian reserve, or previous ART failures. One such approach involves the use of growth hormone (GH). GH supplementation is thought to improve follicular development, oocyte maturation, and embryo quality by augmenting insulin-like growth factor (IGF) activity within the ovary, thereby supporting granulosa cell function and enhancing the intrafollicular environment. Some studies have reported improved oocyte yield and better embryo quality in poor responders, but results are inconsistent, and GH use remains controversial and largely empirical.

Dehydroepiandrosterone (DHEA), an androgen precursor, has also been explored as an adjunct for women with diminished ovarian reserve. DHEA may promote early folliculogenesis, increase the pool of recruitable follicles, and potentially improve oocyte quality by modulating androgen and growth factor signaling within the ovary. While some observational studies and small trials suggest improved ovarian response, higher oocyte numbers, or better pregnancy rates, the overall evidence is mixed, and standardized dosing, timing, and ideal patient selection remain uncertain.

Other adjuvants, including myo-inositol, L-carnitine, and various micronutrients, are under investigation for their potential to support oocyte health through mechanisms such as improving insulin sensitivity, enhancing mitochondrial function, and reducing oxidative stress. Myo-inositol, for example, is widely used in women with PCOS to improve metabolic and ovulatory function, while L-carnitine may support mitochondrial energy metabolism. However, for many of these agents, data are limited and heterogeneous (68–70).

Overall, the efficacy of adjunctive therapies varies, and high-quality, randomized controlled trials are still needed to determine their true benefits, optimal dosing regimens, appropriate indications, and long-term safety. Until more definitive evidence is available, these interventions should be used cautiously, ideally within an individualized, evidence-informed treatment plan and with clear counseling about the current limits of scientific support.

1.4.6.5 Emerging Approaches

As understanding of oocyte biology deepens, a range of emerging strategies is being developed to improve oocyte quality and reproductive outcomes. Nutraceuticals – food-derived products with potential medical or health benefits – are attracting growing interest. These include antioxidants, omega-3 fatty acids, and various plant extracts, which may help modulate oxidative stress, inflammation, and mitochondrial function within oocytes and the surrounding follicular environment. By improving cellular resilience and metabolic balance, nutraceuticals may enhance oocyte competence, although evidence is still evolving and standardization of products and dosing is needed (71).

Closely related are mitochondrial nutrients, such as coenzyme Q10, L-carnitine, and resveratrol, which specifically target mitochondrial health. Because mitochondria provide the energy required for oocyte maturation, fertilization, and early embryonic development, supporting mitochondrial function is a key therapeutic focus, particularly in older women or those with diminished ovarian reserve. These compounds aim to improve ATP production, reduce oxidative damage, and stabilize mitochondrial DNA, thereby potentially enhancing the developmental capacity of oocytes (72).

Personalized medicine represents another major frontier. Advances in genomics, transcriptomics, metabolomics, and molecular diagnostics are enabling clinicians to design individualized treatment protocols based on a woman's unique genetic, metabolic, and environmental profile. By tailoring ovarian stimulation regimens, adjunctive therapies, and lifestyle recommendations to each patient's specific characteristics, personalized approaches seek to optimize both the number and quality of oocytes retrieved during ART while minimizing unnecessary interventions and side effects (73).

Regenerative medicine offers some of the most innovative, though still largely experimental, approaches for women with severely compromised oocyte quality or ovarian failure. Techniques under investigation include ovarian tissue cryopreservation and transplantation to restore endocrine and reproductive function, stem cell–based therapies aimed at regenerating ovarian tissue or supporting folliculogenesis, and mitochondrial transfer procedures designed to improve the energetic capacity of aging or dysfunctional oocytes. While these strategies are not yet part of routine clinical practice and raise important ethical, safety, and regulatory questions, they illustrate the direction of future research and the potential for transformative changes in the management of female infertility (74).

1.5 INTRODUCTION TO NUTRACEUTICALS

1.5.1 Definition and Historical Background

The term nutraceutical is a blend of "nutrition" and "pharmaceutical," first coined in the late 1980s to describe food-derived products that offer medical or health benefits, including the prevention and treatment of disease. Nutraceuticals occupy a unique space between conventional foods and pharmaceuticals, providing bioactive compounds that can influence physiological functions and promote overall health (75).

1.5.2 Categories of Nutraceuticals

Nutraceuticals encompass a broad spectrum of products that bridge the gap between nutrition and medicine and can be grouped into several main categories. Dietary supplements include concentrated sources of nutrients or other substances with nutritional or physiological effects, such as vitamins, minerals, amino acids, and fatty acids, typically provided in forms like capsules, tablets, or powders. Functional foods are conventional foods that have been enhanced with additional ingredients or modified to provide health benefits beyond basic nutrition – for example, cereals fortified with vitamins and minerals, probiotic yogurts designed to support gut and immune health, or beverages enriched with omega-3 fatty acids. Herbal extracts and botanicals comprise plant-derived compounds, including flavonoids, polyphenols, and phytoestrogens, which are known for their antioxidant, anti-inflammatory, or hormone-modulating properties and are often used with the aim of supporting metabolic, cardiovascular, or reproductive health (Table 1.6) (76).

1.5.3 Mechanisms of Action

Nutraceuticals exert their beneficial effects through multiple, often overlapping mechanisms that can influence reproductive health and oocyte quality. A major pathway is antioxidant activity: many nutraceuticals neutralize reactive oxygen species, thereby reducing oxidative stress and protecting key cellular structures such as DNA, proteins, and lipids from damage. This is

Table 1.6: Common Categories and Examples of Nutraceuticals

Category	Examples
Antioxidants	Vitamin C, vitamin E, coenzyme Q10
Omega-3 fatty acids	Fish oil, flaxseed oil
Minerals	Zinc, selenium, magnesium
Herbal extracts	Green tea extract, resveratrol, curcumin
Probiotics	Lactobacillus, Bifidobacterium

particularly important in oocytes, where cumulative oxidative injury contributes to aging and reduced developmental competence. Anti-inflammatory effects represent another important mechanism. Various plant-derived compounds, including flavonoids and polyphenols, can modulate inflammatory signaling pathways and cytokine production. This is especially relevant in reproductive conditions characterized by chronic inflammation, such as endometriosis and polycystic ovary syndrome, where reducing inflammation may help improve the follicular environment and endometrial receptivity. Hormonal modulation is also a key action of some nutraceuticals. Phytoestrogens and other bioactive molecules can interact with estrogen receptors or influence hormone synthesis and metabolism, potentially supporting more balanced endocrine function and menstrual regularity. In addition, certain nutrients, such as coenzyme Q10 and L-carnitine, help improve mitochondrial function by supporting ATP production and stabilizing mitochondrial membranes. Because mitochondria are central to oocyte maturation, fertilization, and early embryonic development, enhancing mitochondrial efficiency can have a direct positive impact on reproductive outcomes. Finally, immune system support is another important mechanism. Probiotics and specific micronutrients, such as vitamins D and B, zinc, and selenium, can modulate immune responses and promote a more balanced immune environment. This may be beneficial for implantation and early pregnancy maintenance, where dysregulated immunity can contribute to implantation failure or early pregnancy loss. Together, these mechanisms illustrate how nutraceuticals can act on oxidative balance, inflammation, hormonal regulation, cellular energetics, and immune function to potentially support fertility and reproductive health (77, 78).

1.5.4 Nutraceuticals in Reproductive Medicine

In recent years, nutraceuticals have gained increasing attention in the field of reproductive medicine. Their potential to modulate physiological processes, reduce oxidative stress, and improve cellular function makes them attractive adjuncts in the management of infertility. Some of the most commonly studied nutraceuticals in reproductive health include:

- *Antioxidants*: Such as vitamins C and E, melatonin, and coenzyme Q10, which may improve oocyte and sperm quality.
- *Omega-3 Fatty Acids*: Known for their anti-inflammatory properties and potential to improve endometrial receptivity and embryo implantation.
- *Vitamins and Minerals*: Including folic acid, vitamin D, zinc, and selenium, which are essential for hormonal balance, DNA synthesis, and cellular health.
- *Herbal Extracts*: Such as resveratrol, curcumin, and green tea polyphenols, which may offer additional antioxidant and anti-inflammatory benefits (79, 80).

1.5.5 Safety and Accessibility

Nutraceuticals offer several advantages in terms of safety and accessibility, which make them attractive as adjuncts in reproductive health and fertility care. In general, they have a more favorable safety profile than many pharmaceutical drugs, particularly when used at physiologic or moderately elevated doses. Most nutraceuticals are derived from foods or plants with a long history of human consumption, and serious adverse effects are relatively uncommon when products are properly manufactured and used as directed. Their wide availability – often over the counter – and the ease with which they can be integrated into daily routines (through diet, supplements, or functional foods) further enhance their practicality for many individuals seeking to support fertility and overall health.

However, their accessibility also comes with important caveats. The quality, purity, and actual content of nutraceutical products can vary substantially between manufacturers and even between batches, especially in settings with limited regulatory oversight. Contamination, adulteration, inaccurate labeling, or subtherapeutic dosing are documented concerns. Moreover, "natural" does not always mean "risk-free": some nutraceuticals can interact with medications, affect hormone levels, or be inappropriate in certain medical conditions or during pregnancy. For these reasons, the use of nutraceuticals should be guided by evidence-based recommendations as much as possible, with preference for products from reputable sources, and ideally under the supervision of healthcare professionals who can consider individual health status, concurrent treatments, and specific reproductive goals (81, 82).

1.5.6 The Role of Nutraceuticals in Reproductive Medicine

The use of nutraceuticals in reproductive medicine has gained significant attention in recent years, driven by growing evidence of their potential to positively influence fertility outcomes. Nutraceuticals, with their diverse bioactive properties, offer a promising adjunct to conventional infertility treatments, particularly in enhancing oocyte quality, supporting hormonal balance, and reducing inflammation – three key factors in successful conception and pregnancy (83).

1.5.6.1 Mechanisms of Action

Nutraceuticals can impact reproductive health through several interconnected mechanisms that act at the cellular, metabolic, and endocrine levels. One major pathway is the reduction of oxidative stress. Many nutraceuticals, including vitamins C and E, coenzyme Q10, and melatonin, function as antioxidants that neutralize reactive oxygen species. When present in excess, ROS can damage DNA, proteins, and lipids in oocytes, sperm, and reproductive tissues. By lowering oxidative stress, these compounds help preserve the structural integrity and functional capacity of gametes and may support better embryo development.

Another key mechanism is the improvement of mitochondrial function. Mitochondria provide the energy required for oocyte maturation, fertilization, and early embryonic cleavage. Nutraceuticals such as coenzyme Q10 and L-carnitine support mitochondrial energy production, enhance ATP synthesis, and protect mitochondrial membranes and DNA from oxidative damage. This can be particularly relevant in older women or those with diminished ovarian reserve, where mitochondrial dysfunction is a major contributor to reduced oocyte competence.

Nutraceuticals can also support hormonal balance. Agents like omega-3 fatty acids, vitamin D, myo-inositol, and certain herbal extracts may modulate hormone synthesis, metabolism, and receptor sensitivity. This is especially important in conditions such as polycystic ovary syndrome and luteal phase defects, where disturbances in insulin signaling, gonadotropins, or sex steroids impair ovulation and endometrial receptivity. By helping to normalize endocrine function, these compounds can improve cycle regularity and ovulatory patterns.

Finally, many nutraceuticals exert anti-inflammatory effects. Chronic, low-grade inflammation is implicated in reproductive disorders such as endometriosis and PCOS, as well as in obesity-related infertility. Omega-3 fatty acids, curcumin, resveratrol, and various polyphenols can downregulate pro-inflammatory cytokines and signaling pathways, thereby reducing inflammation in the reproductive tract and creating a more favorable environment for folliculogenesis, implantation, and early pregnancy. Together, these mechanisms – antioxidant activity, mitochondrial support, hormonal modulation, and anti-inflammatory action – illustrate how nutraceuticals may contribute to improved reproductive health and oocyte quality when used appropriately and in conjunction with evidence-based medical care (84) (Figure 1.6).

1.6 KEY NUTRACEUTICALS STUDIED IN REPRODUCTIVE MEDICINE

Several nutraceuticals have been investigated for their potential to support fertility, improve oocyte quality, and enhance outcomes in assisted reproductive technologies.

Coenzyme Q10 is a vital component of the mitochondrial electron transport chain and a potent lipophilic antioxidant. By supporting mitochondrial energy production and reducing oxidative damage, CoQ10 supplementation has been shown in multiple studies to improve mitochondrial function in oocytes, enhance fertilization rates, and increase embryo quality. These benefits appear particularly relevant in women of advanced reproductive age or those with diminished ovarian reserve, in whom mitochondrial dysfunction and oxidative stress are prominent contributors to reduced oocyte competence.

Melatonin, best known for regulating circadian rhythms, also acts as a powerful antioxidant within the ovarian follicle. It accumulates in follicular fluid, where it scavenges reactive oxygen species and stabilizes cellular structures. Clinical and experimental studies suggest that melatonin supplementation can improve oocyte maturation, decrease oxidative damage to oocytes and surrounding granulosa cells, enhance embryo quality, and in some cases increase pregnancy and live birth rates in women undergoing ART.

Omega-3 fatty acids, primarily eicosapentaenoic acid (EPA) and docosahexaenoic acid (DHA) derived from fish oil, as well as alpha-linolenic acid (ALA) from plant sources such as flaxseed, exert anti-inflammatory and membrane-stabilizing effects. In reproductive medicine, they may improve follicular development, luteal function, and endometrial receptivity by modulating prostaglandin synthesis, cytokine profiles, and cellular membrane composition. Some data also suggest potential improvements in embryo quality and a reduction in inflammation-related reproductive disorders.

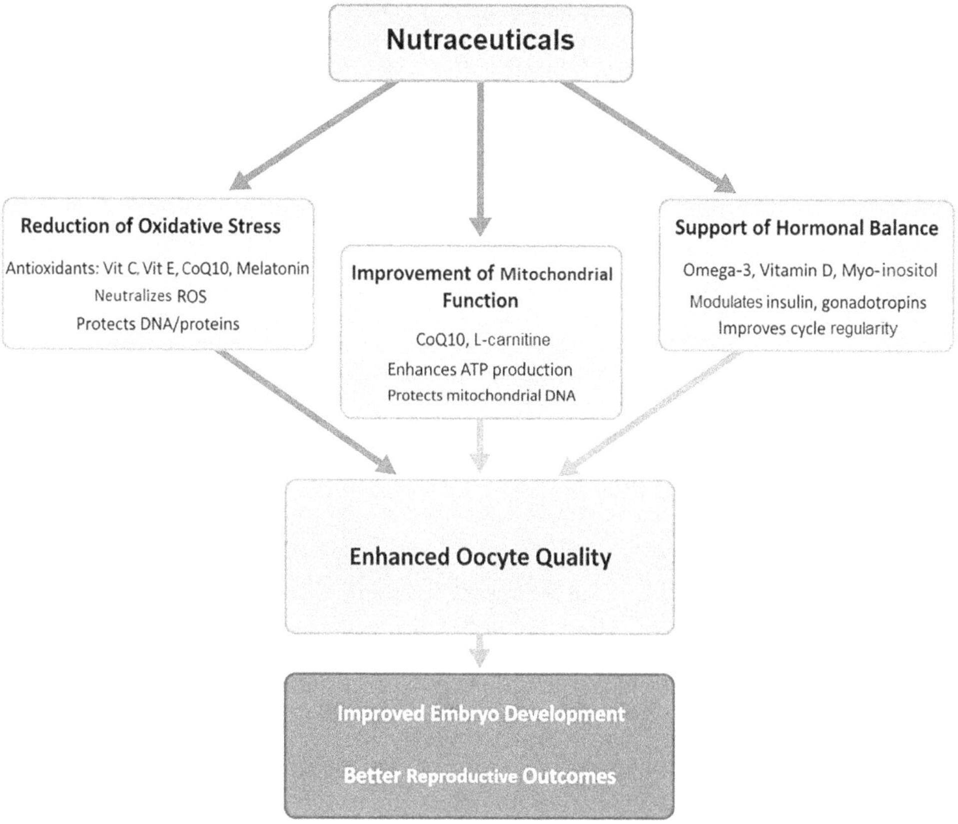

Figure 1.6 Mechanisms of action of nutraceuticals in oocyte quality improvement. (Original figure created by the author, based on data from (84). Licensed under CC BY 4.0.)

Vitamins and minerals are essential micronutrients that support multiple aspects of reproductive physiology. Vitamin D influences ovarian steroidogenesis, anti-Müllerian hormone expression, and endometrial receptivity; deficiency has been associated with poorer ART outcomes in some studies. Folic acid is crucial for DNA synthesis and methylation, supporting proper cell division and reducing the risk of neural tube defects. Zinc plays roles in oocyte maturation, fertilization, and early embryogenesis, while selenium contributes to antioxidant defense via selenoproteins and may help protect gametes from oxidative stress. Adequate intake and correction of deficiencies in these micronutrients are important components of preconception care.

Herbal extracts and plant-derived polyphenols are another growing area of interest. Compounds such as resveratrol, curcumin, and green tea polyphenols (e.g., epigallocatechin gallate, EGCG) have well-documented antioxidant and anti-inflammatory properties. Experimental and early clinical data suggest they may benefit ovarian function, improve insulin sensitivity and inflammatory status in conditions like PCOS, and support endometrial health. However, their effects can be dose dependent and context specific, and robust, large-scale clinical trials are still needed to define optimal dosing, safety in pregnancy, and precise indications. Overall, these key nutraceuticals illustrate the potential of targeted nutritional and bioactive compounds as adjuncts to conventional fertility treatments, while underscoring the need for evidence-based use and professional guidance (85, 86).

1.6.1 Clinical Evidence and Limitations

Although preclinical and early clinical studies on nutraceuticals in reproductive medicine are encouraging, the overall evidence base remains incomplete and heterogeneous. Some randomized controlled trials have reported improvements in oocyte quality, fertilization rates, embryo development, and even pregnancy outcomes with specific agents such as CoQ10, melatonin, myo-inositol, and certain micronutrients. Despite these promising findings, several important limitations constrain interpretation and routine clinical application.

First, there is substantial variability in study design. Differences in patient populations (e.g., age, ovarian reserve, presence of PCOS or endometriosis), inclusion criteria, dosages, duration of supplementation, and specific formulations make direct comparison across studies difficult and limit the ability to perform robust meta-analyses. Second, there is a lack of standardization in the nutraceutical industry. The quality, purity, bioavailability, and actual content of products can vary widely between manufacturers, and even between batches, which can significantly influence both efficacy and safety.

Third, long-term safety data are limited. Most clinical studies focus on short-term outcomes such as cycle parameters, laboratory markers, and immediate ART results. The long-term safety of high-dose or prolonged nutraceutical use – particularly during conception, pregnancy, and lactation – remains uncertain, and potential interactions with medications are often underexplored. Finally, there is a growing recognition that responses to nutraceuticals are likely to be individualized. Genetic polymorphisms, metabolic status, gut microbiota, coexisting medical conditions, and environmental exposures can all influence how a given compound is absorbed, metabolized, and utilized. This underscores the need for more personalized approaches and well-designed trials that stratify patients by relevant biological characteristics, so that clearer, evidence-based recommendations can be made for specific subgroups rather than applying a one-size-fits-all strategy.

1.6.2 Future Directions

Further research is needed to define the optimal dosages, combinations, and treatment durations of nutraceuticals in reproductive medicine. Large-scale, well-designed randomized clinical trials are essential to confirm their efficacy and safety across diverse patient populations and clinical settings. Standardization of product quality, bioavailability, and formulation will also be critical to ensure reproducible outcomes and to allow meaningful comparison between studies. In parallel, advances in personalized medicine – including genomics, metabolomics, and detailed phenotyping – are likely to enable more targeted and efficient use of nutraceuticals based on individual patient profiles, maximizing potential benefits while minimizing risks and unnecessary interventions.

1.6.3 Conclusion

Infertility is a multifactorial condition in which female factors, particularly oocyte quality and quantity, play a central and often limiting role. Women are born with a finite, non-renewable pool of oocytes that decline in both number and competence over time. Age-related deterioration of oocyte quality – driven by chromosomal segregation errors, mitochondrial dysfunction, impaired DNA repair, oxidative damage, and epigenetic alterations – is one of the most robustly documented phenomena in reproductive biology and a key determinant of natural and ART-related reproductive outcomes. Poor oocyte quality underlies many clinical challenges, including failed fertilization, arrested embryonic development, implantation failure, higher miscarriage rates, and reduced likelihood of live birth.

Female infertility arises from a wide range of causes, including ovulatory disorders, tubal pathology, endometriosis, uterine and cervical abnormalities, and diminished ovarian reserve, and is further shaped by lifestyle, environmental exposures, systemic medical conditions, and iatrogenic factors. At the pathophysiological level, hormonal imbalances, chronic inflammation, immune dysregulation, oxidative stress, and structural abnormalities all contribute to impaired gametogenesis, fertilization, and implantation. Beyond its biological dimensions, infertility has profound societal and psychological consequences, often associated with stigma, marital strain, and significant emotional distress. These burdens are amplified by the cost, invasiveness, and uncertainty of current infertility treatments.

Over the past century, major advances in diagnostic tools – hormonal assays, imaging modalities, and sophisticated ART techniques such as IVF, ICSI, and preimplantation genetic testing – have transformed the evaluation and management of infertility. Nonetheless, ART success remains strongly constrained by intrinsic oocyte quality, especially in women of advanced maternal age or with diminished ovarian reserve. This realization has shifted attention from simply increasing oocyte quantity to understanding and improving oocyte competence itself.

Oocyte quality is shaped by an intricate interplay of genetic, metabolic, environmental, and lifestyle factors. Age is the dominant non-modifiable determinant, but oxidative stress, metabolic disorders (e.g., obesity, diabetes, PCOS), exposure to environmental toxins, smoking, alcohol, suboptimal diet, and physical inactivity all negatively affect oocyte structure and function. At the mechanistic level, genetic integrity, mitochondrial function, epigenetic regulation, and cytoplasmic maturation are critical pathways linking oocyte health to ART outcomes, influencing fertilization rates, embryo development, implantation, and miscarriage risk.

Clinically, these insights highlight the importance of early fertility assessment and counseling, particularly for women contemplating delayed childbearing, and underscore the need for targeted strategies to preserve and enhance oocyte quality. Conventional interventions include lifestyle optimization (healthy diet, regular moderate exercise, weight management, avoidance of smoking and excessive alcohol), antioxidant support, and individualized hormonal stimulation protocols designed to maximize both oocyte yield and safety. Adjunctive therapies such as growth hormone, DHEA, myo-inositol, L-carnitine, and other micronutrients are being explored, especially in poor responders, though evidence remains variable and often inconclusive.

Against this background, nutraceuticals have emerged as a promising adjunct in reproductive medicine. Derived largely from foods and plants with favorable safety profiles, nutraceuticals – including antioxidants (vitamins C and E, CoQ10, melatonin), omega-3 fatty acids, vitamins and trace minerals, and a variety of herbal extracts – may influence reproductive outcomes through several interconnected mechanisms: reduction of oxidative stress, improvement of mitochondrial function, modulation of hormonal balance, attenuation of chronic inflammation, and support of immune homeostasis. Key agents such as CoQ10, melatonin, omega-3s, vitamin D, folate, zinc, selenium, resveratrol, and other polyphenols have shown encouraging effects on oocyte quality, embryo development, and, in some studies, pregnancy rates.

However, the current evidence base for nutraceuticals is still evolving. Heterogeneity in study designs, small sample sizes, variability in patient populations, lack of product standardization, and a focus on short-term outcomes limit the strength and generalizability of existing data. Long-term safety, optimal dosing, ideal combinations, and the most appropriate clinical indications remain incompletely defined. Moreover, individual responses to nutraceuticals are likely to be influenced by genetic background, metabolic status, comorbidities, and environmental factors, reinforcing the need for personalized approaches rather than uniform prescriptions.

Looking forward, the field of reproductive medicine is moving toward more precise, mechanism-based, and patient-specific strategies. Future directions include: large, well-designed clinical trials to clarify the efficacy and safety of key nutraceuticals; standardization and quality control of nutraceutical products; identification of robust biomarkers of oocyte competence; and integration of genomics, metabolomics, and other "omics" technologies to enable genuinely personalized treatment plans. Emerging regenerative and experimental techniques – such as ovarian tissue preservation and transplantation, stem cell-based approaches, and mitochondrial transfer – further illustrate the trajectory toward restoring or enhancing ovarian function in women with severely compromised oocyte quality.

In summary, this chapter emphasizes that oocyte quality sits at the heart of female fertility and ART success. While age and intrinsic biological constraints cannot be fully overcome, a combination of early counseling, lifestyle modification, optimized hormonal protocols, and carefully selected adjunctive and nutraceutical interventions offers meaningful opportunities to improve reproductive outcomes. To fully realize the potential of these strategies, especially nutraceuticals, more rigorous, standardized, and individualized research is essential. Ultimately, integrating these insights into clinical practice can help reduce the emotional and financial burden of infertility and increase the likelihood of achieving healthy, sustained pregnancies.

REFERENCES

1. Vander Borght M, Wyns C. Fertility and infertility: Definition and epidemiology. *Clinical Biochemistry*. 2018;62:2–10.
2. Feng J, Wu Q, Liang Y, Liang Y, Bin Q. Epidemiological characteristics of infertility, 1990–2021, and 15-year forecasts: An analysis based on the global burden of disease study 2021. *Reproductive Health*. 2025;22(1):26.
3. Liang Y, Huang J, Zhao Q, Mo H, Su Z, Feng S, et al. Global, regional, and national prevalence and trends of infertility among individuals of reproductive age (15–49 years) from 1990 to 2021, with projections to 2040. *Human Reproduction*. 2025;40(3):529–44.
4. Santi D, Corona G, Salonia A, Ferlin A. Current drawbacks and future perspectives in the diagnosis and treatment of male factor infertility, with a focus on FSH treatment: An expert opinion. *Journal of Endocrinological Investigation*. 2025;48(5):1085–100.

5. Munro MG, Balen AH, Cho S, Critchley HOD, Díaz I, Ferriani R, et al. The FIGO ovulatory disorders classification system. *International Journal of Gynaecology and Obstetrics: The Official Organ of the International Federation of Gynaecology and Obstetrics*. 2022;159(1):1–20.
6. Ambildhuke K, Pajai S, Chimegave A, Mundhada R, Kabra P. A review of tubal factors affecting fertility and its management. *Cureus*. 2022;14(11):e30990.
7. Bonavina G, Taylor HS. Endometriosis-associated infertility: From pathophysiology to tailored treatment. *Frontiers in Endocrinology*. 2022;13:1020827.
8. de Ziegler D, Pirtea P, Carbonnel M, Poulain M, Cicinelli E, Bulletti C, et al. Assisted reproduction in endometriosis. *Best Practice & Research Clinical Endocrinology & Metabolism*. 2019;33(1):47–59.
9. Vitale SG, De Angelis MC, Della Corte L, Saponara S, Carugno J, Laganà AS, et al. Uterine cervical stenosis: From classification to advances in management. Overcoming the obstacles to access the uterine cavity. *Archives of Gynecology and Obstetrics*. 2024;309(3):755–64.
10. Liu X, Zhao Y, Feng Y, Wang S, Zhang J. Ovarian aging: Mechanisms, age-related disorders, and therapeutic interventions. *MedComm*. 2025;6(12):e70481.
11. Houeis L, Donnez J, Dolmans M-M. Premature ovarian insufficiency and diminished ovarian reserve: From diagnosis to current management and treatment. *Journal of Clinical Medicine*. 2025;14(21):7473.
12. Zhu Z, Xu W, Liu L. Ovarian aging: Mechanisms and intervention strategies. *Medical Review*. 2022;2(6):590–610.
13. Jirge PR. Poor ovarian reserve. *Journal of Human Reproductive Sciences*. 2016;9(2):63–9.
14. Feng K, Zhang Z, Wu L, Zhu L, Li X, Li D, et al. Predictive factors for the formation of viable embryos in subfertile patients with diminished ovarian reserve: A clinical prediction study. *Reproductive Sciences*. 2024;31(6):1747–56.
15. Wu D, Liu C, Ding L. Follicular metabolic dysfunction, oocyte aneuploidy and ovarian aging: A review. *Journal of Ovarian Research*. 2025;18(1):53.
16. Skoracka K, Ratajczak AE, Rychter AM, Dobrowolska A, Krela-Kaźmierczak I. Female Fertility and the nutritional approach: The most essential aspects. *Advances in Nutrition (Bethesda, Md)*. 2021;12(6):2372–86.
17. de Angelis C, Nardone A, Garifalos F, Pivonello C, Sansone A, Conforti A, et al. Smoke, alcohol and drug addiction and female fertility. *Reproductive Biology and Endocrinology: RB&E*. 2020;18(1):21.
18. Kumar M, Sarma DK, Shubham S, Kumawat M, Verma V, Prakash A, et al. Environmental endocrine-disrupting chemical exposure: Role in non-communicable diseases. *Frontiers in Public Health*. 2020;8:553850.
19. Hannah Himabindu P, Swathi G, Padmavathi K, Penumalla S, Kandimalla R. Hypothyroidism and its impact on menstrual irregularities in reproductive-age women: A comprehensive analysis at a tertiary care center. *Cureus*. 2024;16(6):e63158.
20. Kim S, Kim SW, Han SJ, Lee S, Park HT, Song JY, et al. Molecular mechanism and prevention strategy of chemotherapy- and radiotherapy-induced ovarian damage. *International Journal of Molecular Sciences*. 2021;22(14).
21. Vigil P, Meléndez J, Soto H, Petkovic G, Bernal YA, Molina S. Chronic stress and ovulatory dysfunction: Implications in times of COVID–19. *Frontiers in Global Women's Health*. 2022;3:866104.
22. Bendarska-Czerwińska A, Zmarzły N, Morawiec E, Panfil A, Bryś K, Czarniecka J, et al. Endocrine disorders and fertility and pregnancy: An update. *Frontiers in Endocrinology*. 2022;13:970439.
23. Bosch E, Alviggi C, Lispi M, Conforti A, Hanyaloglu AC, Chuderland D, et al. Reduced FSH and LH action: Implications for medically assisted reproduction. *Human Reproduction (Oxford, England)*. 2021;36(6):1469–80.
24. Ou Y, Wang H, Zhou C, Chen Y, Lyu J, Feng M, et al. Endometriosis-associated infertility: Multi-omics insights into pathogenesis and precision therapeutics. *Frontiers in Endocrinology*. 2025;16:1613334.
25. Moustakli E, Zikopoulos A, Katopodis P, Dafopoulos S, Paraschos VS, Zachariou A, et al. Dietary and lifestyle interventions to mitigate oxidative stress in male and female fertility: Practical insights for infertility management-a narrative review. *Metabolites*. 2025;15(6).
26. Hosseinirad H, Yadegari P, Falahieh FM, Shahrestanaki JK, Karimi B, Afsharzadeh N, et al. The impact of congenital uterine abnormalities on pregnancy and fertility: A literature review. *JBRA Assisted Reproduction*. 2021;25(4):608–16.
27. Behude YT, Sendo EG, Tamir HH. Psycho-social experiences and coping strategies of infertile couples attending infertility clinics in Saint Paul's Hospital Millennium Medical College, Addis Ababa, Ethiopia: A qualitative study. *BMJ Open*. 2025;15(9):e095313.
28. de Castro MHM, Mendonça CR, Noll M, de Abreu Tacon FS, do Amaral WN. Psychosocial aspects of gestational grief in women undergoing infertility treatment: A systematic review of qualitative and quantitative evidence. *International Journal of Environmental Research and Public Health*. 2021;18(24):13143.
29. Vignozzi L, Cipriani S, Lippi D. Why couple infertility is historically a female-driven problem? *Andrology*. 2025;13(4):675–80.
30. Wang T, Dong T, Nie F. Clinical applications, advances, and future directions in hysterosalpingography. *Frontiers in Medicine*. 2025;12.

31. Chamayou S, Giacone F, Cannarella R, Guglielmino A. What does intracytoplasmic sperm injection change in embryonic development? The spermatozoon contribution. *J Clin Med.* 2023;12(2).
32. Ubaldi FM, Cimadomo D, Vaiarelli A, Fabozzi G, Venturella R, Maggiulli R, et al. Advanced maternal age in IVF: Still a challenge? The present and the future of its treatment. *Frontiers in Endocrinology.* 2019;10:94.
33. Conti M, Franciosi F. Acquisition of oocyte competence to develop as an embryo: Integrated nuclear and cytoplasmic events. *Human Reproduction Update.* 2018;24(3):245–66.
34. Chian RC, Guan YC, He XJ, Xu J, Shu JH, Li JH. The quality of human eggs and its pre-IVF incubation. *Reproductive Medicine and Biology.* 2025;24(1):e12652.
35. Wasielak-Politowska M, Kordowitzki P. Chromosome segregation in the oocyte: What goes wrong during aging. *International Journal of Molecular Sciences.* 2022;23(5).
36. Baldini GM, Ferri D, Malvasi A, Laganà AS, Vimercati A, Dellino M, et al. Genetic abnormalities of oocyte maturation: Mechanisms and clinical implications. *International Journal of Molecular Sciences.* 2024;25(23):13002.
37. Fan W, Yuan Z, Li M, Zhang Y, Nan F. Decreased oocyte quality in patients with endometriosis is closely related to abnormal granulosa cells. *Frontiers in Endocrinology.* 2023;14:1226687.
38. Sreerangaraja Urs DB, Wu WH, Komrskova K, Postlerova P, Lin YF, Tzeng CR, et al. Mitochondrial function in modulating human granulosa cell steroidogenesis and female fertility. *International Journal of Molecular Sciences.* 2020;21(10).
39. Chian R-C, Guan Y-C, He X-J, Xu J, Shu J-H, Li J-H. The quality of human eggs and its pre-IVF incubation. *Reproductive Medicine and Biology.* 2025;24(1):e12652.
40. Kordowitzki P, Graczyk S, Haghani A, Klutstein M. Oocyte aging: A multifactorial phenomenon in a unique cell. *Aging and Disease.* 2024;15(1):5–21.
41. Moghadam ARE, Moghadam MT, Hemadi M, Saki G. Oocyte quality and aging. *JBRA Assisted Reproduction.* 2022;26(1):105–22.
42. Wang X, Wang L, Xiang W. Mechanisms of ovarian aging in women: A review. *Journal of Ovarian Research.* 2023;16(1):67.
43. Bertoldo MJ, Listijono DR, Ho W-HJ, Riepsamen AH, Goss DM, Richani D, et al. NAD+ Repletion rescues female fertility during reproductive aging. *Cell Reports.* 2020;30(6):1670–81.e7.
44. Massarotti C, Cimadomo D, Spadoni V, Conforti A, Zacà C, Carosso AR, et al. Female fertility preservation for family planning: A position statement of the Italian Society of Fertility and Sterility and Reproductive Medicine (SIFES-MR). *Journal of Assisted Reproduction and Genetics.* 2024;41(9):2521–35.
45. Moaya M, Shahali S, Lamyian M, Azin SM, Milanifar A. Exploring the fertility needs of women before and after oocyte freezing for medical and non-medical reasons: A scoping review. *International Journal of Women's Health.* 2025;17:3361–74.
46. Hussain A, Abbas M, Zain-ul A, Mustafa G, Lateef M, Mansoor A, et al. Innovations and challenges in modern infertility treatment: Bridging technology and psychosocial care. *Middle East Fertility Society Journal.* 2025;30(1):44.
47. Scantamburlo VM, Von Linsingen R, Centa LJR, Dal Toso KF, Scaraboto D, Júnior EA, et al. Association between decreased ovarian reserve and poor oocyte quality. *Obstetrics & Gynecology Science.* 2021;64(6):532–9.
48. Song SY. Integrative approaches to ovulation induction in polycystic ovary syndrome: A narrative review of conventional and complementary therapies. *Biomedicines.* 2025;13(11).
49. Hwang YJ, Lee J, Hwang J, Sim H, Kim N, Kim TS. Psychiatric considerations of infertility. *Psychiatry Investigation.* 2024;21(11):1175–82.
50. Rebar RW. What are the risks of the assisted reproductive technologies (ART) and how can they be minimized? *Reproductive Medicine and Biology.* 2013;12(4):151–8.
51. Molla G, Bitew M. Revolutionizing personalized medicine: Synergy with multi-omics data generation, main hurdles, and future perspectives. *Biomedicines.* 2024;12(12).
52. Reddy B. The impact of age on oocyte quality and reproductive potential. *African Journal of Biomedical Research.* 2024;27:571–9.
53. Ribeiro S, Sousa M. In vitro fertilisation and intracytoplasmic sperm injection predictive factors: A review of the effect of female age, ovarian reserve, male age, and male factor on IVF/ICSI treatment outcomes. *JBRA Assisted Reproduction.* 2023;27(1):97–111.
54. Fan Y, Yang Q, Lin Y, Fu X, Shu J. The effect of endometriosis on oocyte quality: Mechanisms, diagnosis and treatment. *Archives of Gynecology and Obstetrics.* 2025;311(3):841–50.
55. Guimarães RM, Ribeiro LM, Sasaki LP, Nakagawa HM, Cabral IO. Oocyte morphology and reproductive outcomes – case report and literature review. *JBRA Assisted Reproduction.* 2021;25(3):500–7.
56. Ahmad MF, Elias MH, Mat Jin N, Abu MA, Syafruddin SE, Zainuddin AA, et al. Oocytes quality assessment – The current insight: A systematic review. *Biology.* 2024;13(12):978.
57. Mtango N, Potireddy S, Latham K. Oocyte quality and maternal control of development. *International Review of Cell and Molecular Biology.* 2008;268:223–90.

58. Petrogiannis N, Filippa M, Chatzovoulou K, Petrogiannis S, Filippas I, Grimbizis G, et al. Add-on technologies that aim to improve oocyte quality and embryo implantation potential. *Medicina (Kaunas, Lithuania)*. 2025;61(3).
59. Chicea E, Chicea R, Teacoe D, Chicea L, Radu I, Chicea D, et al. Advancements in sonication-based extraction techniques for ovarian follicular fluid analysis: Implications for infertility diagnostics and assisted reproductive technologies. *International Journal of Molecular Sciences*. 2025;26:10368.
60. Chen Y, Yang J, Zhang L. The impact of follicular fluid oxidative stress levels on the outcomes of assisted reproductive therapy. *Antioxidants (Basel, Switzerland)*. 2023;12(12).
61. Sharma R, Biedenharn KR, Fedor JM, Agarwal A. Lifestyle factors and reproductive health: Taking control of your fertility. *Reproductive Biology and Endocrinology: RB&E*. 2013;11:66.
62. Barraza-Ortega E, Gómez-Gil B, García-Gasca T, Lizárraga D, Díaz N, García-Gasca A. The impact of lifestyle on reproductive health: Microbial complexity, hormonal dysfunction, and pregnancy outcomes. *International Journal of Molecular Sciences*. 2025;26(17):8574.
63. Agarwal A, Maldonado Rosas I, Anagnostopoulou C, Cannarella R, Boitrelle F, Munoz LV, et al. Oxidative stress and assisted reproduction: A comprehensive review of its pathophysiological role and strategies for optimizing embryo culture environment. *Antioxidants (Basel, Switzerland)*. 2022;11(3).
64. Voros C, Athanasiou D, Papapanagiotou I, Mavrogianni D, Varthaliti A, Bananis K, et al. Cracking the code of oocyte quality: The oxidative stress link to IVF success. *International Journal of Molecular Sciences*. 2025;26(13):6377.
65. Liu H, Jin L, Wang X, Shi J, He Y, Sun N, et al. Reactive oxygen species in polycystic ovary syndrome: Mechanistic insights into pathogenesis and therapeutic opportunities. *Redox Biology*. 2025;85:103776.
66. Leão Rde B, Esteves SC. Gonadotropin therapy in assisted reproduction: An evolutionary perspective from biologics to biotech. *Clinics (Sao Paulo, Brazil)*. 2014;69(4):279–93.
67. Koloda Y, Korsak V, Rozenson O, Anshina M, Sagamonova K, Baranov I, et al. Use of a recombinant human follicle-stimulating hormone: Recombinant human luteinizing hormone (r-hFSH:r-hLH) 2:1 combination for controlled ovarian stimulation during assisted reproductive technology treatment: A real-world study of routine practice in the Russian Federation. *Best Practice & Research Clinical Obstetrics & Gynaecology*. 2022;85:134–48.
68. Conforti A, Carbone L, Di Girolamo R, Iorio GG, Guida M, Campitiello MR, et al. Therapeutic management in women with a diminished ovarian reserve: A systematic review and meta-analysis of randomized controlled trials. *Fertility and Sterility*. 2025;123(3):457–76.
69. Etrusco A, Agrifoglio V, Castillo Farfán JC, Bernabeu Garcia A, Laganà AS, Moliner Renau B, et al. Effectiveness of hormone add-on strategies in ovarian stimulation for women with poor ovarian response: A systematic review and network meta-analysis of randomized controlled trials. *J Assist Reprod Genet*. 2025;42(10):3231–52.
70. Xu Z, Tong W, Yang Z, Zhang H, Chen X. Comparative efficacy of different growth hormone supplementation protocols in improving clinical outcomes in women with poor ovarian response undergoing assisted reproductive therapy: A network meta-analysis. *Scientific Reports*. 2024;14(1):3377.
71. Chen H, Wang S, Song M, Yang D, Li H. Oocyte and dietary supplements: A mini review. *Frontiers in Cell and Developmental Biology*. 2025;13:1619758.
72. Gałęska E, Kowalczyk A, Wrzecińska M, García MC, Czerniawska-Piątkowska E, Gwoździewicz S, et al. The importance of mitochondrial processes in the maturation and acquisition of competences of oocytes and embryo culture. *International Journal of Molecular Sciences*. 2025;26(9).
73. Jamalinia M, Weiskirchen R. Advances in personalized medicine: Translating genomic insights into targeted therapies for cancer treatment. *Annals of Translational Medicine*. 2025;13(2):18.
74. Zhang S, Zhu D, Mei X, Li Z, Li J, Xie M, et al. Advances in biomaterials and regenerative medicine for primary ovarian insufficiency therapy. *Bioactive Materials*. 2021;6(7):1957–72.
75. Kalra EK. Nutraceutical – definition and introduction. *AAPS PharmSci*. 2003;5(3):E25.
76. Tomar S, Musyuni P, Aggarwal G. An overview of regulation for nutraceuticals and concept of personalized nutraceuticals. *Journal of Generic Medicines*. 2023;19(2):66–74.
77. Manful CF, Fordjour E, Subramaniam D, Sey AA, Abbey L, Thomas R. Antioxidants and reactive oxygen species: Shaping human health and disease outcomes. *International Journal of Molecular Sciences*. 2025;26(15):7520.
78. Gulcin İ. Antioxidants: A comprehensive review. *Archives of Toxicology*. 2025;99(5):1893–997.
79. Street ME, Casadei F, Di Bari ER, Ferraboschi F, Montani AG, Mele MC, et al. The role of nutraceuticals and probiotics in addition to lifestyle intervention in the management of childhood obesity – Part 2: Comorbidities. *Nutrients*. 2025;17(9):1487.
80. Liu X, Zeng T, Zhang E, Bin C, Liu Q, Wu K, et al. Plant-based bioactives and oxidative stress in reproduction: Anti-inflammatory and metabolic protection mechanisms. *Frontiers in Nutrition*. 2025;12:1650347.
81. Liu X, Zeng T, Zhang E, Bin C, Liu Q, Wu K, et al. Plant-based bioactives and oxidative stress in reproduction: Anti-inflammatory and metabolic protection mechanisms. *Frontiers in Nutrition*. 2025;12:1650347.

82. Marcianò G, Rania V, Vocca C, Palleria C, Crudo M, Evangelista M, et al. The role and safety of plant-derived nutraceuticals as adjuvant treatments for pain management: A narrative review. *Nutraceuticals*. 2025;5(4):38.
83. Alrashidi AS, Feraih Aljaghwani L, Saleh AlMohimeed R. The effect of nutrient supplementation on female fertility: A systematic review. *Cureus*. 2024;16(8):e67028.
84. Farina M, Maugeri A, Rapisarda A, Navarra M. The impact of food and nutraceuticals on human fertility. *Food Nutrition*. 2025;1(2):100021.
85. Rodríguez-Varela C, Labarta E. Does coenzyme Q10 supplementation improve human oocyte quality? *International Journal of Molecular Sciences*. 2021;22(17).
86. Solati A, Taghvimi S, Jamali Z, Vahedi F, Moazamfard M, Bahmyari S, et al. The effect of antioxidants on increased oocyte competence in IVM: A review. *Reproductive and Developmental Medicine*. 2023;7(3).

2 Inositol's Impact on Infertility Treatment

Samaneh Harimi, Amir Masoud Firouzabadi, Maryam Azizi-Kutenaei, and Farzaneh Fesahat

2.1 INTRODUCTION

In the landscape of nutritional interventions for female infertility, few compounds have garnered as much scientific interest as inositol. Inositols are a group of nine distinct carbocyclic sugar stereoisomers that belong to the vitamin B complex, playing fundamental roles as structural components of cell membranes and as precursors for intracellular second messengers (1). Among these, myo-inositol (MI) is the most abundant isoform in the human body, with D-chiro-inositol (DCI) being its most studied epimer (2) (Figure 2.1).

The primary mechanism of action for inositols lies in their role within the phosphoinositide signaling pathway. MI is a key component of phosphatidy linositols, which, upon hormonal stimulation at the cell surface, are cleaved to generate second messengers like inositol trisphosphate (IP3) and diacylglycerol (DAG) (1). These molecules are critical for modulating intracellular calcium ($Ca2+$) levels and activating protein kinase C, thereby mediating the signals of numerous hormones, including follicle-stimulating hormone (FSH), thyroid-stimulating hormone (TSH), and insulin (3). DCI, on the other hand, is primarily involved in a separate pathway as a mediator of insulin's action on glycogen synthesis (4). The body maintains a specific, tissue-dependent ratio of MI to DCI, regulated by an insulin-dependent epimerase that converts MI to DCI (5, 6) (Figure 2.2).

This intricate biochemical system has profound implications for female reproductive physiology. MI is found in high concentrations within follicular fluid, and its levels are considered a biomarker for good-quality oocytes (8, 9). It is integral to FSH signaling in granulosa cells, which is essential for proper follicular maturation and oocyte development (10). A disruption in the physiological balance between MI and DCI, often seen in metabolic disorders like polycystic ovary syndrome (PCOS), can lead to impaired insulin signaling and contribute to the hyperandrogenism and ovulatory dysfunction characteristic of the condition (5, 6). This phenomenon, sometimes termed the "inositol paradox," highlights that an excess of DCI relative to MI at the ovarian level can be detrimental to oocyte quality (11, 12). This chapter will synthesize the evidence from randomized controlled trials (RCTs) regarding the clinical applications of inositol, particularly MI, in the treatment of female infertility, with a primary focus on PCOS and assisted reproductive technologies (ARTs), alongside complementary applications in conditions like gestational diabetes.

2.2 INOSITOL IN INFERTILITY TREATMENT: MECHANISMS AND PHYSIOLOGICAL ROLES

Inositol's impact on infertility treatment is multifactorial, targeting the core physiological disturbances that underpin many cases of anovulation and subfertility. Its therapeutic has been extensively investigated in clinical settings, primarily focusing on women with PCOS and those undergoing ART. The evidence from a large body of RCTs supports its use for improving both metabolic and reproductive outcomes (13).

PCOS is the most common endocrinopathy in reproductive-aged women and a leading cause of anovulatory infertility (14). Its pathophysiology is intrinsically linked to insulin resistance (IR) and hyperandrogenism, making it a prime target for inositol therapy (15). The therapeutic efficacy of inositols, particularly MI, has been validated across numerous randomized controlled trials, showing significant improvements in the core metabolic, hormonal, and clinical features of the syndrome (16).

2.2.1 Metabolic and Clinical Improvements (Insulin Sensitivity and Menstrual Cyclicity)

A foundational aspect of many infertility cases, especially in the context of PCOS, is insulin resistance and the resultant compensatory hyperinsulinemia (14). This is consistently measured by a decrease in the homeostasis model assessment of insulin resistance (HOMA-IR) index and fasting insulin levels. Elevated insulin levels act synergistically with LH to stimulate excess androgen production by ovarian theca cells, which disrupt follicular development and lead to anovulation (4, 17, 18).

DOI: 10.1201/9781003741541-2

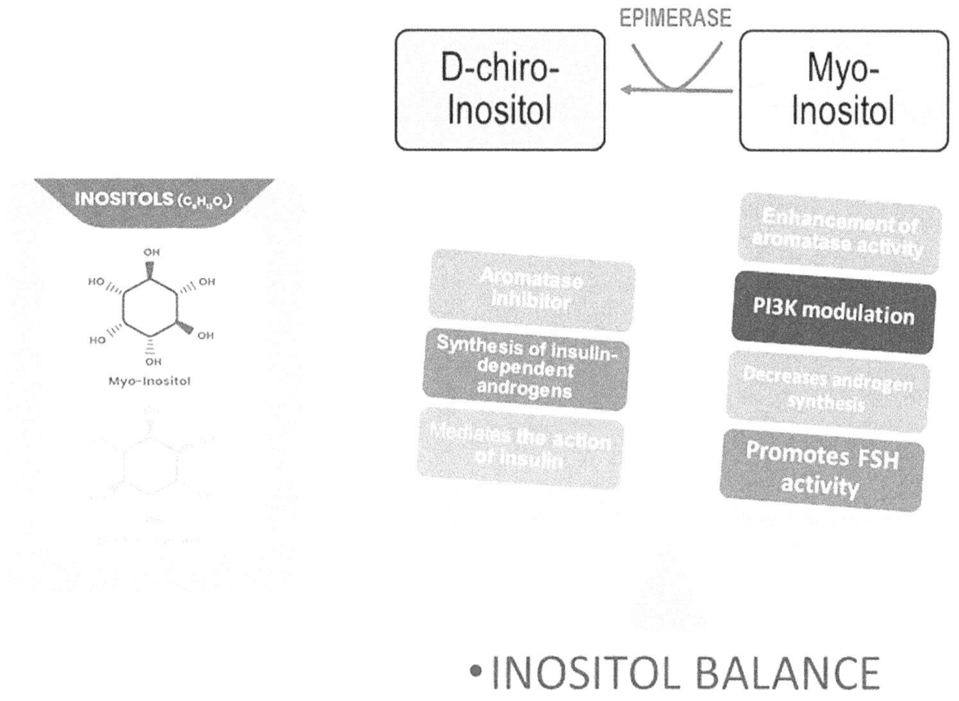

Figure 2.1 Comparing myo-inositol with D-chiro-inositol. D-chiro-inositol inhibits aromatase synthesis and increases androgen synthesis under insulin stimulation. Myo-inositol modulates PI3K activity while increasing aromatase and FSH receptor synthesis in granulosa cells. In addition, myo-inositol reduces androgen release from theca cells. (Under Creative Commons Attribution License [2].)

Inositol stereoisomers, particularly MI and DCI, function as insulin-sensitizing agents (17). They are precursors to inositol phosphoglycans (IPGs), which are second messengers that mediate insulin's metabolic actions, such as cellular glucose uptake (19). By improving the body's sensitivity to insulin, inositol supplementation effectively lowers circulating insulin levels (20, 21). This reduction in hyperinsulinemia alleviates the excessive stimulation of the ovaries, leading to decreased androgen production and the restoration of spontaneous ovulatory cycles in a significant proportion of anovulatory women (22, 23).

Some RCT studies confirm that taking 4 g/day of MI can improve insulin sensitivity, restore fasting insulin levels and normal menstrual cycles, and improve ovulation (18, 20, 22–24). In a double-blind trial by Costantino et al. on 42 PCOS women, 4 g/day of MI (plus folic acid) for 12–16 weeks resulted in a significant decrease in the area under the plasma insulin curve (AUC) after an oral glucose tolerance test (OGTT) ($P = 0.03$) with an 84% increase in the composite whole-body insulin sensitivity index (ISIcomp) ($P < 0.002$), effects not seen in the placebo group (23). This metabolic correction translated directly to clinical outcomes: 69.5% (16 out of 23) of women in the MI group ovulated, compared to only 21% (4 out of 19) in the placebo group ($P = 0.001$) (23). In one trial, 88% of patients restored at least one spontaneous menstrual cycle, with 72% maintaining normal ovulatory activity (22). However, some RCT studies confirm that taking 2 g/day of MI can similarly reduce insulin levels, improve HOMA index and glucose-to-insulin ratio, leading to restoration of menstrual cycles in all subjects with amenorrhea and oligomenorrhea (9, 21, 25).

Several RCTs have directly compared the efficacy of MI to metformin, the conventional insulin-sensitizing drug used in PCOS (3, 17, 20, 24, 26). These studies have consistently found that 4 g/day of MI is at least as effective as metformin in improving insulin sensitivity, reducing BMI, and restoring menstrual cyclicity (17, 24), but with a significantly better safety profile, most notably the absence of gastrointestinal side effects commonly associated with metformin (24). Furthermore, MI upregulates the gene expression of PPAR-γ ($P = 0.002$), a key regulator of insulin and lipid metabolism, suggesting a more profound mechanistic benefit than metformin (20).

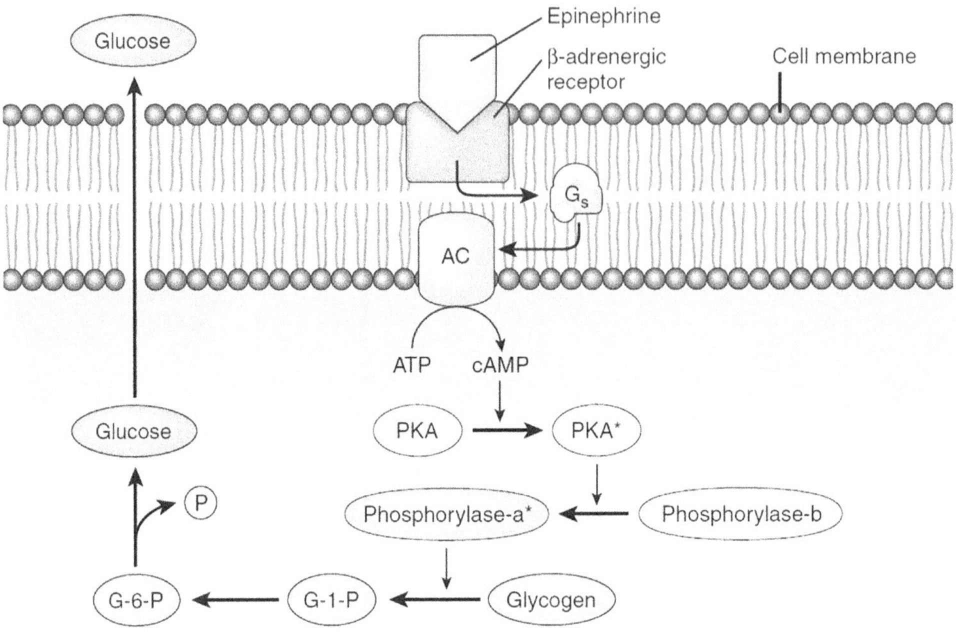

Figure 2.2 Schematic of the inositol signaling pathway. Schematic representation of the action of a chemical regulator working through a Gq-protein to activate the enzyme phopholipase C (PLC) and generating the second messenger inositol trisphosphate (IP3) and diacylglycerol (DAG) from phosphatidylinositol bisphosphate (PIP2). IP3 releases intracellular Ca^{2+}, which may interact with secretory vesicles and induce exocytosis of some product (e.g., hormone, secretory protein). DAG may activate phosphokinase C (PKC*) and produce additional phosphorylations and various effects (7). (From [7], under Creative Commons Attribution License.)

2.2.2 Role in Oocyte Maturation and Hormonal Regulation

The quality of an oocyte is a critical determinant of fertilization, embryo development, and successful implantation (8, 9). Myo-inositol is a key player in this process. As a precursor to IP3, MI mediates the intracellular calcium oscillations that are essential for the meiotic progression of oocytes (3, 22). Clinical studies have consistently shown that higher concentrations of MI in the follicular fluid correlate positively with the retrieval of mature, high-quality oocytes (8, 9, 27). Supplementation with 4 g/day of MI has been demonstrated to improve oocyte and subsequent embryo quality in women undergoing ART, particularly those with PCOS (8, 10, 28). One study also provided mechanistic insight, showing that MI supplementation significantly upregulated the gene expression of oocyte quality markers PGK1, RGS2, and CDC42 in granulosa cells (10).

Furthermore, MI is the second messenger for FSH, and the primary gonadotropin responsible for follicular recruitment and growth (22, 28). In PCOS, where hormonal imbalances such as elevated luteinizing hormone (LH) and hyperandrogenism are common, impaired FSH signaling can lead to follicular arrest (4, 26). By improving the cellular response to FSH, MI may help overcome this arrest, promoting normal folliculogenesis (22, 26). RCTs have shown that both 2 g/day (4, 25) and 4 g/day MI (23, 29) administration can lead to a significant reduction in serum LH, testosterone, and prolactin levels, while improving the LH/FSH ratio, thereby helping to normalize the hormonal milieu required for ovulation.

The correction of hyperinsulinemia directly leads to the second major benefit of inositol: the significant reduction of hyperandrogenism. By lowering the insulin stimulus on the ovaries, MI supplementation compared to metformin effectively breaks the vicious cycle of androgen overproduction. This is reflected in significant reductions in serum total and free testosterone, androstenedione, and LH levels, often accompanied by a beneficial increase in sex hormone-binding globulin (SHBG) (3, 4, 23, 25, 30). A study by Formuso et al. also noted that MI treatment in

137 overweight PCOS women led to significant improvements in acne scores, another clinical sign of hyperandrogenism (14).

Some RCTs demonstrated that 4 g/day of MI was superior to metformin in significantly decreasing total testosterone, mF-G hirsutism scores, and the inflammatory marker hs-CRP (3, 17, 26). When compared to oral contraceptive pills (OCPs), the combination of MI with an OCP was more effective in controlling metabolic and endocrine profiles than OCPs alone (15, 31).

2.2.3 Role in Assisted Reproductive Technologies

Beyond restoring natural fertility, inositols have been studied for their role in improving outcomes for women undergoing ART procedures like in vitro fertilization (IVF) and intracytoplasmic sperm injection (ICSI). The focus in this context is on enhancing oocyte and embryo quality, which is often compromised in PCOS patients (8, 28).

Oocyte and Embryo Quality: MI supplementation prior to and during controlled ovarian stimulation has been shown to increase the number of mature (metaphase II) oocytes retrieved while reducing the number of immature oocytes (8, 9, 28, 32, 33). This leads to a higher yield of top-quality embryos available for transfer (8, 27, 33). Mechanistic studies suggest this is due to MI's role in modulating the expression of genes related to apoptosis in cumulus cells, creating a more favorable environment for oocyte development (34).

Pregnancy and Live Birth Rates: The improvement in gamete and embryo quality often translates to better clinical outcomes. Several RCTs have reported higher clinical pregnancy and implantation rates in women treated with inositol (27, 28, 35, 36). The benefits are particularly pronounced when MI is used in combination therapies. A study by Mendoza et al. found that a combination of MI and a high dose of DCI (3.6:1 ratio) resulted in significantly higher pregnancy (65.5% vs. 25.9%) and live birth rates (55.2% vs. 14.8%) in PCOS women undergoing ICSI compared to a low-DCI combination (40:1 ratio) (37). Similarly, another trial comparing metformin alone to a combination of metformin plus MI found a significantly higher live birth rate in the combination group (55% vs. 26.67%) (36). Furthermore, inositol supplementation may reduce the risk of ovarian hyperstimulation syndrome (OHSS), a potential complication of ovarian stimulation, by promoting more controlled follicular development (35). Finally, the large trial by Pacchiarotti et al. showed a clear trend of higher clinical pregnancy rates in the inositol-treated groups (41.4% for MI+Melatonin and 36.7% for MI alone) compared to the control group (31.0%), further supporting the role of inositol-based therapies in improving successful ART outcomes (28).

The robust evidence from these clinical trials is summarized in Tables 2.1 and 2.2 (Table 2.1 for PCOS; Table 2.2 for ART).

2.3 COMBINATION THERAPIES

The efficacy of inositol is often enhanced when combined with other compounds that target related or complementary physiological pathways. Research into these formulations is aimed at creating synergistic effects to improve overall treatment outcomes (53).

2.3.1 Myo-Inositol and D-Chiro-Inositol

The co-administration of MI and DCI is perhaps the most debated and studied combination. The rationale is based on the physiological tissue-specific ratios of these two isomers. While plasma maintains an MI/DCI ratio of approximately 40:1, this ratio varies significantly in different tissues based on their function (6). The ovary, a high glucose-utilizing organ, requires a very high MI/DCI ratio (around 100:1) for proper FSH signaling and oocyte development (33). In PCOS, hyperinsulinemia can overstimulate the epimerase enzyme in the ovary, excessively converting MI to DCI and creating an MI deficiency that impairs oocyte quality (5, 33).

Based on this, several RCTs have found that administering MI and DCI in the physiological plasma ratio of 40:1 is more effective than MI alone for improving metabolic parameters in overweight PCOS patients (54) and is superior to other ratios for restoring ovulation (6). However, the optimal ratio may be context-dependent. A landmark RCT in the ART setting by Mendoza et al. demonstrated that a much lower ratio of 3.6:1 (higher DCI dose) led to significantly better pregnancy and live birth rates in ICSI cycles compared to a 40:1 ratio (35). This suggests that while a 40:1 ratio may be ideal for restoring natural ovulation and systemic metabolic balance, a different formulation might be more beneficial in the context of controlled ovarian stimulation.

Table 2.1: Summary of Key Randomized Controlled Trials of Inositol in Polycystic Ovary Syndrome

Study Population	Intervention(s) & Dosage	Comparator	Key Outcomes	Ref
137 Overweight PCOS women	MI (4 g/day) or DCI (1 g/day)	Placebo	Both MI and DCI improved menstrual regularity, acne, and metabolic parameters.	(14)
50 PCOS women with insulin resistance	MI (4 g/day)	Metformin (1500 mg/day)	MI and metformin were equally effective in improving BMI, insulin sensitivity, and menstrual cycles; MI had better tolerability.	(24)
66 PCOS women (normal & overweight)	MI (4 g/day)	Metformin (1500 mg/day)	Both treatments showed similar beneficial effects on BMI, body composition, hormones, and glucose metabolism.	(17)
50 PCOS women	MI (4 g/day)	DCI (1 g/day)	MI showed a more marked effect on the metabolic profile, while DCI was better at reducing hyperandrogenism.	(29)
60 PCOS women	MI (4 g/day)	Metformin (1500 mg/day)	MI was superior in decreasing testosterone, hirsutism score, hs-CRP, and inflammatory gene expression.	(3)
53 PCOS women	MI (4 g/day)	Metformin (1500 mg/day)	MI was superior in improving glycemic control (FPG, insulin, HOMA-IR), triglycerides, and upregulating PPAR-γ.	(20)
25 PCOS women with anovulation	MI (4 g/day)	N/A (Observational)	88% of patients restored at least one menstrual cycle, and 40% achieved pregnancy.	(22)
42 Obese PCOS patients	MI (2 g/day)	N/A (Pre-post)	MI was more effective in reducing insulin levels in patients with higher baseline fasting insulin (>12 μU/mL).	(21)
42 PCOS women	MI (4 g/day)	Placebo (folic acid)	MI significantly improved insulin sensitivity, reduced androgens, blood pressure, and triglycerides, and increased ovulation rate (69.5% vs. 21%).	(23)
20 Overweight PCOS patients	MI (2 g/day)	Placebo (folic acid)	MI significantly improved insulin sensitivity, reduced LH, PRL, T, and insulin levels, and restored menstrual cyclicity.	(4)

(Continued)

Table 2.1: (Continued)

Study Population	Intervention(s) & Dosage	Comparator	Key Outcomes	Ref
26 Normal-weight PCOS women	MI (1.2 g/day)	Placebo	MI treatment significantly reduced hormonal, metabolic, and oxidative stress abnormalities by improving insulin resistance.	(38)
50 Overweight PCOS patients	MI (2 g/day)	Placebo	After 12 weeks, MI group showed significant reductions in LH, PRL, T, insulin, and LH/FSH.	(25)
120 PCOS women	MI (4 g/day)	Metformin (1500 mg/day)	65% of patients on MI restored ovulation vs. 50% on metformin. Total pregnancy rate was higher with MI (48.4% vs. 36.6%).	(39)
20 Lean PCOS women	DCI (600 mg/day)	Placebo	DCI significantly reduced insulin AUC, free testosterone, blood pressure, and triglycerides; 60% ovulated vs. 20% in placebo.	(40)
150 Infertile PCOS women resistant to letrozole	MI (4 g/day) or metformin (1500 mg/day)	Placebo	Adding MI or metformin to letrozole improved ovarian function, with MI being more effective in patients with normal BMI.	(41)
283 Women with oligomenorrhea & PCO	Inositol (200 mg/day)	Placebo	Inositol group had a significantly higher ovulation frequency (23% vs. 13%) and significant weight loss.	(42)
Overweight/obese PCOS patients	DCI (500 mg/day)	N/A (Pre-post)	DCI improved insulin sensitivity and hormonal patterns, particularly in patients with diabetic relatives.	(5)
50 PCOS women	MI (4 g/day)	DCI (1 g/day)	Myo-inositol showed a more marked effect on the metabolic profile, whereas D-chiro-inositol reduced hyperandrogenism better.	(43)
11 PCOS women	DCI	Placebo	Showed a positive correlation between the change in DCI-IPG release and the change in insulin sensitivity.	(37)

Table 2.2: Summary of Key Randomized Controlled Trials of Inositol in Assisted Reproductive Technology

Study Population	Intervention(s) & Dosage	Comparator	Key Outcomes	Ref
526 PCOS women undergoing IVF	MI (4 g/day) + Melatonin (3 mg/day)	MI (4 g/day) alone/placebo	The combination of MI + melatonin was superior to MI alone in improving oocyte and embryo quality.	(28)
PCOS Patients undergoing IVF	DCI (1 g/day)	N/A (Pre-post)	DCI administration appeared to reduce the oxidation of thiol groups in follicular fluid, suggesting a reduction in oxidative stress.	(44)
60 PCOS women undergoing ICSI	MI + DCI (3.6:1 ratio)	MI + DCI (40:1 ratio)	The high-DCI ratio group had significantly higher pregnancy and live birth rates.	(35)
60 Infertile PCOS women undergoing ICSI	MI (4 g/day)	Placebo	MI administration improved the expression of apoptosis-related genes in cumulus cells, which correlated with good-quality embryos.	(34)
60 Infertile PCOS women undergoing ICSI	MI (4 g/day)	Placebo	MI improved hormonal profiles, oxidative stress markers in follicular fluid, cleavage rate, and good embryo quality.	(8)
PCOS patients undergoing IVF	MI (4 g/day)	Placebo	MI group had a significantly greater number of follicles >15 mm, more oocytes recovered, and a reduced number of immature oocytes.	(32)
50 Infertile PCOS patients undergoing ART	MI (4 g/day)	Placebo	MI significantly improved MII oocyte percentage, fertilization rate, and embryo quality.	(10)
172 Oocytes from 11 PCOS women undergoing ICSI	MI (550 mg) + DCI (300 mg) / day	MI (550 mg) + DCI (27.6 mg)/ day	High doses of DCI in combination with MI had a positive influence on the quality of the oocyte cytoplasm.	(45)
196 Infertile PCOS patients undergoing IUI	MI (4 g / day) + rFSH	rFSH alone	MI administration increased clinical pregnancy rates (18.6% vs. 12.2%), lowered the total rFSH dose, and shortened the duration of stimulation.	(9)
PCOS Women undergoing IVF-ET	MI + DCI (40:1 ratio)	DCI alone	The 40:1 combination improved IVF outcome, whereas DCI alone was not effective.	(33)
84 Euglycemic PCOS patients undergoing ICSI	MI (4 g/day)	DCI (1.2 g/day)	MI was superior to DCI in increasing the number of mature oocytes and top-quality embryos, and resulted in more pregnancies.	(46)

(Continued)

Table 2.2: (Continued)

Study Population	Intervention(s) & Dosage	Comparator	Key Outcomes	Ref
19 Women undergoing IVF	N/A (Observational)	N/A	A higher MI/DCI ratio in follicular fluid was significantly correlated with better blastocyst quality.	(12)
65 Women undergoing IVF	MI + Folic Acid + Melatonin	MI + folic acid	The addition of melatonin significantly increased the number of mature oocytes and top-quality embryos.	(47)
112 Poor ovarian responders undergoing ICSI	MI (4 g/day)	Placebo	MI treatment significantly increased the number of Grade A embryos and the fertilization rate.	(48)
60 Poor ovarian responders undergoing ART	MI (4 g/day)	Placebo	MI significantly improved the ovarian sensitivity index and fertilization rate and reduced the required dose of gonadotropins.	(49)
46 Women with prior IVF failure due to poor oocyte quality	MI (4 g / day) + Melatonin (3 mg / day)	N/A (Pre-post)	The combination improved the number of mature oocytes, fertilization rate, and number of top-quality embryos transferred.	(50)
100 Women undergoing ICSI	MI + Alpha – Lactalbumin + Melatonin + Vitamin D3	Placebo	The complex supplementation significantly improved blastocyst and oocyte quality and achieved a higher clinical pregnancy rate (42% vs. 24%).	(51)
120 Infertile women undergoing IVF	MI + Melatonin + Folic Acid + Vitamin D3	MI + melatonin + folic acid	The addition of vitamin D3 significantly increased implantation rate (37.1% vs. 19.2%).	(52)
149 Patients undergoing ICSI	MI + Folic acid	Folic acid alone	MI group had significantly higher numbers of excellent/good-quality oocytes, more grade A embryos transferred, and a significantly higher clinical pregnancy rate.	(27)

2.3.2 Inositol with Melatonin, Folic Acid, and Other Antioxidants

Melatonin: Melatonin is a potent antioxidant that is naturally present in follicular fluid and protects oocytes from oxidative stress, a key factor in poor oocyte quality (28, 47, 50). RCTs have shown that combining MI (4 g/day) with melatonin (3 mg/day) acts synergistically to improve oocyte and embryo quality, particularly in PCOS patients and women with a history of poor oocyte quality in previous IVF cycles (28, 47, 50).

Folic Acid: Folic acid is almost universally co-administered with inositol in clinical trials, primarily for its established role in preventing neural tube defects (55). However, it should be noted that no data from the literature report the metabolic or hormonal effect of folic acid in women of reproductive age (56).

Alpha-Lipoic Acid (ALA) and Alpha-Lactalbumin: ALA is another powerful antioxidant and insulin-sensitizing agent. A combination of MI and ALA has been shown to effectively reduce markers of inflammation (HMGB1) and improve insulin sensitivity in adolescents with PCOS (57). Alpha-lactalbumin is a protein that has been studied for its ability to improve the intestinal absorption of MI. In patients identified as "MI-resistant" (i.e., those who do not ovulate on MI alone), the addition of alpha-lactalbumin was able to overcome this resistance, significantly increasing MI plasma levels and successfully restoring ovulation (58, 59).

These combination therapies highlight a move toward multi-targeted approaches, addressing not just insulin resistance but also oxidative stress, inflammation, and nutrient absorption to optimize the reproductive environment (Table 2.3).

2.4 COMPLEMENTARY APPLICATION

2.4.1 Complementary Application in Gestational Diabetes Mellitus

Beyond its primary application in fertility and PCOS management, a significant body of research has explored the role of myo-inositol in the prevention and management of gestational diabetes mellitus (GDM), a condition characterized by abnormal glucose tolerance with onset or first recognition during pregnancy (68). Insulin resistance is a key pathophysiological feature of GDM, making insulin-sensitizing agents like MI a logical therapeutic candidate (68, 69).

Several randomized controlled trials have demonstrated the efficacy of MI supplementation in reducing GDM incidence, particularly in high-risk populations. A consistent finding across multiple studies is that a daily dose of 4 grams of myo-inositol, often combined with 400 mcg of folic acid and initiated in the first trimester, yields significant preventive effects. For example, in a trial involving 220 pregnant women with a family history of type 2 diabetes, MI supplementation significantly reduced the GDM rate to 6%, compared to 15.3% in the placebo group ($P = 0.04$) (70). This risk reduction was even more pronounced in populations stratified by BMI. Another study by the same research group on 220 obese pregnant women (BMI ≥ 30) found that MI treatment lowered the GDM rate to 14.0%, a stark contrast to the 33.6% observed in the control group ($P = 0.001$) (69). Similarly, in a cohort of 220 overweight women (BMI 25–29.9), GDM incidence was significantly lower in the MI group (11.6% vs. 27.4%, $P = 0.004$) (71). A smaller study on non-obese women with elevated first-trimester fasting glucose further corroborated these findings, reporting a significant reduction in GDM incidence ($P = 0.001$) and a decreased need for subsequent insulin therapy in the MI group (72). A trial using a lower dose of 2 g/day MI also found a noticeable reduction in GDM incidence in overweight pregnant women (RR = 0.29, $P = 0.037$) (73). These findings suggest that starting MI supplementation from the first trimester can be an effective preventive strategy.

The primary mechanism underlying these benefits is the improvement of insulin sensitivity. The trial on obese women demonstrated a significantly greater reduction in the HOMA-IR index in the MI-treated group compared to controls (-1.0 ± 3.1 vs. 0.1 ± 1.8, $P = 0.048$) (69). This was supported by Asimakopoulos et al., who not only confirmed a lower HOMA-IR in their MI group but also showed significantly higher insulin sensitivity as measured by the Matsuda Index ($P = 0.037$) (68).

The choice of inositol isomer and dosage has also been a subject of investigation. A study compared MI, DCI, and a combination in high-risk pregnant women, concluding that the largest benefit in preventing GDM was observed in the MI-only group (74). Another study in women already diagnosed with GDM found that 4000 mg of MI was superior to other isomers or lower doses in decreasing HOMA-IR and reducing the need for intensified insulin therapy (75). Furthermore, combining MI with alpha-lactalbumin in GDM patients significantly reduced HOMA-IR values after 2 months (3.1 ± 1.4 vs. 6.1 ± 3.4, $p = 0.0002$) and decreased the rate of women requiring insulin (6.7% vs. 20.3%, $p = 0.03$) (76).

However, the evidence is not uniformly positive, highlighting the complexity of GDM and patient response. The large-scale NiPPeR international trial, which used a combined supplement containing 4 g/day MI, probiotics, and micronutrients, did not find a significant difference in gestational glycemia or GDM rates between the intervention and control groups (24.8% vs. 22.6%) (77). Similarly, a randomized controlled trial using a 40:1 combination of MI and DCI in 240 women with a family history of diabetes found no preventive effect on GDM incidence (23.3% in the intervention group vs. 18.3% in the control group, $P = 0.34$) (78). These conflicting results may be due to differences in study populations (e.g., general preconception vs. high-risk pregnant cohorts), the specific formulation used (MI alone vs. complex combinations), and the timing of the intervention. Nonetheless, a strong body of evidence points to a promising role for MI, particularly when administered early in pregnancy at a dose of 4 g/day to at-risk populations, for improving glycemic control and reducing the incidence of GDM.

Table 2.3: Summary of Key Randomized Controlled Trials on Combination Therapies with Inositol

Study Population	Intervention(s) & Dosage	Comparator	Key Outcomes	Ref
1729 Women planning conception	MI + Probiotics + Micronutrients	Standard micronutrients	No overall effect on time-to-conception, but shortened it in overweight women and lengthened it in non-White obese women.	(60)
Lean PCOS teenagers	MI + OCP	OCP alone or MI alone	In older teens (17–19), combining MI with OCP prevented weight gain and improved metabolic/hormonal profiles more than either alone.	(15)
70 Young PCOS women	MI (1100 mg) + DCI (300 mg) / day (3.6:1 ratio)	Combined hormonal contraceptive (CHC)	MI+DCI restored spontaneous menses in 84.85% and improved HOMA-IR ($P < 0.001$).	(30)
56 PCOS patients	Various MI/DCI ratios (4 g/day total)	Other ratios	The 40:1 MI/DCI ratio was most effective for restoring ovulation and normalizing parameters.	(6)
53 overweight/ obese PCOS women	Metformin + MI / DCI	Metformin alone	The combination was significantly better for improving menstrual regularity and quality of life.	(61)
60 PCOS women	MI + DCI (40:1 ratio)	Metformin	Both treatments were effective, but metformin showed slightly better outcomes in Phenotype A patients, while MI+DCI was hypothesized to be better for Phenotypes C and D.	(26)
37 anovulatory PCOS women	MI (4 g/day), then MI + Alpha-lactalbumin for non-responders	N/A	Adding alpha-lactalbumin to MI in "MI-resistant" patients restored ovulation in 86% of them by increasing MI plasma levels.	(58)
168 PCOS women	Acarbose + MI (2 g / day)	Acarbose + metformin/ metformin alone	The Acarbose + MI group showed significant reductions in fasting insulin, triglycerides, and LDL, indicating cardio-metabolic benefits.	(62)
34 PCOS women (Mexican & Italian)	MI (4 g / day) + Alpha-lactalbumin	N/A (Pre-post)	The combination improved key parameters (insulin, HOMA, LH, Androstenedione) in both populations despite different baseline metabolic profiles.	(59)

(Continued)

Table 2.3: Summary of Key Randomized Controlled Trials on Combination Therapies with Inositol (Continued)

Study Population	Intervention(s) & Dosage	Comparator	Key Outcomes	Ref
50 Anovulatory PCOS women with IR	MI (4 g / day), then MI + Clomiphene for non-responders	N/A	61.7% ovulated on MI alone. Adding clomiphene citrate to MI non-responders induced ovulation in another 72.2%.	(18)
50 Overweight PCOS women	MI + DCI (40:1 ratio)	MI alone	The combined therapy was more effective after 3 months in improving metabolic parameters compared to MI monotherapy.	(54)
15 PCOS patients	MI (1.75 g / day) + DCI (0.25 g / day) + Glucomannan (4 g / day)	Healthy controls	The treatment significantly decreased BMI and altered the metabolomic profile, affecting pathways of fatty acid, amino acid, and glucose metabolism.	(63)
23 Adolescent PCOS patients	MI (2 g / day) + ALA (800 mg / day)	Healthy controls	The combination normalized elevated HMGB1 levels (an inflammatory marker) and significantly reduced insulin and HOMA-IR.	(57)
40 PCOS women	Inositol + Glucomannan	Inositol alone/ glucomannan alone	The combination therapy showed a more significant reduction in blood glucose and insulin levels.	(64)
30 PCOS women with IR	MI + Monacolin K + Lipoic Acid (two dosages)	Lower vs. higher dose	The higher dosage showed a significantly greater improvement in lipid and hyperandrogenism parameters.	(65)
155 PCOS patients	OCP + MI (4 g / day)	OCP alone	The combined therapy was more effective in reducing hirsutism, hyperinsulinemia, androgens, and improving lipid profiles.	(31)
60 PCOS women with chronic periodontitis	MI + SRP (scaling and root planning)	MI alone	The combination of periodontal therapy and MI resulted in a greater reduction of systemic inflammation (hsCRP).	(66)
Obese PCOS women	Metformin + MI + ALA	Metformin alone	The combination therapy showed significantly better improvement in hyperandrogenism, BMI, and HOMA index.	(67)
120 Infertile PCOS women	Metformin + MI (1800 mg / day)	Metformin alone	The combination group had a significantly higher live birth rate (55% vs. 26.67%).	(36)
26 PCOS patients	MI + Clomiphene Citrate (CC)	Historical cohort on CC alone	The ovulation rate was significantly higher with the combination therapy (65.5% vs. 42%).	(56)

2.4.2 Complementary Application in Postmenopausal Women

Beyond its primary application in fertility, inositol's role as a potent insulin-sensitizing agent has led to its investigation in other related conditions. Notably, a significant body of evidence from randomized controlled trials suggests a beneficial effect on the metabolic parameters of postmenopausal women. For instance, in a 6-month randomized, placebo-controlled on 80 postmenopausal women with metabolic syndrome, supplementation with 4 g/day of myo-inositol (2 g b.i.d.) led to dramatic improvements compared to placebo. The MI group demonstrated a decrease in diastolic blood pressure (–11%), a substantial 75% reduction in the HOMA index, a 20% decrease in serum triglycerides, and a 22% improvement in HDL-cholesterol (79). A follow-up 12-month study on a similar population confirmed these findings, showing significant improvements in serum glucose, insulin, HOMA-IR, triglycerides, and cholesterol levels compared to the placebo group (80). Furthermore, D'Anna et al. explored combining MI with melatonin, noting that while MI alone (4 g/day) appeared to improve thyroid function, the combination positively affected glucose metabolism in women during the menopausal transition (81). This underscores its broad importance in female endocrine and metabolic health throughout the lifespan.

The robust evidence from these clinical trials is summarized in Table 2.4.

Table 2.4: Summary of Key Randomized Controlled Trials of Inositol in Complementary Application

Study Population	Intervention(s) & Dosage	Comparator	Key Outcomes	Ref
200 Pregnant women at 11–13 weeks	MI (4 g/day)	Placebo	Incidence of GDM was significantly lower in the MI group (14.9% vs. 28.5%). MI group also had lower HOMA-IR and higher insulin sensitivity.	(68)
220 Overweight pregnant women	MI (4 g/day)	Placebo	GDM incidence was significantly lower in the MI group (11.6% vs. 27.4%).	(71)
198 Pregnant women at high risk for GDM	MI (4 g/day)	Placebo	Pilot trial showed feasibility. HOMA-IR and serum insulin levels were lower in the MI group, suggesting a signal for efficacy.	(82)
220 Obese pregnant women	MI (4 g/day)	Placebo	GDM rate was significantly reduced in the MI group (14.0% vs. 33.6%), and HOMA-IR was significantly reduced.	(69)
223 Overweight pregnant women	MI (2 g/day)	Placebo	GDM incidence was significantly reduced in the MI group.	(83)
75 Non-obese pregnant women with elevated fasting glucose	MI	Placebo	GDM incidence was significantly reduced in the MI group. MI group required less insulin therapy and had smaller babies.	(72)
1729 Women planning conception	MI + Probiotics + Micronutrients	Standard micronutrients	Did not lower gestational glycemia or GDM rates, but did reduce preterm birth.	(77)
60 Overweight pregnant women	MI (2 g/day)	Placebo	GDM incidence was significantly minimized in the MI group (RR = 0.29).	(73)
High-risk pregnant women	MI, DCI, or MI/DCI combo	Placebo	The MI-only group had the lowest incidence of abnormal OGTT and the largest benefit in preventing GDM.	(74)

(Continued)

Table 2.4: Summary of Key Randomized Controlled Trials of Inositol in Complementary Application (Continued)

Study Population	Intervention(s) & Dosage	Comparator	Key Outcomes	Ref
80 Women with GDM	MI (4 g/day), DCI, or MI/DCI combo	Placebo	MI (4 g/day) group showed a significant decrease in HOMA-IR and required less insulin treatment.	(75)
220 Pregnant women with family history of T2D	MI (4 g/day)	Placebo	GDM incidence was significantly reduced in the MI group (6% vs. 15.3%).	(70)
120 Women with GDM	MI + Alpha-Lactalbumin	Placebo	The combination significantly reduced insulin resistance (HOMA-IR) and excessive fetal growth after 2 months.	(76)
240 Pregnant women with family history of diabetes	MI + DCI (40 : 1 ratio)	Placebo	The inositol combination did *not* prevent GDM (23.3% in intervention vs. 18.3% in control).	(78)
40 Women in menopausal transition	MI (4 g/day) or MI (4 g/day) + Melatonin (3 mg/day)	N/A	MI alone seemed to improve thyroid function, while the combination positively affected glucose metabolism.	(81)
80 Postmenopausal women with metabolic syndrome	MI (4 g/day)	Placebo	After 12 months, MI significantly improved all metabolic parameters except BMI and waist circumference.	(80)
80 Postmenopausal women with metabolic syndrome	MI (4 g/day)	Placebo	After 6 months, MI improved blood pressure, HOMA index, cholesterol, and triglyceride levels.	(79)

2.5 SAFETY, DOSAGE, AND EFFICACY

Across the extensive body of clinical research, inositols, particularly myo-inositol, have demonstrated an excellent safety profile.

2.5.1 Recommended Dosages

Based on the reviewed RCTs, the most commonly studied and effective dosage for myo-inositol is 4 grams per day, typically administered as 2 grams twice daily (22, 24, 28, 32). For combination therapies involving MI and DCI, the 40:1 ratio is frequently used to mimic physiological plasma levels (6, 54), though other ratios have shown efficacy in specific contexts like ART (35). Dosages for adjunctive therapies like melatonin are typically 3 mg/day (28, 47).

2.5.2 Safety and Side Effect Profile

A significant advantage of inositol therapy is its high tolerability. Unlike metformin, which frequently causes gastrointestinal side effects such as nausea, diarrhea, and abdominal pain, leading to discontinuation in some patients, inositol is virtually free of such adverse events at standard therapeutic doses (17, 24). The US Food and Drug Administration (FDA) has classified myo-inositol as a "generally recognized as safe" (GRAS) substance, reinforcing its safety for use as a nutritional supplement (84). This favorable safety profile makes it a highly acceptable first-line or adjunctive therapy for long-term management of conditions like PCOS.

2.6 CHALLENGES AND CONTROVERSIES

Despite the largely positive evidence, the use of inositol is not without its complexities and areas of ongoing debate. The "one prescription fits all" approach is challenged by findings of differential patient responses and conflicting data on optimal formulations. Also, there is a lack of research on the effectiveness of inositol in other causes of infertility, such as endometriosis or unexplained infertility.

2.6.1 Heterogeneity of Patient Response

A major challenge in inositol therapy is the variability in patient response. Not all women with PCOS respond equally.

Impact of BMI and Ethnicity: The large-scale NiPPeR trial, while not finding an overall improvement in time-to-conception for the general population, revealed a significant interaction with BMI. The inositol-based supplement shortened time-to-conception in overweight women, bringing it to a level comparable to normal-weight women. However, it paradoxically *lengthened* the time-to-conception in women with obesity, an effect predominantly observed in non-White women (60). This suggests that the underlying metabolic dysregulation in obesity may be too severe to be corrected by the supplement alone or that different ethnic groups may have different metabolic responses.

Inositol Resistance: A subset of patients, termed "inositol-resistant," fail to respond to standard MI therapy. This may be due to factors impairing intestinal absorption, such as gut dysbiosis, or other underlying genetic factors (18, 58). Research into combination therapies with absorption enhancers like alpha-lactalbumin aims to address this issue (58, 59).

2.6.2 The Myo-Inositol vs. D-Chiro-Inositol Ratio Debate

The optimal ratio of MI to DCI remains a point of significant controversy. While many studies support the physiological 40:1 ratio for restoring systemic metabolic balance and natural ovulation (6, 54), evidence from the ART setting complicates this picture. The finding by Mendoza et al. that a 3.6:1 ratio (higher in DCI) yielded superior pregnancy and live birth rates in ICSI cycles suggests that the needs of the ovary under controlled stimulation may differ from those during a natural cycle (35). Conversely, other studies in ART have concluded that MI is superior to DCI for improving oocyte quality, and that high doses of DCI may even be detrimental (12, 33). This highlights the need for context-specific recommendations rather than a single universal ratio.

2.6.3 Inconclusive Evidence and Research Gaps

Not all studies have yielded positive results. The NiPPeR trial, the largest RCT to date, found no overall effect on its primary outcomes of gestational glycemia or the secondary outcome of time-to-conception in the general population planning pregnancy (60, 77). Similarly, some trials investigating inositol for the prevention of gestational diabetes have reported no significant benefit (78). These null findings underscore that inositol may not be a panacea and its efficacy is likely concentrated in specific patient populations, particularly those with underlying insulin resistance and ovulatory dysfunction like PCOS.

2.7 FUTURE DIRECTIONS

The growing body of research on inositol continues to open new avenues for its application in female reproductive health. Future investigations should aim to refine its use through personalization, deeper mechanistic understanding, and innovative therapeutic strategies.

2.7.1 Personalized, Phenotype-Specific Approaches

Given the clear evidence of differential responses based on BMI, ethnicity, and underlying pathology, the future of inositol therapy lies in a more personalized approach. Future RCTs should be designed to stratify patients by PCOS phenotype (e.g., hyperandrogenic vs. non-hyperandrogenic), degree of insulin resistance, and BMI. This would allow for the development of tailored therapeutic strategies, optimizing the type (MI, DCI, or combination) and dosage of inositol for individual patient profiles to maximize efficacy and avoid potential negative effects in certain subgroups.

2.7.2 Elucidating Molecular Mechanisms

While the role of inositol as insulin sensitizers and second messengers is well-established, their full range of molecular effects is still being uncovered. Emerging research using metabolomics, proteomics, and genomics is beginning to shed light on how inositol modulates complex cellular networks. Future studies should continue to explore their impact on gene expression in granulosa and cumulus cells, oxidative stress markers, and inflammatory pathways to provide a more complete picture of their mechanism of action and identify novel biomarkers to predict patient response. Understanding the basis of "inositol resistance" at a molecular level is a critical research gap that needs to be addressed.

2.7.3 Novel Formulations and Combination Therapies

The success of combining inositol with agents like melatonin (28, 47, 50, 51) and alpha-lactalbumin (58, 59) suggests that multi-component formulations hold significant promise. Future research should explore other synergistic combinations, potentially including other antioxidants (e.g., coenzyme Q10), vitamins, and compounds that modulate the gut microbiome. Furthermore, developing novel delivery systems or formulations, such as those that enhance intestinal absorption, could improve bioavailability and overcome inositol resistance, broadening the population of women who can benefit from this safe and effective therapy.

2.8 CONCLUSION

The extensive body of evidence synthesized in this chapter positions inositol, particularly myo-inositol, as a safe, well-tolerated, and effective therapeutic agent in the management of female infertility. Its efficacy is most pronounced in women with polycystic ovary syndrome, where it addresses the core pathophysiological drivers of insulin resistance and hyperandrogenism. By restoring metabolic and hormonal balance, inositol supplementation has been shown in numerous randomized controlled trials to improve insulin sensitivity, reduce androgen levels, restore spontaneous ovulation, and enhance oocyte and embryo quality in assisted reproductive technologies. Furthermore, its utility extends to complementary applications, such as the prevention of gestational diabetes in high-risk pregnancies and the management of metabolic syndrome in postmenopausal women. However, inositol's application faces complexities. Challenges include heterogeneous patient responses, linked to factors like BMI, ethnicity, and "inositol resistance." Furthermore, the optimal MI/DCI ratio remains unresolved, with different needs suggested for natural ovulation versus ART contexts. The future of inositol therapy lies in personalization, requiring patient stratification by phenotype and degree of insulin resistance. Elucidating the mechanisms of inositol resistance and developing novel formulations, such as those with absorption-enhancers like alpha-lactalbumin, are critical. In conclusion, inositol is a cornerstone nutritional intervention that requires further refinement.

REFERENCES

1. Chatree S, Thongmaen N, Tantivejkul K, Sitticharoon C, Vucenik I. Role of inositols and inositol phosphates in energy metabolism. *Molecules*. 2020;25(21):5079.
2. Bizzarri M, Monti N, Piombarolo A, Angeloni A, Verna R. Myo-inositol and D-chiro-inositol as modulators of ovary steroidogenesis: A narrative review. *Nutrients*. 2023;15(8):1875.
3. Jamilian M, Farhat P, Foroozanfard F, Afshar Ebrahimi F, Aghadavod E, Bahmani F, Badehnoosh B, Jamilian H, Asemi Z. Comparison of myo-inositol and metformin on clinical, metabolic and genetic parameters in polycystic ovary syndrome: A randomized controlled clinical trial. *Clin Endocrinol (Oxf)*. 2017;87(2):194–200.
4. Genazzani AD, Lanzoni C, Ricchieri F, Jasonni VM. Myo-inositol administration positively affects hyperinsulinemia and hormonal parameters in overweight patients with polycystic ovary syndrome. *Gynecological Endocrinology*. 2008;24(3):139–44.
5. Genazzani AD, Santagni S, Rattighieri E, Chierchia E, Despini G, Marini G, et al. Modulatory role of D-chiro-inositol (DCI) on LH and insulin secretion in obese PCOS patients. *Gynecological Endocrinology*. 2014;30(6):438–43.
6. Nordio M, Basciani S, Camajani E. The 40: 1 myo-inositol/D-chiro-inositol plasma ratio is able to restore ovulation in PCOS patients: Comparison with other ratios. *European Review for Medical & Pharmacological Sciences*. 2019;23(12).
7. Norris D, Carr J. Chapter 3 – Synthesis, Metabolism, and Actions of Bioregulators. *Vertebrate Endocrinology*. San Diego: Academic Press; 2013.
8. Yazdanpanah Z, Cheraghi E, Nasrabadi MH, Salehipour M. Improvement in biochemical manifestations of the serum and follicular fluid and ICSI outcomes in PCOS patients with myo-inositol administration: Prospective randomized research. *Naunyn-Schmiedeberg's Archives of Pharmacology*. 2025;398(6):7187–98.

9. Emekçi Özay Ö, Özay AC, Çağlıyan E, Okyay RE, Gülekli B. Myo-inositol administration positively effects ovulation induction and intrauterine insemination in patients with polycystic ovary syndrome: A prospective, controlled, randomized trial. *Gynecological Endocrinology.* 2017;33(7):524–8.
10. Akbari Sene A, Tabatabaie A, Nikniaz H, Alizadeh A, Sheibani K, Mortezapour Alisaraie M, et al. The myo-inositol effect on the oocyte quality and fertilization rate among women with polycystic ovary syndrome undergoing assisted reproductive technology cycles: A randomized clinical trial. *Archives of Gynecology and Obstetrics.* 2019;299(6):1701–7.
11. Carlomagno G, Unfer V, Roseff S. The D-chiro-inositol paradox in the ovary. *Fertility and Sterility.* 2011;95(8):2515–6.
12. Ravanos K, Monastra G, Pavlidou T, Goudakou M, Prapas N. Can high levels of D-chiro-inositol in follicular fluid exert detrimental effects on blastocyst quality? *European Review for Medical & Pharmacological Sciences.* 2017;21(23).
13. Pundir J, Psaroudakis D, Savnur P, Bhide P, Sabatini L, Teede H, et al. Inositol treatment of anovulation in women with polycystic ovary syndrome: A meta-analysis of randomised trials. *BJOG: An International Journal of Obstetrics & Gynaecology.* 2018;125(3):299–308.
14. Formuso C, Stracquadanio M, Ciotta L. Myo-inositol vs. D-chiro inositol in PCOS treatment. *Minerva Ginecol.* 2015;67(4):321–5.
15. Pkhaladze L, Russo M, Unfer V, Nordio M, Basciani S, Khomasuridze A, et al. Treatment of lean PCOS teenagers: A follow-up comparison between myo-inositol and oral contraceptives. *European Review for Medical & Pharmacological Sciences.* 2021;25(23).
16. Unfer V, Facchinetti F, Orrù B, Giordani B, Nestler J. Myo-inositol effects in women with PCOS: A meta-analysis of randomized controlled trials. *Endocrine Connections.* 2017;6(8):647–58.
17. Soldat-Stanković V, Popović-Pejičić S, Stanković S, Prtina A, Malešević G, Bjekić-Macut J, et al. The effect of metformin and myoinositol on metabolic outcomes in women with polycystic ovary syndrome: Role of body mass and adiponectin in a randomized controlled trial. *Journal of Endocrinological Investigation.* 2022;45(3):583–95.
18. Kamenov Z, Kolarov G, Gateva A, Carlomagno G, Genazzani A. Ovulation induction with myo-inositol alone and in combination with clomiphene citrate in polycystic ovarian syndrome patients with insulin resistance. *Gynecological Endocrinology.* 2015;31(2):131–5.
19. DiNicolantonio J, O'Keefe J. Myo-inositol for insulin resistance, metabolic syndrome, polycystic ovary syndrome and gestational diabetes. *Open Heart.* 2022;9(1):e001989.
20. Shokrpour M, Foroozanfard F, Afshar Ebrahimi F, Vahedpoor Z, Aghadavod E, Ghaderi A, et al. Comparison of myo-inositol and metformin on glycemic control, lipid profiles, and gene expression related to insulin and lipid metabolism in women with polycystic ovary syndrome: A randomized controlled clinical trial. *Gynecological Endocrinology.* 2019;35(5):406–11.
21. Genazzani AD, Prati A, Santagni S, Ricchieri F, Chierchia E, Rattighieri E, et al. Differential insulin response to myo-inositol administration in obese polycystic ovary syndrome patients. *Gynecological Endocrinology.* 2012;28(12):969–73.
22. Papaleo E, Unfer V, Baillargeon J-P, De Santis L, Fusi F, Brigante C, et al. Myo-inositol in patients with polycystic ovary syndrome: A novel method for ovulation induction. *Gynecological Endocrinology.* 2007;23(12):700–3.
23. Costantino D, Minozzi G, Minozzi F, Guaraldi. Metabolic and hormonal effects of myo-inositol in women with polycystic ovary syndrome: A double-blind trial. *European Review for Medical & Pharmacological Sciences.* 2009;13(2).
24. Fruzzetti F, Perini D, Russo M, Bucci F, Gadducci A. Comparison of two insulin sensitizers, metformin and myo-inositol, in women with polycystic ovary syndrome (PCOS). *Gynecological Endocrinology.* 2017;33(1):39–42.
25. Artini PG, Di Berardino O, Papini F, Genazzani A, Simi G, Ruggiero M, et al. Endocrine and clinical effects of myo-inositol administration in polycystic ovary syndrome. A randomized study. *Gynecological Endocrinology.* 2013;29(4):375–9.
26. Gul M, Khan H, Rauf B, Bukhari SMS, Ehtesham E, Malik MO, et al. Comparative efficacy of combined myo-inositol and D-chiro inositol versus metformin across PCOS phenotypes: Enhancing ovarian function, ovulation, and stress response in a prospective clinical trial. *Naunyn-Schmiedeberg's Archives of Pharmacology.* 2025:1–12.
27. Brusco G, Mariani M. Inositol: Effects on oocyte quality in patients undergoing ICSI. An open study. *European Review for Medical & Pharmacological Sciences.* 2013;17(22).
28. Pacchiarotti A, Carlomagno G, Antonini G, Pacchiarotti A. Effect of myo-inositol and melatonin versus myo-inositol, in a randomized controlled trial, for improving in vitro fertilization of patients with polycystic ovarian syndrome. *Gynecological Endocrinology.* 2016;32(1):69–73.

29. Pizzo A, Lagana AS, Barbaro L. Comparison between effects of myo-inositol and D-chiro-inositol on ovarian function and metabolic factors in women with PCOS. *Gynecological Endocrinology*. 2014;30(3):205–8.
30. Kachhawa G, Senthil Kumar KV, Kulshrestha V, Khadgawat R, Mahey R, Bhatla N. Efficacy of myo-inositol and d-chiro-inositol combination on menstrual cycle regulation and improving insulin resistance in young women with polycystic ovary syndrome: A randomized open-label study. *International Journal of Gynecology & Obstetrics*. 2022;158(2):278–84.
31. Minozzi M, Costantino D, Guaraldi C, Unfer V. The effect of a combination therapy with myo-inositol and a combined oral contraceptive pill versus a combined oral contraceptive pill alone on metabolic, endocrine, and clinical parameters in polycystic ovary syndrome. *Gynecological Endocrinology*. 2011;27(11):920–4.
32. Ciotta L, Stracquadanio M, Pagano I, Carbonaro A, Palumbo M, Gulino F. Effects of myo-inositol supplementation on oocyte's quality in PCOS patients: A double blind trial. *European Review for Medical & Pharmacological Sciences*. 2011;15(5).
33. Unfer V, Carlomagno G, Rizzo P, Raffone E, Roseff S. Myo-inositol rather than D-chiro-inositol is able to improve oocyte quality in intracytoplasmic sperm injection cycles. A prospective, controlled, randomized trial. *European Review for Medical & Pharmacological Sciences*. 2011;15(4).
34. Yazdanpanah Z, Nasrabadi MH, Cheraghi E, Salehipour M. The ameliorative effect of myo-inositol on apoptosis-related genes expression in cumulus cells of women with polycystic ovary syndrome undergoing ICSI and its relationship with the quality of oocyte and embryo. *Naunyn-Schmiedeberg's Archives of Pharmacology*. 2025:1–10.
35. Mendoza N, Diaz-Ropero MP, Aragon M, Maldonado V, Llaneza P, Lorente J, Mendoza-Tesarik R, Maldonado-Lobon J, Olivares M, Fonolla J. Comparison of the effect of two combinations of myo-inositol and D-chiro-inositol in women with polycystic ovary syndrome undergoing ICSI: A randomized controlled trial. *Gynecol Endocrinol*. 2019;35(8):695–700.
36. Agrawal A, Mahey R, Kachhawa G, Khadgawat R, Vanamail P, Kriplani A. Comparison of metformin plus myoinositol vs metformin alone in PCOS women undergoing ovulation induction cycles: Randomized controlled trial. *Gynecological Endocrinology*. 2019;35(6):511–4.
37. Cheang KI, Baillargeon J-P, Essah PA, Ostlund Jr RE, Apridonize T, Islam L, et al. Insulin-stimulated release of D-chiro-inositol–containing inositol phosphoglycan mediator correlates with insulin sensitivity in women with polycystic ovary syndrome. *Metabolism*. 2008;57(10):1390–7.
38. Dona G, Sabbadin C, Fiore C, Bragadin M, Giorgino FL, Ragazzi E, et al. Inositol administration reduces oxidative stress in erythrocytes of patients with polycystic ovary syndrome. *European Journal of Endocrinology*. 2012;166(4):703–10.
39. Raffone E, Rizzo P, Benedetto V. Insulin sensitiser agents alone and in co-treatment with r-FSH for ovulation induction in PCOS women. *Gynecological Endocrinology*. 2010;26(4):275–80.
40. Iuorno MJ, Jakubowicz DJ, Baillargeon J-P, Dillon P, Gunn RD, Allan G, et al. Effects of D-chiro-inositol in lean women with the polycystic ovary syndrome. *Endocrine Practice*. 2002;8(6):417–23.
41. Pourghasem S, Bazarganipour F, Taghavi SA, Kutenaee MA. The effectiveness of inositol and metformin on infertile polycystic ovary syndrome women with resistant to letrozole. *Archives of Gynecology and Obstetrics*. 2019;299(4):1193–9.
42. Gerli S, Mignosa M, Di Renzo. Effects of inositol on ovarian function and metabolic factors in women with PCOS: A randomized double blind placebo-controlled trial. *European Review for Medical and Pharmacological Sciences*. 2003;7(6):151–9.
43. Le Donne M, Alibrandi A, Giarrusso R, Lo Monaco I, Muraca U. Diet, metformin and inositol in overweight and obese women with polycystic ovary syndrome: Effects on body composition. *Minerva Ginecologica*. 2012;64(1):23–9.
44. De Leo V, La Marca A, Cappelli V. Evaluation of the treatment with D-chiroinositol on levels of oxidative stress in PCOS patients. *Reproduktivnaa Endokrinologia*. 2019;2019(49):67–72.
45. Mendoza N, Galan MI, Molina C, Mendoza-Tesarik R, Conde C, Mazheika M, et al. High dose of d-chiro-inositol improves oocyte quality in women with polycystic ovary syndrome undergoing ICSI: A randomized controlled trial. *Gynecological Endocrinology*. 2020;36(5):398–401.
46. Colazingari S, Treglia M, Najjar R, Bevilacqua A. The combined therapy myo-inositol plus D-chiro-inositol, rather than D-chiro-inositol, is able to improve IVF outcomes: Results from a randomized controlled trial. *Archives of Gynecology and Obstetrics*. 2013;288(6):1405–11.
47. Rizzo P, Raffone E, Benedetto V. Effect of the treatment with myo-inositol plus folic acid plus melatonin in comparison with a treatment with myo-inositol plus folic acid on oocyte quality and pregnancy outcome in IVF cycles. A prospective, clinical trial. *European Review for Medical & Pharmacological Sciences*. 2010;14(8).
48. Nazari L, Salehpour S, Hosseini S, Saharkhiz N, Azizi E, Hashemi T, et al. Effect of myo-inositol supplementation on ICSI outcomes among poor ovarian responder patients: A randomized controlled trial. *Journal of Gynecology Obstetrics and Human Reproduction*. 2020;49(5):101698.

49. Mohammadi S, Eini F, Bazarganipour F, Taghavi SA, Kutenaee M. The effect of Myo-inositol on fertility rates in poor ovarian responder in women undergoing assisted reproductive technique: A randomized clinical trial. *Reproductive Biology and Endocrinology.* 2021;19(1):61.
50. Unfer V, Raffone E, Rizzo P, Buffo S. Effect of a supplementation with myo-inositol plus melatonin on oocyte quality in women who failed to conceive in previous in vitro fertilization cycles for poor oocyte quality: A prospective, longitudinal, cohort study. *Gynecological Endocrinology.* 2011;27(11):857–61.
51. Wdowiak A, Filip M. The effect of myo-inositol, vitamin D3 and melatonin on the oocyte quality and pregnancy in in vitro fertilization: A randomized prospective controlled trial. *European Review for Medical & Pharmacological Sciences.* 2020;24(16).
52. Bezerra Espinola MS, Bilotta G, Aragona C. Positive effect of a new supplementation of vitamin D3 with myo-inositol, folic acid and melatonin on IVF outcomes: A prospective randomized and controlled pilot study. *Gynecological Endocrinology.* 2021;37(3):251–4.
53. Sortino MA, Salomone S, Carruba MO, Drago F. Polycystic ovary syndrome: Insights into the therapeutic approach with inositols. *Front Pharmacol.* 2017;8:341.
54. Nordio M, Proietti E. The combined therapy with myo-inositol and D-chiro-inositol reduces the risk of metabolic disease in PCOS overweight patients compared to myo-inositol supplementation alone. *Eur Rev Med Pharmacol Sci.* 2012;16(5):575–81.
55. Greene ND, Leung K-Y, Gay V, Burren K, Mills K, Chitty LS, et al. Inositol for the prevention of neural tube defects: A pilot randomised controlled trial. *British Journal of Nutrition.* 2016;115(6):974–83.
56. Rolland A, Peigné M, Plouvier P, Dumont A, Catteau-Jonard S, Dewailly D, et al. Could myo-inositol soft gel capsules outperform clomiphene in inducing ovulation? Results of a pilot study. *European Review for Medical & Pharmacological Sciences.* 2017;21.
57. Cirillo F, Catellani C, Lazzeroni P, Sartori C, Tridenti G, Vezzani C, et al. HMGB1 is increased in adolescents with polycystic ovary syndrome (PCOS) and decreases after treatment with myo-inositol (MYO) in combination with alpha-lipoic acid (ALA). *Gynecological Endocrinology.* 2020;36(7):588–93.
58. Montanino Oliva M, Buonomo G, Calcagno M, Unfer V. Effects of myo-inositol plus alpha-lactalbumin in myo-inositol-resistant PCOS women. *Journal of Ovarian Research.* 2018;11(1):38.
59. Hernandez Marin I, Picconi O, Laganà A, Costabile L, Unfer V. A multicenter clinical study with myo-inositol and alpha-lactalbumin in Mexican and Italian PCOS patients. *European Review for Medical & Pharmacological Sciences.* 2021;25(8).
60. Chan S-Y, Barton SJ, Loy SL, Chang HF, Titcombe P, Wong J-T, et al. Time-to-conception and clinical pregnancy rate with a myo-inositol, probiotics, and micronutrient supplement: Secondary outcomes of the NiPPeR randomized trial. *Fertility and Sterility.* 2023;119(6):1031–42.
61. Nazirudeen R, Sridhar S, Priyanka R, Sumathi B, Natarajan V, Subbiah E, et al. A randomized controlled trial comparing myoinositol with metformin versus metformin monotherapy in polycystic ovary syndrome. *Clinical Endocrinology.* 2023;99(2):198–205.
62. Andavar M, Kamaraj R, Vijayakumar TM, Murugesan A. Effectiveness of dual combination therapy of acarbose plus metformin and acarbose plus myo-inositol in ameliorating the metabolic and endocrinologic complications of polycystic ovary syndrome–a randomized controlled trial. *European Journal of Obstetrics & Gynecology and Reproductive Biology.* 2024;300:6–11.
63. Troisi J, Cinque C, Giugliano L, Symes S, Richards S, Adair D, et al. Metabolomic change due to combined treatment with myo-inositol, D-chiro-inositol and glucomannan in polycystic ovarian syndrome patients: A pilot study. *Journal of Ovarian Research.* 2019;12(1):25.
64. De Leo V, Tosti C, Cappelli V, Morgante G, Cianci E. Combination inositol and glucomannan in PCOS patients. *Minerva Ginecologica.* 2014;66(6):527–33.
65. Morgante G, Cappelli V, Di Sabatino A, Massaro M, De Leo V. Polycystic ovary syndrome (PCOS) and hyperandrogenism: The role of a new natural association. *Minerva Ginecologica.* 2015;67(5):457–63.
66. Deepti, Tewari S, Narula SC, Singhal SR, Sharma RK. Effect of non-surgical periodontal therapy along with myo-inositol on high-sensitivity C-reactive protein and insulin resistance in women with polycystic ovary syndrome and chronic periodontitis: A randomized controlled trial. *Journal of Periodontology.* 2017;88(10):999–1011.
67. Cappelli V, Di Sabatino A, Musacchio M, De Leo V. Evaluation of a new association between insulin-sensitizers and α-lipoic acid in obese women affected by PCOS. *Minerva Ginecologica.* 2013;65(4):425–33.
68. Asimakopoulos G, Pergialiotis V, Anastasiou E, Antsaklis P, Theodora M, Vogiatzi E, et al. Effect of dietary myo-inositol supplementation on the insulin resistance and the prevention of gestational diabetes mellitus: Study protocol for a randomized controlled trial. *Trials.* 2020;21(1):633.
69. D'Anna R, Di Benedetto A, Scilipoti A, Santamaria A, Interdonato ML, Petrella E, et al. Myo-inositol supplementation for prevention of gestational diabetes in obese pregnant women: A randomized controlled trial. *Obstetrics & Gynecology.* 2015;126(2):310–5.
70. D'Anna R, Scilipoti A, Giordano D, Caruso C, Cannata ML, Interdonato ML, et al. myo-Inositol supplementation and onset of gestational diabetes mellitus in pregnant women with a family history of type 2 diabetes: A prospective, randomized, placebo-controlled study. *Diabetes Care.* 2013;36(4):854–7.

71. Santamaria A, Di Benedetto A, Petrella E, Pintaudi B, Corrado F, D'Anna R, et al. Myo-inositol may prevent gestational diabetes onset in overweight women: A randomized, controlled trial. *Journal of Maternal-Fetal & Neonatal Medicine*. 2016;29(19):3234–7.
72. Matarrelli B, Vitacolonna E, D'Angelo M, Pavone G, Mattei PA, Liberati M, et al. Effect of dietary myo-inositol supplementation in pregnancy on the incidence of maternal gestational diabetes mellitus and fetal outcomes: A randomized controlled trial. *Journal of Maternal-Fetal & Neonatal Medicine*. 2013;26(10):967–72.
73. Esmaeilzadeh S, Ghadimi R, Mashayekh-Amiri S, Delavar MA, Basirat Z. The effect of myo-inositol supplementation on the prevention of gestational diabetes in overweight pregnant women: a randomized, double-blind, controlled trial. *Minerva Obstet Gynecol*. 2023;75(4):357–64.
74. Celentano C, Matarrelli B, Pavone G, Vitacolonna E, Mattei PA, Berghella V, et al. The influence of different inositol stereoisomers supplementation in pregnancy on maternal gestational diabetes mellitus and fetal outcomes in high-risk patients: A randomized controlled trial. *Journal of Maternal-Fetal & Neonatal Medicine*. 2020;33(5):743–51.
75. Fraticelli F, Celentano C, Zecca IA, Di Vieste G, Pintaudi B, Liberati M, et al. Effect of inositol stereoisomers at different dosages in gestational diabetes: An open-label, parallel, randomized controlled trial. *Acta Diabetologica*. 2018;55(8):805–12.
76. D'Anna R, Corrado F, Loddo S, Gullo G, Giunta L, Di Benedetto A. Myoinositol plus α-lactalbumin supplementation, insulin resistance and birth outcomes in women with gestational diabetes mellitus: A randomized, controlled study. *Scientific Reports*. 2021;11(1):8866.
77. Godfrey KM, Barton SJ, El-Heis S, Kenealy T, Nield H, Baker PN, et al. Myo-inositol, probiotics, and micronutrient supplementation from preconception for glycemia in pregnancy: NiPPeR international multicenter double-blind randomized controlled trial. *Diabetes Care*. 2021;44(5):1091–9.
78. Farren M, Daly N, McKeating A, Kinsley B, Turner MJ, Daly S. The prevention of gestational diabetes mellitus with antenatal oral inositol supplementation: A randomized controlled trial. *Diabetes Care*. 2017;40(6):759–63.
79. Giordano D, Corrado F, Santamaria A, Quattrone S, Pintaudi B, Di Benedetto A, et al. Effects of myo-inositol supplementation in postmenopausal women with metabolic syndrome: A perspective, randomized, placebo-controlled study. *Menopause*. 2011;18(1):102–4.
80. Santamaria A, Giordano D, Corrado F, Pintaudi B, Interdonato ML, Vieste GD, et al. One-year effects of myo-inositol supplementation in postmenopausal women with metabolic syndrome. *Climacteric*. 2012;15(5):490–5.
81. D'Anna R, Santamaria A, Giorgianni G, Vaiarelli A, Gullo G, Di Bari F, et al. Myo-inositol and melatonin in the menopausal transition. *Gynecological Endocrinology*. 2017;33(4):279–82.
82. Amaefule CE, Drymoussi Z, Carreras FJG, Llorente MdCP, Lanz D, Dodds J, et al. Myo-inositol nutritional supplement for prevention of gestational diabetes (EMmY): A randomised, placebo-controlled, double-blind pilot trial with nested qualitative study. *BMJ Open*. 2022;12(3):e050110.
83. Vitale SG, Corrado F, Caruso S, Di Benedetto A, Giunta L, Cianci A, et al. Myo-inositol supplementation to prevent gestational diabetes in overweight non-obese women: Bioelectrical impedance analysis, metabolic aspects, obstetric and neonatal outcomes – A randomized and open-label, placebo-controlled clinical trial. *International Journal of Food Sciences and Nutrition*. 2021;72(5):670–9.
84. Zarezadeh M, Dehghani A, Faghfouri AH, Radkhah N, Naemi Kermanshahi M, Hamedi Kalajahi F, et al. Inositol supplementation and body mass index: A systematic review and meta-analysis of randomized clinical trials. *Obesity Science & Practice*. 2022;8(3):387–97.

3 Clinical Applications and Evidence of Melatonin in Infertility Treatment

Ali Afrasiabi, Amir Masoud Firouzabadi, Maryam Azizi-Kutenaei, and Farzaneh Fesahat

3.1 INTRODUCTION

3.1.1 Melatonin: Overview and Functions

Melatonin, an indoleamine neurohormone predominantly synthesized by the pineal gland, serves essential functions in circadian rhythm synchronization, reproductive physiology, and sleep-wake cycle regulation. Beyond these regulatory roles, it demonstrates extensive antioxidant properties as a wide-ranging free radical neutralizer, providing cytoprotective effects against oxidative stress. In ovarian tissue, melatonin participates in critical reproductive mechanisms such as steroid hormone production, follicular development, and oocyte maturation. Experimental evidence indicates its protective capacity against reactive oxygen species-mediated damage in developing oocytes (1). Additionally, melatonin upregulates the expression of both MT1 and MT2 melatonin receptors alongside p53 receptor enhancement, potentially optimizing uterine receptivity and significantly supporting embryonic implantation processes (2).

3.1.2 Female Infertility: Definitions and Key Disorders

Infertility is clinically characterized by the inability to achieve conception following a minimum of 12 months of regular unprotected coitus (3). The etiological spectrum of female infertility encompasses diverse pathological conditions, with polycystic ovary syndrome (PCOS) and diminished ovarian reserve (DOR) representing significant diagnostic entities within this classification.

1. Polycystic ovary syndrome represents a prevalent endocrine disorder within gynecological practice, affecting 7–10% of women during their reproductive years and responsible for approximately 80% of anovulatory infertility cases. Diagnostic criteria established by the Rotterdam consensus require the presence of at least two of three cardinal features: ovulatory dysfunction (manifested as oligo-ovulation or anovulation with irregular menstrual cycles including oligomenorrhea or amenorrhea), clinical or biochemical hyperandrogenism (presenting as hirsutism, acne, or androgenetic alopecia), and polycystic ovarian morphology on ultrasonographic examination. While the precise pathogenic mechanisms remain incompletely elucidated, PCOS is characterized by chronic low-grade inflammatory states and oxidative stress, which correlate with additional clinical manifestations and metabolic disturbances. Affected individuals typically demonstrate elevated concentrations of C-reactive protein (CRP), tumor necrosis factor-α (TNF-α), and malondialdehyde (MDA), concurrent with diminished total antioxidant capacity (TAC). The underlying pathophysiology may involve deficiencies in antioxidant compounds and essential micronutrients including melatonin and magnesium, potentially amplifying oxidative damage in PCOS patients (1).
2. Diminished ovarian reserve describes a clinical condition marked by the quantitative reduction and qualitative decline in the ovarian follicular pool, resulting in compromised reproductive potential (4).

3.1.3 Role of Micronutrients and Antioxidants in Female Fertility

Several micronutrients play vital roles in female fertility, notably magnesium and selenium.

1. *Magnesium*: Magnesium is the second most abundant intracellular cation in the human body and serves critical functions in maintaining health. It acts as a key antioxidant cofactor for various enzymatic reactions, contributes to cell membrane stabilization, and attenuates oxidative stress (1).
2. *Selenium*: Selenium, a nonmetal element, has essential physiological roles, including antioxidant activity, despite its toxicity at high concentrations (5).

3.1.4 Antioxidant Classification and Therapeutic Approaches

Antioxidants are generally classified into enzymatic and non-enzymatic types. Enzymatic antioxidants are endogenously produced to combat oxidative stress, with the primary enzymes

DOI: 10.1201/9781003741541-3

including superoxide dismutase, catalase, and glutathione peroxidase (GPx). A combination therapy approach incorporating antioxidants and micronutrients is critical for managing several infertility-related disorders (1).

3.2 CURRENT CLINICAL EVIDENCE AND APPLICATIONS OF MELATONIN IN REPRODUCTIVE MEDICINE

3.2.1 Mechanistic Insights on Melatonin in Reproduction

Melatonin serves as a pleiotropic regulator in human reproductive physiology, exerting its effects partially through myo-inositol (MI), which functions as the intracellular secondary messenger for follicle-stimulating hormone (FSH). Experimental evidence indicates that MI-mediated signaling pathways contribute to FSH-stimulated anti-Müllerian hormone (AMH) synthesis within granulosa cells (6). During oocyte development, increased melatonin levels stimulate progesterone secretion and enhance ovarian follicular responsiveness to luteinizing hormone (LH). The hormone mediates its actions via multiple pathways: two G-protein-coupled membrane receptors (MT1-R and MT2-R), nuclear receptor interactions, and direct intracellular antioxidant activity. These receptor systems are distributed throughout reproductive tissues, including gonadotropin-releasing hypothalamic neurons, anterior pituitary gland, and both male and female gonads (6). Additionally, melatonin demonstrates selective estrogen-regulatory properties through aromatase inhibition and estrogen receptor modulation, providing a mechanistic basis for its therapeutic application in polycystic ovary syndrome. This includes documented reductions in circulating androgens and clinical improvements in hyperandrogenic manifestations and ovarian dysfunction. While supplementation with magnesium, melatonin, or their combination showed no significant effect on high-sensitivity C-reactive protein (hs-CRP) or malondialdehyde (MDA) concentrations, all interventions significantly enhanced systemic total antioxidant capacity (TAC) (1).

3.2.2 Clinical Trial Evidence on Melatonin Supplementation

Melatonin has been extensively studied as an adjunct in assisted reproductive techniques (ART), with evidence from randomized controlled trials (RCTs) highlighting its multifaceted benefits on oocyte maturation, oxidative stress modulation, and pregnancy outcomes. These studies can be categorized based on treatment composition and target populations.

3.2.2.1 Melatonin Combined with Myo-Inositol and Folic Acid

Multiple randomized controlled trials have investigated melatonin when administered within combination therapies incorporating myo-inositol and folic acid.

Pacchiarotti et al. (2015) established that adjuvant melatonin (3 mg) combined with myo-inositol (4000 mg) and folic acid (400 μg) significantly elevated serum estradiol concentrations, circulating melatonin levels, and the yield of Grade I metaphase II oocytes relative to the control regimen without melatonin. These outcomes substantiate melatonin's role in augmenting luteinizing hormone responsiveness and promoting progesterone synthesis during follicular development (6).

Corroborating these findings, Rizzo et al. (2010) documented enhanced clinical pregnancy and implantation rates (as statistical trends), decreased proportions of germinal vesicle and degenerated oocytes, and increased numbers of mature oocytes and high-grade embryos following melatonin supplementation to myo-inositol and folic acid base therapy, despite comparable total oocyte retrieval between groups (7).

In a separate investigation, Jiménez Tuñón et al. (2017) demonstrated that pretreatment with a quadri-therapy containing folic acid, myo-inositol, melatonin, and selenium (Seidivid) favorably modulated embryo quality distribution – diminishing low-grade (C) embryos while augmenting high-quality (A and B) embryos. Although biochemical and clinical pregnancy rates were numerically elevated in the melatonin cohort, these differences failed to achieve statistical significance (5).

3.2.2.2 Melatonin Monotherapy in ART Cycles

A distinct series of investigations has focused on melatonin monotherapy as an antioxidant intervention in infertile women undergoing assisted reproductive technology. Eryilmaz et al. (2011) demonstrated that melatonin administration significantly enhanced oocyte yield and the number of Grade 1 embryos, alongside improved ratios of metaphase II oocytes, indicating optimized follicular conditions despite comparable fertilization and implantation outcomes between groups (8). In accordance with these results, Batıoğlu et al. (2012) observed elevated proportions of mature oocytes and Grade 1 embryos following melatonin treatment, accompanied by a non-significant increase in clinical pregnancy rates (9). Complementing these findings, Tamura et al. (2007) established that supplementation with 3 mg/day melatonin significantly improved fertilization rates in patients with previous unsuccessful in vitro fertilization attempts, highlighting its potential for restoring follicular developmental competence (10).

3.2.2.3 Melatonin and Oxidative Stress Modulation

Espino et al. (2019) conducted a dose-dependent study (3 mg vs. 6 mg/day for 40 days) in infertile women, showing significant improvements in total antioxidant capacity and superoxide dismutase (SOD) activity, along with reduced lipid peroxidation and oxidative DNA damage. Treated groups exhibited higher rates of mature and fertilized oocytes and transferable embryos, with overall ART success increasing to 30% (3).

3.2.2.4 Melatonin in Women with Diminished Ovarian Reserve

Two randomized controlled trials have specifically investigated melatonin administration in women with diminished ovarian reserve. Jahromi et al. (2017) reported that melatonin supplementation resulted in increased numbers of metaphase II oocytes and high-quality embryos (grades 1 and 2), although clinical pregnancy and miscarriage rates showed no significant differences compared to the control group (4). Conversely, Sadeghpour et al. (2025) documented more pronounced therapeutic effects, with melatonin administration significantly enhancing oocyte retrieval numbers, fertilization rates, and embryo quality scores. The treatment also improved oxidative stress parameters, including elevated reduced glutathione (rGSH) and total antioxidant capacity (TAC). Of particular note, TAC measurements demonstrated a strong inverse correlation with ovarian stimulation duration, indicating improved ovarian responsiveness. Furthermore, the melatonin group exhibited a statistically significant increase in clinical pregnancy rates (11).

3.2.2.5 Melatonin in Women with Polycystic Ovary Syndrome

Akter et al. (2023) investigated melatonin's metabolic and reproductive effects in PCOS patients. After 8 weeks, melatonin treatment reduced serum testosterone, luteinizing hormone, and HOMA-IR, while improving glucose tolerance, follicle maturation, and endometrial thickness, though anti-Müllerian hormone levels remained unchanged (12). These findings indicate melatonin's potential to modulate both oxidative and endocrine imbalances in PCOS.

3.2.2.6 Clinical and Morphological Improvements in Folliculogenesis

Mokhtari et al. (2019) reported that melatonin administration significantly increased chemical and clinical pregnancy rates (~30% vs. 18%), enhanced follicle size ($p = 0.002$), and improved endometrial thickness in infertile women undergoing ART (2). Collectively, these findings emphasize melatonin's supportive role in endometrial receptivity and follicular development.

3.2.2.7 Summary

Across diverse populations – including women with DOR, PCOS, or idiopathic infertility – melatonin supplementation consistently improved oocyte and embryo quality, enhanced antioxidant defenses, and modestly increased pregnancy outcomes. When combined with agents such as myo-inositol and folic acid, melatonin's synergistic effects on follicular microenvironment and oxidative balance appear even more pronounced, establishing it as a promising adjunct in reproductive medicine.

3.3 SUCCESSFUL SYNERGISM OF MELATONIN AND MYO-INOSITOL IN ASSISTED REPRODUCTIVE TECHNOLOGIES

Myo-inositol and melatonin are endogenously produced molecules recognized as effective predictors of oocyte quality and in vitro fertilization (IVF) outcomes. Elevated concentrations of these molecules have been positively correlated with improved oocyte quality (6). Several clinical trials have demonstrated that supplementation with MI alone or in combination with melatonin significantly improves oocyte quality and IVF success rates, both in patients with polycystic ovary syndrome and in normo-ovulatory women (7, 13).

Table 3.1: Results of RCTs Based on Dosage and Drug Combinations

Author	Year of Publication	Study Design	Number of Enrollments	Dose, Combination, Time	Key Findings
Pacchiarotti	2015	RCT	*N* = 526	Myo-inositol 4000 mg, folic acid 400 mcg, and melatonin 3 mg twice daily	↑ E2, melatonin, Grade I MII embryos.
Jiménez Tuñón	2017	RCT	*N* = 101	Two daily oral sachets, each containing 2 g myo-inositol, 0.975 mg melatonin, 200 µg folic acid, and 27.5 µg selenium (Seidivid)	↑ Biochemical & clinical pregnancy;↑ quality A/B embryos; ↓ quality C embryos.
Rizzo	2010	RCT	*N* = 65	2 g Myo-inositol twice daily combined with 200 mcg folic acid and 3 mg melatonin	↑ Mature oocytes, ↑ top-quality embryos; ↓ degenerated oocytes.
Mokhtari	2019	RCT	*N* = 198	Melatonin 3 mg tablets	↑ Chemical & clinical pregnancy;↑ follicle size, ↑ endometrial thickness.
Jahromi	2017	Double-blind RCT	*N* = 66	3 mg melatonin capsules	↑ MII oocytes, ↑ top-quality embryos; no difference in pregnancy rates.
Espino	2019	RCT	*N* = 40	Melatonin 3 mg or 6 mg daily	↑ TAC, ↑ SOD (6mg), ↓ oxidative stress; ↑ mature/fertilized oocytes.
Eryilmaz	2011	RCT	*N* = 60	Melatonin 3 mg daily	↑ Retrieved oocytes & Grade 1 embryos;↑ MII ratio; pregnancy rates similar.
Batıoğlu	2012	RCT	*N* = 85	Melatonin 3 mg daily	↑ Mature oocytes & Grade 1 embryos; clinical pregnancy trend ↑ (NS).
Tamura	2007	RCT	-	Melatonin 3 mg daily	3 mg/day melatonin improved fertilization in IVF failures.
Akter	2023	RCT	*N* = 74	Melatonin 3 mg nightly by co-treatment with letrozole ovulation induction	↓ Testosterone, LH, HOMA-IR;↑ follicles & endometrial thickness.

3.3.1 Clinical Evidence from Randomized Controlled Trials

Rizzo et al., 2010: In a randomized clinical trial involving 65 in vitro fertilization patients, participants were allocated to two intervention arms: Group A received combined myo-inositol, folic acid, and melatonin ($n = 32$), while Group B received myo-inositol and folic acid without melatonin ($n = 33$). The melatonin-supplemented cohort demonstrated non-significant trends toward improved clinical and implantation rates. Oocyte evaluation revealed decreased proportions of germinal vesicle and degenerated oocytes alongside increased morphologically mature oocytes at retrieval, despite comparable total oocyte yields between groups. A statistically significant enhancement in top-quality embryo production was observed in the melatonin-treated group (7).

Wdowiak et al., 2020: In a randomized controlled trial involving 100 women undergoing intracytoplasmic sperm injection (ICSI), participants were equally allocated to either an intervention or control group. The intervention group received a comprehensive supplementation regimen consisting of: 2 g myo-inositol, 50 mg alpha-lactalbumin, and 200 mcg folic acid daily in powder form for 6 months (3 months pre-oocyte retrieval and 3 months post-ICSI), supplemented with 600 mg myo-inositol, 1 mg melatonin, and 200 mcg folic acid nightly for 3 months preceding oocyte retrieval. This was subsequently modified to 600 mg myo-inositol, 200 mcg folic acid, 1 mg melatonin, and 50 mcg vitamin D3 until the 12th gestational week. The control group received 200 mcg folic acid twice daily. The supplemented cohort demonstrated significantly improved outcomes, including higher oocyte yield, elevated estradiol levels (2392.64 pg/mL versus control), and increased endometrial thickness at recombinant hCG administration (12.4 mm versus control). Furthermore, the intervention group exhibited enhanced oocyte and blastocyst quality metrics, along with a substantially higher clinical pregnancy rate (42% versus 24%). While no significant differences emerged in pregnancy progression, the control group experienced shorter gestational durations (16). Collectively, these studies highlight the beneficial synergy of melatonin and myo-inositol supplementation in ART cycles – enhancing oocyte maturation, embryo quality, endometrial receptivity, and pregnancy outcomes. These findings support the integration of combined melatonin and myo-inositol supplementation into standard IVF protocols, particularly for women with a history of poor oocyte quality or PCOS.

3.3.2 Effect of Melatonin on Antioxidant Capacity and Inflammation

Reactive oxygen species (ROS) participate in essential physiological functions, yet their excessive accumulation induces cellular damage. Elevated ROS concentrations have been associated with compromised reproductive outcomes, including spontaneous abortion, unexplained recurrent pregnancy loss, and embryonic developmental abnormalities (5).

Magnesium supplementation may attenuate oxidative stress through dual mechanisms: suppression of ROS generation and potentiation of glutathione peroxidase activity, thereby strengthening endogenous antioxidant systems. Concurrently, melatonin emerges as a multifunctional antioxidant with broad-spectrum free radical scavenging capacity and direct anti-inflammatory properties, especially significant for ovarian physiology (1). It actively participates in regulating ovulatory processes, follicular maturation, corpus luteum activity, and oocyte development.

Polycystic ovary syndrome represents a chronic inflammatory state characterized by elevated oxidative stress. Melatonin counteracts these pathophysiological processes through multiple pathways: direct neutralization of free radicals, suppression of nuclear factor-kappa B (NF-κB) signaling, and stimulation of glutathione production. Clinical evidence demonstrates that melatonin supplementation in PCOS patients reduces hirsutism severity, decreases circulating total testosterone, diminishes inflammatory markers (hs-CRP and malondialdehyde), and downregulates tumor necrosis factor-alpha gene expression, while simultaneously enhancing total antioxidant capacity and glutathione concentrations (1).

Additionally, melatonin upregulates key endogenous antioxidant enzymes such as superoxide dismutase and glutathione peroxidase, further strengthening its protective role against oxidative damage (6). These comprehensive antioxidant and anti-inflammatory characteristics position melatonin as a promising therapeutic intervention for enhancing ovarian function and managing oxidative stress-associated infertility conditions.

3.3.3 Effect of Melatonin on Psychosexual Status in Infertility and ART

Assisted reproductive technology serves as the ultimate therapeutic approach for numerous couples facing infertility. This treatment paradigm involves intensive protocols comprising daily hormonal injections, repeated ultrasonographic evaluations, seminal fluid assessments, and invasive clinical procedures. These demanding medical interventions frequently correlate with heightened psychological distress, anxiety manifestations, sleep disturbances, depressive symptoms, and alterations in sexual health parameters among patients (8).

Melatonin, while primarily recognized for circadian rhythm modulation and soporific effects, demonstrates additional therapeutic utility in ART settings through its robust antioxidant and radical-scavenging capacities. Through modification of tissue redox equilibrium, melatonin potentially mitigates oxidative damage associated with reactive oxygen species, which are established contributors to oxidative stress and impaired reproductive function.

A randomized controlled investigation enrolling 60 infertile women evaluated melatonin's effects on sleep parameters and reproductive outcomes during in vitro fertilization cycles (8). The trial documented sleep improvement in 7 of 30 participants receiving melatonin, compared to 2 of 30 in the control arm. This intergroup difference, however, failed to achieve statistical significance, suggesting that melatonin administration throughout IVF treatment may not sufficiently alleviate sleep disruptions in this population.

Although current evidence regarding melatonin's direct impact on psychological and sexual parameters remains limited, its established influences on sleep architecture, affective regulation, and oxidative stress reduction indicate potential ancillary benefits that merit systematic exploration through methodologically rigorous studies. The management of psychological well-being and sexual health continues to represent an essential consideration for optimizing success rates in fertility interventions.

3.4 SAFETY, DOSAGE, AND EFFICACY OF MELATONIN SUPPLEMENTATION IN REPRODUCTIVE MEDICINE

3.4.1 Dosage and Therapeutic Effects

Melatonin supplementation at 10 mg/day was shown to improve C-reactive protein levels in participants with non-alcoholic fatty liver disease (1).

In patients with polycystic ovary syndrome, co-administration of two melatonin tablets (each 3 mg) plus 250 mg magnesium oxide daily for 8 weeks had restorative effects on fertility characteristics (1).

A randomized controlled trial involving administration of two daily oral sachets, each containing 2 g myo-inositol, 0.975 mg melatonin, 200 µg folic acid, and 27.5 µg selenium (Seidivid), for at least 2 months before ovarian puncture significantly improved embryonic quality (5).

In IVF cycles, melatonin 3 mg/day starting from the day of GnRH administration until oocyte retrieval improved clinical pregnancy rates without statistical significance, while biochemical pregnancy rates were similar between melatonin-treated and control groups (9).

PCOS patients were treated orally from the first day of the menstrual cycle until 14 days after embryo transfer with myo-inositol 4000 mg, folic acid 400 mcg, and melatonin 3 mg twice daily. This combination proved effective as predictors of positive IVF outcomes, correlating with enhanced oocyte quality compared to control groups receiving only folic acid or myo-inositol with folic acid. The study suggested synergistic effects of myo-inositol and melatonin (6).

In another IVF study, patients received 2 g myo-inositol twice daily combined with 200 mcg folic acid and 3 mg melatonin, administered from GnRH stimulation until oocyte retrieval. Melatonin was found to enhance the effectiveness of myo-inositol and folic acid by improving oocyte quality and pregnancy outcomes in women with a history of poor oocyte quality (7).

A RCT on ovulation induction using letrozole in PCOS patients incorporated melatonin 3 mg tablets daily from cycle day 3 until hCG administration on cycle day 10, significantly improving chemical pregnancy rates (2).

Women with diminished ovarian reserve received 3 mg melatonin capsules nightly from cycle day 5 before gonadotropin stimulation, resulting in higher serum estradiol on trigger day and improved oocyte and embryo quality, though other ART outcomes did not differ (4).

Unexplained infertility patients treated with melatonin 3 mg or 6 mg daily from first appointment through follicular puncture showed improved intrafollicular oxidative balance, oocyte quality, and a modest increase in pregnancy rates/live births (3).

In IVF-ET patients with sleep disturbances, melatonin 3 mg daily was administered from menstrual cycle days 3–5 until hCG injection, resulting in significantly higher numbers of retrieved and mature MII oocytes and Grade 1 embryos, though sleep quality changes were insignificant (8).

PCOS infertile women receiving melatonin 3 mg nightly for 8 weeks pretreatment followed by co-treatment with letrozole ovulation induction for 3 cycles showed improved biochemical and ovarian responses (12).

Another DOR ART study involved melatonin 3 mg daily starting on cycle day 5, showing potential improvements in oocyte quality and reproductive technology outcomes, possibly via reducing oxidative stress (13).

Women undergoing ICSI received 2 g myo-inositol, 50 mg alpha-lactalbumin, and 200 mcg folic acid daily for 6 months (3 months before and 3 months after oocyte pick-up) along with melatonin and vitamin D3, representing an innovative support strategy (14).

Across multiple randomized controlled trials, melatonin doses ranging from 0.975 mg to 10 mg per day have demonstrated safety and therapeutic benefits in improving antioxidant capacity, reducing inflammation, enhancing oocyte quality, and promoting better pregnancy outcomes in women with PCOS, diminished ovarian reserve, and other infertility issues. The dosing regimens vary depending on the clinical context but commonly span from the early follicular phase to oocyte retrieval or through ovulation induction cycles. Combining melatonin with complementary agents such as myo-inositol, folic acid, magnesium, selenium, and vitamin D3 often yields synergistic effects.

3.4.2 Safety Profiles and Potential Side Effects of Melatonin

Melatonin is widely regarded as safe when administered orally across various dosages and durations; however, some adverse effects have been reported. These include nausea, headache, dizziness, drowsiness, abdominal pain, and transient feelings of depression. Such side effects are generally mild and self-limiting but should be considered when recommending melatonin supplementation (3, 15).

Regarding its use in reproductive technologies, recent findings have raised concerns about the potential toxicity of high melatonin concentrations in embryo culture media. Fernando et al. demonstrated that elevated melatonin levels in the culture environment may exert toxic effects on embryos, impacting their viability. This toxicity is thought to arise from melatonin's dose-dependent activity, which at high concentrations could disrupt embryo development (15).

Conversely, other studies have shown that melatonin supplementation at optimal concentrations in culture media can protect embryos by reducing oxidative stress and preventing mitochondrial dysfunction induced by toxic agents such as mycotoxins (Zearalenone) or lipopolysaccharides. Melatonin's antioxidant properties mitigate reactive oxygen species, DNA damage, and oxidative stress-induced autophagy in early embryos, fostering improved developmental outcomes (6).

Taken together, while oral melatonin administration is largely safe with minimal side effects, caution should be exercised with its concentration in embryo culture media during assisted reproductive techniques to avoid potential embryotoxicity. Further research is necessary to define safe and effective dosing ranges for melatonin use in reproductive biotechnologies.

3.5 COMBINING MELATONIN WITH CONVENTIONAL TREATMENTS

3.5.1 Melatonin and Magnesium Co-Supplementation in PCOS

The effect of concurrent melatonin and magnesium supplementation on hirsutism and biomarkers of inflammation and oxidative stress among patients with polycystic ovary syndrome was assessed for the first time in a randomized controlled trial involving 76 participants who completed the study. Co-administration of melatonin and magnesium for 8 weeks resulted in significantly greater improvements in hirsutism scores and total antioxidant capacity levels compared to melatonin or magnesium supplementation alone. This combined treatment also led to significant reductions in tumor necrosis factor-alpha and increased serum magnesium levels. Notably, these effects were shown to be dose-dependent, underscoring the importance of optimized dosing for therapeutic efficacy (1).

Additional studies support the synergistic impact of these agents in PCOS management. For example, co-supplementation has been demonstrated to improve metabolic and hormonal markers, including reductions in testosterone levels, improvement in insulin resistance, and favorable lipid profile changes.

3.5.2 Melatonin, Selenium, and Folic Acid Co-Administration

The combined use of melatonin, selenium, and folic acid has exhibited positive effects on both biochemical and clinical pregnancy rates (5). This combination leverages the antioxidant and

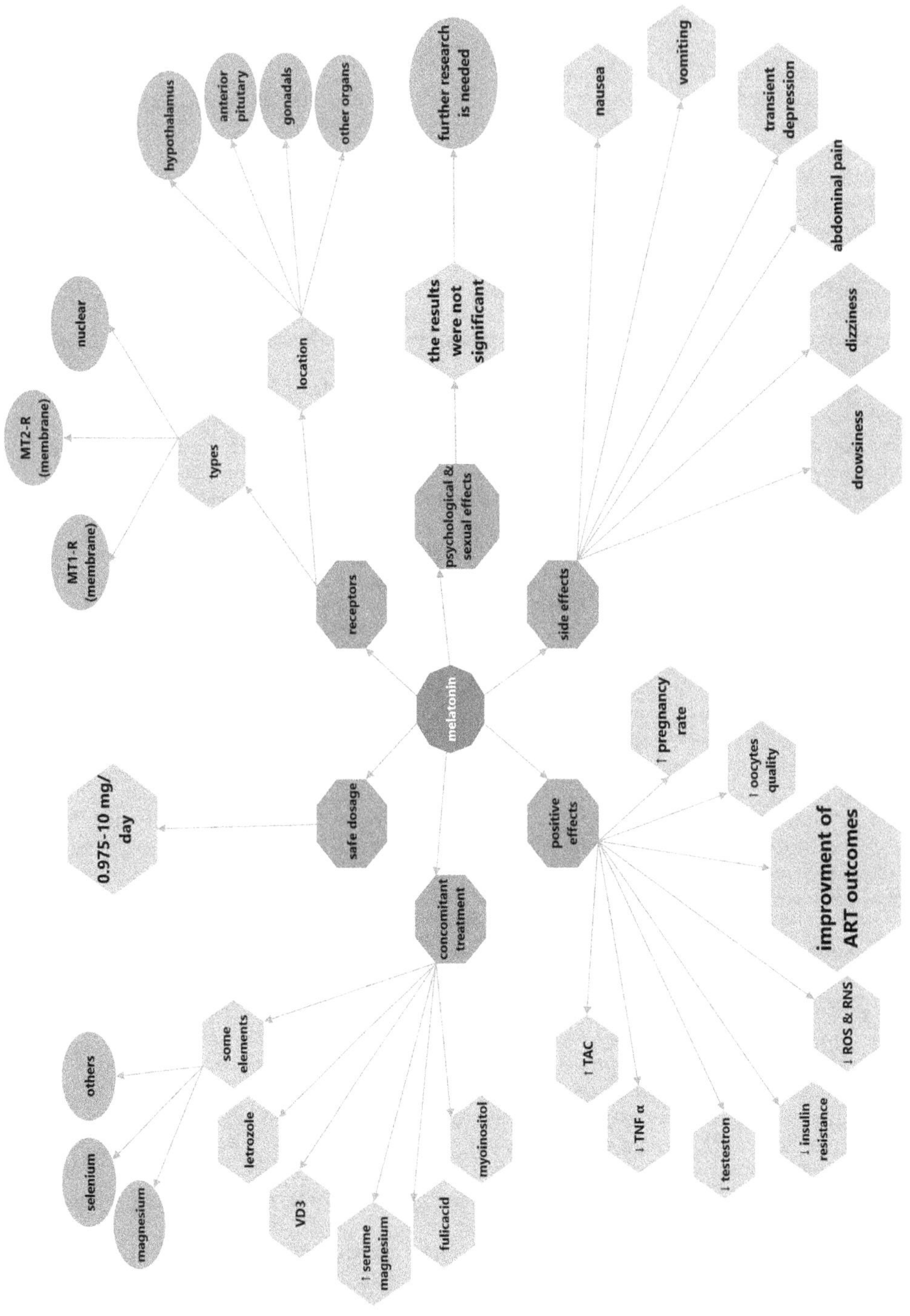

Figure 3.1 A mind map of mechanisms and effects of melatonin on women infertility and some extra information. (From the Authors.)

anti-inflammatory properties of melatonin and selenium alongside folic acid's role in DNA synthesis and repair, contributing to enhanced reproductive outcomes.

3.5.3 Myo-Inositol, Melatonin, and Vitamin D3 in Assisted Reproductive Technologies

Supplementation protocols incorporating myo-inositol, melatonin, and vitamin D3 have shown improvements in the efficacy of intracytoplasmic sperm injection (ICSI) procedures. Specifically, such combined treatments facilitated better ovarian response, oocyte quality, and pregnancy rates (14, 16).

3.5.4 Melatonin with Ovulation Induction Agents

According to Akter et al. (2023), after 8 weeks of pretreatment with melatonin and co-treatment through three ovulation induction cycles using letrozole, patients exhibited enhanced biochemical and ovarian responses. This suggests melatonin's beneficial role in augmenting the effectiveness of conventional ovulation induction protocols in women with infertility (12).

3.6 CHALLENGES AND CONTROVERSIES

Despite growing evidence from randomized controlled trials supporting the beneficial effects of melatonin supplementation in female reproductive medicine, several challenges and controversies remain. Variability in study designs, including differences in melatonin dosages (ranging from 0.975 mg to 10 mg daily); treatment durations; and combinations with other agents such as myo-inositol, magnesium, selenium, and folic acid, complicates the establishment of standardized therapeutic protocols. Additionally, some trials report improvements in biochemical and clinical pregnancy rates without achieving statistical significance, highlighting the need for larger, well-powered studies to confirm efficacy. The potential dose-dependent toxicity of melatonin, particularly in embryo culture media, raises safety concerns that warrant cautious optimization of concentration thresholds to avoid embryotoxic effects. Furthermore, inconsistencies in measuring clinical endpoints such as live birth rates, implantation rates, and oocyte quality, alongside variable reporting of oxidative stress markers, contribute to difficulties in interpreting and comparing outcomes. Psychological and psychosexual benefits of melatonin remain underexplored, with current data insufficient to draw definitive conclusions. Therefore, while melatonin shows promise as an adjunct in assisted reproductive technologies, further rigorous, standardized investigations are necessary to resolve these controversies and fully delineate its clinical role and safety profile (Figure 3.1).

REFERENCES

1. Mousavi R, Alizadeh M, Asghari Jafarabadi M, Heidari L, Nikbakht R, Babaahmadi Rezaei H, et al. Effects of melatonin and/or magnesium supplementation on biomarkers of inflammation and oxidative stress in women with polycystic ovary syndrome: A randomized, double-blind, placebo-controlled trial. *Biol Trace Elem Res*. 2022;200(3):1010–9.
2. Mokhtari F, Akbari Asbagh F, Azmoodeh O, Bakhtiyari M, Almasi-Hashiani A. Effects of melatonin administration on chemical pregnancy rates of polycystic ovary syndrome patients undergoing intrauterine insemination: A randomized clinical trial. *Int J Fertil Steril*. 2019;13(3):225–9.
3. Espino J, Macedo M, Lozano G, Ortiz Á, Rodríguez C, Rodríguez AB, et al. Impact of melatonin supplementation in women with unexplained infertility undergoing fertility treatment. *Antioxidants (Basel)*. 2019;8(9).
4. Jahromi BN, Sadeghi S, Alipour S, Parsanezhad ME, Alamdarloo SM. Effect of melatonin on the outcome of assisted reproductive technique cycles in women with diminished ovarian reserve: A double-blinded randomized clinical trial. *Iran J Med Sci*. 2017;42(1):73–8.
5. Jiménez Tuñón JM, Trilles PP, Molina MG, Duvison MH, Pastor BM, Martín PS, et al. A double-blind, randomized prospective study to evaluate the efficacy of previous therapy with melatonin, myo-inositol, folic acid, and selenium in improving the results of an assisted reproductive treatment. *Clinical Medicine Insights: Therapeutics*. 2017;9:1179559X17742902.
6. Pacchiarotti A, Carlomagno G, Antonini G, Pacchiarotti A. Effect of myo-inositol and melatonin versus myo-inositol, in a randomized controlled trial, for improving in vitro fertilization of patients with polycystic ovarian syndrome. *Gynecol Endocrinol*. 2016;32(1):69–73.
7. Rizzo P, Raffone E, Benedetto V. Effect of the treatment with myo-inositol plus folic acid plus melatonin in comparison with a treatment with myo-inositol plus folic acid on oocyte quality and pregnancy outcome in IVF cycles. A prospective, clinical trial. *Eur Rev Med Pharmacol Sci*. 2010;14(6):555–61.
8. Eryilmaz OG, Devran A, Sarikaya E, Aksakal FN, Mollamahmutoğlu L, Cicek N. Melatonin improves the oocyte and the embryo in IVF patients with sleep disturbances, but does not improve the sleeping problems. *J Assist Reprod Genet*. 2011;28(9):815–20.

9. Batıoğlu AS, Sahin U, Gürlek B, Oztürk N, Unsal E. The efficacy of melatonin administration on oocyte quality. *Gynecol Endocrinol.* 2012;28(2):91–3.
10. Tamura H, Takasaki A, Miwa I, Taniguchi K, Maekawa R, Asada H, et al. Oxidative stress impairs oocyte quality and melatonin protects oocytes from free radical damage and improves fertilization rate. *J Pineal Res.* 2008;44(3):280–7.
11. Sadeghpour S, Ghasemnejad-Berenji M, Maleki F, Behroozi-Lak T, Bahadori R, Ghasemnejad-Berenji H. The effects of melatonin on follicular oxidative stress and art outcomes in women with diminished ovarian reserve: A randomized controlled trial. *Journal of Ovarian Research.* 2025;18(1):5.
12. Akter S, Banu J, Ishrat S, Rani C, Jahan S, Nazneen S, et al. Melatonin enhances ovarian response in infertile women with polycystic ovary syndrome. *Bangladesh Journal of Medical Science.* 2023;22(4):850–8.
13. Unfer V, Raffone E, Rizzo P, Buffo S. Effect of a supplementation with myo-inositol plus melatonin on oocyte quality in women who failed to conceive in previous in vitro fertilization cycles for poor oocyte quality: A prospective, longitudinal, cohort study. *Gynecol Endocrinol.* 2011;27(11):857–61.
14. Wdowiak A, Filip M. The effect of myo-inositol, vitamin D3 and melatonin on the oocyte quality and pregnancy in in vitro fertilization: A randomized prospective controlled trial. *Eur Rev Med Pharmacol Sci.* 2020;24(16):8529–36.
15. Fernando S, Wallace EM, Vollenhoven B, Lolatgis N, Hope N, Wong M, et al. Melatonin in assisted reproductive technology: A pilot double-blind randomized placebo-controlled clinical trial. *Front Endocrinol (Lausanne).* 2018;9:545.
16. Bezerra Espinola MS, Bilotta G, Aragona C. Positive effect of a new supplementation of vitamin D (3) with myo-inositol, folic acid and melatonin on IVF outcomes: A prospective randomized and controlled pilot study. *Gynecol Endocrinol.* 2021;37(3):251–4.

4 Alpha-Lipoic Acid

A Therapeutic Antioxidant in the Treatment of Women's Infertility

Samaneh Harimi, Amir Masoud Firouzabadi, Maryam Azizi-Kutenaei, and Farzaneh Fesahat

4.1 INTRODUCTION TO ALPHA-LIPOIC ACID

Alpha-lipoic acid (ALA), also known as thioctic acid, is an endogenous, sulfur-containing fatty acid that has garnered significant scientific and clinical interest for its potent antioxidant and metabolic regulatory properties. First discovered in the 1930s, it was initially identified as a growth factor for microorganisms before its endogenous synthesis in human mitochondria was understood (1). Structurally, ALA's unique feature is its dithiolane ring, which allows it to function in both aqueous (cytosolic) and lipid (membranous) environments, a trait that distinguishes it from many other antioxidants (2).

Biochemically, ALA serves as an essential cofactor for key mitochondrial enzyme complexes, including the pyruvate dehydrogenase complex (PDC) and the α-ketoglutarate dehydrogenase complex (KGDHC), which are critical hubs in cellular energy production via the Krebs cycle. Beyond this fundamental metabolic role, ALA's therapeutic potential is largely attributed to its powerful and multifaceted mechanisms of action (3).

ALA exists as two stereoisomers (enantiomers): R-(+)-lipoic acid (R-ALA) and S-(-)-lipoic acid (S-ALA). R-ALA is the naturally occurring, biologically active form that functions as the mitochondrial cofactor. S-ALA is a synthetic byproduct of chemical synthesis, and most commercially available supplements consist of a 50/50 racemic mixture of the two. While R-ALA is more efficiently utilized by the body, the racemic mixture has been used in the majority of clinical trials and has demonstrated significant efficacy (4).

The pharmacokinetic profile of ALA is characterized by rapid absorption and metabolism, with a relatively low oral bioavailability of approximately 30–40%, which can be further reduced by the presence of food. This has led to research into more stable and bioavailable formulations, but standard oral supplements remain the most studied form (2) (Figure 4.1).

4.1.1 Key Mechanisms of Action

The therapeutic utility of ALA is not derived from a single action but from its ability to modulate multiple, interconnected cellular pathways.

Multifaceted Antioxidant Activity: ALA exerts its antioxidant effects through several pathways. It directly scavenges a wide range of reactive oxygen species (ROS), including hydroxyl radicals and hypochlorous acid. Furthermore, its reduced form, dihydrolipoic acid (DHLA), is a potent antioxidant that can regenerate other crucial endogenous antioxidants, such as glutathione, vitamin C, vitamin E, and coenzyme Q10 (3). This ability to participate in the antioxidant network makes it a uniquely powerful agent in mitigating cellular oxidative stress.

Insulin Sensitization: A key aspect of ALA's clinical utility is its ability to improve insulin sensitivity. This is primarily achieved through the activation of the AMP-activated protein kinase (AMPK) pathway in skeletal muscle and adipose tissue. AMPK activation enhances glucose uptake via the translocation of GLUT4 transporters to the cell membrane, thereby improving glucose disposal and ameliorating insulin resistance. This mechanism is particularly relevant for the management of metabolic disturbances in conditions like polycystic ovary syndrome (PCOS) (6).

Anti-inflammatory Effects: Chronic low-grade inflammation is a key driver of many gynecological disorders, including endometriosis and PCOS. ALA exhibits significant anti-inflammatory properties by inhibiting the activation of the master inflammatory transcription factor, nuclear factor-kappa B (NF-κB). By suppressing NF-κB, ALA downregulates the expression of pro-inflammatory cytokines (e.g., TNF-α, IL-6) and other inflammatory mediators, thereby dampening the inflammatory cascade (3).

4.2 OXIDATIVE STRESS: THE HIDDEN ENEMY OF FEMALE FERTILITY

Oxidative stress (OS) arises from an imbalance between the production of ROS and the capacity of the body's antioxidant defense systems to neutralize them. In the female

DOI: 10.1201/9781003741541-4

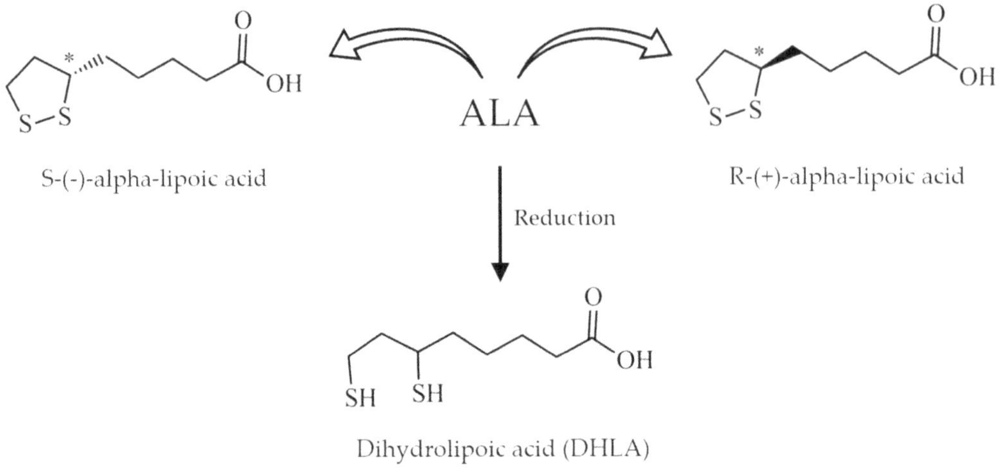

Figure 4.1 Chemical structures of R- and S-lipoic acid (5). The core structure of ALA features a five-membered dithiolane ring containing a disulfide bond. The key difference between the R- and S-enantiomers lies in the 3D spatial arrangement (stereochemistry) at the chiral carbon atom (C6). Upon reduction, ALA generates dihydrolipoic acid (DHLA). (From [5], under Creative Commons Attribution License.)

reproductive system, this imbalance is a critical, often overlooked factor contributing to subfertility and infertility. While a certain level of ROS is necessary for normal physiological processes like ovulation, excessive ROS production – driven by conditions such as PCOS, endometriosis, aging, or environmental factors – can overwhelm the oocyte's delicate microenvironment (7).

The oocyte is particularly vulnerable to oxidative damage. Elevated ROS can inflict harm on all major cellular components:

Genomic Instability: ROS-induced DNA strand breaks and base modifications can compromise the oocyte's genetic integrity, leading to fertilization failure, embryonic arrest, or aneuploidy (8).

Mitochondrial Dysfunction: Oxidative damage to mitochondrial DNA and respiratory chain components cripple ATP production, depriving the oocyte of the immense energy required for completing meiosis and supporting early embryonic cleavage (9).

Cellular and Structural Damage: Lipid peroxidation weakens the oocyte's plasma membrane, while ROS-induced damage to the cytoskeleton can disrupt the formation of the meiotic spindle, a structure essential for correct chromosome segregation.

Cumulatively, this damage severely compromises oocyte quality, leading to impaired maturation, fertilization failure, poor embryonic development, and early pregnancy loss. Therefore, antioxidant interventions that can restore redox balance within the follicular environment represent a logical and promising therapeutic strategy to improve fertility outcomes (10).

4.3 CLINICAL APPLICATIONS OF ALA IN INFERTILITY TREATMENT

4.3.1 Polycystic Ovary Syndrome

Scientific Background: PCOS is the most common endocrine disorder in women of reproductive age, characterized by hyperandrogenism, chronic anovulation, and, in the majority of cases, insulin resistance (IR) (11). IR and the resultant compensatory hyperinsulinemia are central to PCOS pathophysiology, driving increased ovarian androgen production and disrupting normal follicular development. This adverse metabolic and hormonal milieu, combined with high levels of oxidative stress and chronic low-grade inflammation, severely impairs oocyte quality, presenting a major challenge in both natural conception and assisted reproductive technologies (ART) (10, 11).

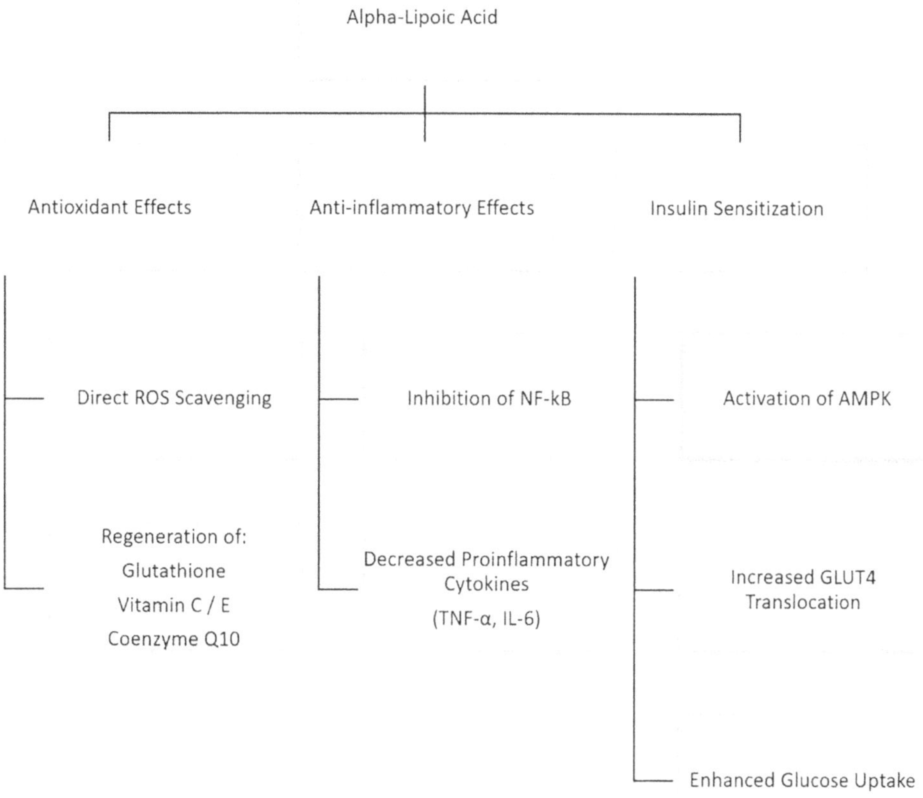

Figure 4.2 Simplified diagram of ALA's key mechanisms of action. This flowchart outlines the three primary therapeutic pathways of Alpha-Lipoic Acid. It acts as a multifaceted antioxidant, an anti-inflammatory agent by inhibiting NF-κB, and an insulin-sensitizing molecule through the activation of AMPK, leading to enhanced glucose uptake. (From the Authors.)

4.3.1.1 Clinical Evidence

Enhanced Oocyte and Embryo Quality in ART: The most definitive evidence for ALA's efficacy in PCOS comes from a robust triple-blind randomized controlled trial (RCT) involving 70 women with PCOS undergoing IVF treatment (12). The intervention group received 600 mg/day of ALA for 12 weeks prior to oocyte retrieval. The study reported remarkable improvements in the ALA group compared to placebo:

The number of mature (MII) oocytes retrieved was significantly higher (11.83 ± 6.27 vs. 7.91 ± 4.88, $p = 0.02$).

Oocyte quality was profoundly improved, with the percentage of good-quality oocytes more than doubling (71.0% vs. 32.7%, $p = 0.01$). Strikingly, **zero poor-quality oocytes** were observed in the ALA group, compared to 45.5% in the control group ($p = 0.0005$).

This translated to a significantly higher number of moderate-quality embryos (3.57 ± 3.61 vs. 1.54 ± 1.56, $p = 0.02$).

Furthermore, serum estradiol levels on the day of hCG trigger were significantly lower in the ALA group, suggesting a more controlled ovarian response and a potentially lower risk of ovarian hyperstimulation syndrome (OHSS) (12).

Metabolic and Inflammatory Modulation: In a study on adolescents with PCOS, a combination of myo-inositol (4g) and ALA (400 mg) for 6 months led to a significant decrease in serum levels of HMGB1, a key pro-inflammatory marker, indicating a reduction in the chronic inflammatory state associated with PCOS (13). Another clinical trial investigated an antioxidant combination including ALA (600 mg), N-acetylcysteine, vitamin B6, and SAMe. This combination demonstrated improvements in metabolic parameters, including a reduction in HOMA-IR, and clinical signs like hirsutism, further supporting its role in addressing the underlying metabolic dysfunction of PCOS (14).

4.3.2 Endometriosis and Chronic Pelvic Pain

Scientific Background: Endometriosis is a chronic, estrogen-dependent inflammatory disease characterized by the growth of endometrial-like tissue outside the uterus. This ectopic tissue incites a significant inflammatory response, leading to chronic pelvic pain, dyspareunia, adhesions, and infertility. Oxidative stress is known to be elevated in the peritoneal fluid of women with endometriosis and is thought to promote the proliferation and survival of ectopic endometrial cells while also sensitizing nerve fibers, thereby contributing to pain (15).

4.3.2.1 Clinical Evidence

A multicenter clinical trial evaluated the efficacy of a combination therapy containing N-acetylcysteine (600 mg), ALA (200 mg), bromelain, and zinc, administered twice daily to 136 women with endometriosis-associated pelvic pain. After 3 and 6 months, patients reported a highly significant and continuous reduction in pain scores (VAS) for dysmenorrhea, dyspareunia, and chronic pelvic pain ($p < 0.001$). The use of rescue analgesics was also significantly reduced (15).

Another study investigated the combination of palmitoylethanolamide (PEA, 400 mg) and ALA (400 mg), taken twice daily for 6 months, for the management of chronic pelvic pain. PEA is a fatty acid amide known for its neuro-inflammatory modulating effects. This combination therapy resulted in a significant reduction in chronic pelvic pain, dysmenorrhea, and dyspareunia ($p < 0.001$), which was accompanied by marked improvements in quality of life and sexual function scores (16).

4.3.3 ALA as a Component of Embryo Culture Media in ART

Beyond maternal supplementation, the antioxidant properties of ALA have been used directly within the IVF laboratory to protect the developing embryo from the inherent stresses of the in vitro environment. The process of removing oocytes and embryos from the protective maternal environment and culturing them in the lab exposes them to higher oxygen tension and artificial conditions, which can increase oxidative stress and impair development (17).

4.3.3.1 Clinical Evidence

A randomized multicenter trial investigated this very application. The study was designed to determine if supplementing a standard embryo culture media system with a trio of antioxidants – acetyl-L-carnitine, N-acetyl-L-cysteine, and ALA – could improve embryo development. The study analyzed over 1500 sibling oocytes from 133 patients. While the overall results showed no significant difference in blastocyst development rates for the entire patient population, a pre-defined subgroup analysis of women aged 35 to 40 revealed significant benefits. In this age group, oocytes cultured in the antioxidant-enriched media had a significantly higher usable blastocyst rate (38.8% vs. 27.8%, $p = 0.01$) and superior Day 3 embryo quality (72.8% vs. 61.2%, $p = 0.03$) compared to their sibling oocytes in the standard media. This evidence strongly suggests that directly adding ALA as part of an antioxidant cocktail to the culture medium can mitigate age-related oxidative stress on the embryo, improving its developmental potential, particularly in an older patient demographic (17).

4.4 APPLICATIONS OF ALA IN OTHER GYNECOLOGICAL CONDITIONS

Threatened Miscarriage and Subchorionic Hematoma: A subchorionic hematoma is a common cause of first-trimester bleeding and a risk factor for miscarriage. The anti-inflammatory and immunomodulatory properties of ALA have been successfully used in this context. A randomized trial compared 10 mg of vaginal ALA, vaginal progesterone, and no treatment in 62 women with threatened miscarriage and subchorionic hematoma. The ALA group showed significantly faster reabsorption of the hematoma compared to both the progesterone group ($p \leq 0.05$) and the no-treatment group ($p < 0.01$) (18). Another RCT found that adding oral ALA (600 mg) to standard progesterone therapy also accelerated healing. The proposed mechanism is ALA's potent local anti-inflammatory and immunomodulatory activity (19).

Prevention of Preterm Birth: Preterm cervical shortening is a primary predictor of preterm birth and is mechanistically linked to inflammation. A pilot RCT in women at risk for preterm birth found that daily administration of 400 mg of vaginal ALA after primary tocolysis prevented further cervical shortening, whereas the placebo group experienced significant shortening ($p = 0.03$). This protective effect was associated with a significant local increase in the anti-inflammatory cytokine IL-4 (20).

Primary Dysmenorrhea: Characterized by painful menstrual cramps driven by prostaglandins and inflammation, primary dysmenorrhea can be debilitating. An RCT showed that adding 400 mg of ALA to standard therapy with mefenamic acid significantly reduced both the severity (VAS score) and duration of pain compared to mefenamic acid alone ($p < 0.001$) (21).

4.5 SAFETY, DOSAGE, AND PRACTICAL CONSIDERATIONS

Across all the reviewed clinical trials, ALA has demonstrated an excellent safety profile. It is generally well-tolerated, and no serious adverse events attributable to the substance have been reported. Minor side effects are rare and may include mild gastrointestinal upset or skin rashes (Table 4.1).

4.6 CHALLENGES, CONTROVERSIES, AND FUTURE DIRECTIONS

Despite the promising results, several key areas require further investigation before ALA can be universally integrated into standard clinical protocols.

Confounder of Combination Therapies: A critical methodological limitation in much of the current literature is the use of ALA within multi-ingredient formulations. While these combinations may reflect a sound clinical strategy to achieve synergistic effects, they make it scientifically difficult to attribute the observed benefits solely to ALA. Future studies should include arms with ALA monotherapy to dissect its specific contribution.

Need for Large-Scale RCTs with Hard Endpoints: Much of the existing research relies on surrogate endpoints such as oocyte quality, inflammatory markers, or pain scores. While valuable, the ultimate goal in fertility treatment is a healthy live birth. There is a pressing need for large, adequately powered RCTs that use live birth rate as the primary endpoint to definitively establish ALA's role in improving reproductive success.

Table 4.1: Summary of Dosages and Designs from Key Clinical Trials of ALA

Indication	ALA Dosage & Route	Key Combination Agent(s)	Primary Finding	Reference
PCOS (ART)	600 mg/day, oral	None	Improved oocyte quality & number	(12)
PCOS (Adolescents)	400 mg/day, oral	Myo-inositol	Reduced inflammatory markers (HMGB1)	(13)
PCOS (Metabolic)	600 mg/day, oral	NAC, Vit B6, SAMe	Improved HOMA-IR & hirsutism	(14)
Endometriosis Pain	400 mg/day, oral	N-acetylcysteine, bromelain	Reduced pelvic pain scores	(15)
Chronic Pelvic Pain	800 mg/day, oral	Palmitoylethanolamide (PEA)	Reduced pelvic pain & dyspareunia	(16)
Subchorionic Hematoma	10 mg/day, vaginal	None	Accelerated hematoma reabsorption	(18)
Cervical Shortening	400 mg/day, vaginal	None	Stabilized cervical length	(20)
Primary Dysmenorrhea	400 mg/day, oral	Mefenamic Acid	Reduced pain severity & duration	(21)

Bioavailability and Formulation: The bioavailability of standard oral ALA supplements can be variable and is often reduced by food. Furthermore, the debate continues regarding the potential superiority of purified R-ALA over the more common racemic mixture. Future research should focus on optimizing formulations to enhance bioavailability and comparing the clinical efficacy of different enantiomers.

Exploring New Populations: The potential benefits of ALA could extend to other challenging patient groups, such as women with diminished ovarian reserve, poor responders in ART, unexplained infertility, or recurrent pregnancy loss, conditions where oxidative stress and mitochondrial dysfunction are also increasingly recognized as key pathological factors.

4.7 CONCLUSION

Alpha-lipoic acid has emerged as a compelling, multi-target therapeutic agent in the fields of gynecology and reproductive medicine. As a powerful antioxidant, insulin sensitizer, and anti-inflammatory molecule, it directly addresses the core pathophysiological mechanisms underlying prevalent conditions like PCOS and endometriosis. The clinical evidence strongly supports its use as a safe and effective adjuvant therapy for significantly improving oocyte and embryo quality in women with PCOS, as well as for managing debilitating pain associated with various gynecological disorders. Considering that eight RCTs conducted on ALA has been published to date, further research with hard clinical endpoints is necessary to solidify its place in standard treatment algorithms, the existing body of evidence strongly suggests that ALA is a valuable tool for clinicians seeking to enhance fertility outcomes and improve the overall reproductive health of their patients.

REFERENCES

1. Gomes MB, Negrato CA. Alpha-lipoic acid as a pleiotropic compound with potential therapeutic use in diabetes and other chronic diseases. *Diabetology & Metabolic Syndrome.* 2014;6(1):80.
2. Salehi B, Berkay Yılmaz Y, Antika G, Boyunegmez Tumer T, Fawzi Mahomoodally M, Lobine D, et al. Insights on the use of α-lipoic acid for therapeutic purposes. *Biomolecules.* 2019;9(8):356.
3. Shahid A, Nasir K, Bhatia M. Therapeutic potential of alpha-lipoic acid: Unraveling its role in oxidative stress and inflammatory conditions. *Current Issues in Molecular Biology.* 2025;47(5):322.
4. Dugbartey GJ, Alornyo KK, Dapaa-Addo CO, Botchway E, Kwashie EK, Harley Y. Alpha-lipoic acid: A promising pharmacotherapy seen through the lens of kidney diseases. *Current Research in Pharmacology and Drug Discovery.* 2024;7:100206.
5. Viana MDM, Lauria PSS, Lima AAd, Opretzka LCF, Marcelino HR, Villarreal CF. Alpha-lipoic acid as an antioxidant strategy for managing neuropathic pain. *Antioxidants.* 2022;11(12):2420.
6. Capece U, Moffa S, Improta I, Di Giuseppe G, Nista EC, Cefalo CM, et al. Alpha-lipoic acid and glucose metabolism: A comprehensive update on biochemical and therapeutic features. *Nutrients.* 2022;15(1):18.
7. Agarwal A, Aponte-Mellado A, Premkumar BJ, Shaman A, Gupta S. The effects of oxidative stress on female reproduction: A review. *Reproductive Biology and Endocrinology.* 2012;10(1):49.
8. Musson R, Gąsior Ł, Bisogno S, Ptak GE. DNA damage in preimplantation embryos and gametes: Specification, clinical relevance and repair strategies. *Human Reproduction Update.* 2022;28(3):376–99.
9. Wang T, Xu P, Yuan J, Chen H, Guo X, Gao J, et al. Mitochondrial dysfunction in oocytes: Implications for fertility and ageing. *Journal of Ovarian Research.* 2025;18(1):186.
10. Voros C, Athanasiou D, Papapanagiotou I, Mavrogianni D, Varthaliti A, Bananis K, et al. Cracking the code of oocyte quality: The oxidative stress link to IVF success. *International Journal of Molecular Sciences.* 2025;26(13):6377.
11. Zhao H, Zhang J, Cheng X, Nie X, He B. Insulin resistance in polycystic ovary syndrome across various tissues: An updated review of pathogenesis, evaluation, and treatment. *Journal of Ovarian Research.* 2023;16(1):9.
12. Azizi-Kutenaei M, Aminpour M, Fesahat F, Salehi E. Alpha-lipoic acid supplementation enhances oocyte quality and reduces hormonal hyper-response in PCOS patients undergoing ART: A randomized controlled trial. 2024. *(Unpublished data)*
13. Cirillo F, Catellani C, Lazzeroni P, Sartori C, Tridenti G, Vezzani C, et al. HMGB1 is increased in adolescents with polycystic ovary syndrome (PCOS) and decreases after treatment with myo-inositol (MYO) in combination with alpha-lipoic acid (ALA). *Gynecological Endocrinology.* 2020;36(7):588–93.
14. Pingarrón Santofímia C, Poyo Torcal S, Lopez Verdu H, Henriquez Linares A, Calvente Aguilar V, Terol Sanchez P, et al. Evaluation of the efficacy of an antioxidant combination for the modulation of metabolic, endocrine, and clinical parameters in patients with polycystic ovary syndrome. *Gynecological Endocrinology.* 2023;39(1):2227277.

15. Lete I, Mendoza N, de la Viuda E, Carmona F. Effectiveness of an antioxidant preparation with N-acetyl cysteine, alpha lipoic acid and bromelain in the treatment of endometriosis-associated pelvic pain: LEAP study. *European Journal of Obstetrics & Gynecology and Reproductive Biology.* 2018;228:221–4.
16. Caruso S, Sareri I, Casella E, Ventura B, Fava V, Cianci A. Chronic pelvic pain, quality of life and sexual health of women treated with palmitoylethanolamide and α-lipoic acid. *Minerva Ginecologica.* 2015;67(5):413–9.
17. Gardner DK, Kuramoto T, Tanaka M, Mitzumoto S, Montag M, Yoshida A. Prospective randomized multicentre comparison on sibling oocytes comparing G-Series media system with antioxidants versus standard G-Series media system. *Reproductive Biomedicine Online.* 2020;40(5):637–44.
18. Costantino M, Guaraldi C, Costantino D. Resolution of subchorionic hematoma and symptoms of threatened miscarriage using vaginal alpha lipoic acid or progesterone: Clinical evidences. *European Review for Medical & Pharmacological Sciences.* 2016;20(9).
19. Porcaro G, Brillo E, Giardina I, Di Iorio R. Alpha lipoic acid (ALA) effects on subchorionic hematoma. Preliminary clinical results. *European Review for Medical and Pharmacological Sciences.* 2015;19(18):3426–32.
20. Grandi G, Pignatti L, Ferrari F, Dante G, Neri I, Facchinetti F. Vaginal alpha-lipoic acid shows an anti-inflammatory effect on the cervix, preventing its shortening after primary tocolysis. A pilot, randomized, placebo-controlled study. *Journal of Maternal-Fetal & Neonatal Medicine.* 2017;30(18):2243–9.
21. Yousefi M, Kavianpour M, Hesami S, Rashidi Nooshabadi M, Khadem Haghighian H. Effect of alpha-lipoic acid at the combination with mefenamic acid in girls with primary dysmenorrhea: Randomized, double-blind, placebo-controlled clinical trial. *Gynecol Endocrinol.* 2019;35(9):782–86.

5 Coenzyme Q10

A Mitochondrial Energizer for Enhancing Female Fertility

Samaneh Harimi, Maryam Azizi-Kutenaei, and Farzaneh Fesahat

5.1 INTRODUCTION TO COENZYME Q10

Coenzyme Q10 (CoQ10), also known as ubiquinone, is a lipid-soluble, vitamin-like substance that is endogenously synthesized and present in virtually all human cells. It plays a central and indispensable role in cellular bioenergetics and antioxidant defense (1, 2). Biochemically, CoQ10 exists in two primary forms: the oxidized form, ubiquinone, and the reduced form, ubiquinol. This capacity to cycle between oxidized and reduced states allows it to perform its two fundamental functions (3).

First, as a mobile electron carrier within the inner mitochondrial membrane, CoQ10 is a critical component of the electron transport chain (ETC), where it plays a crucial role in driving oxidative phosphorylation to generate adenosine triphosphate (ATP), the primary energy molecule of the cell (4). Second, in its reduced form (ubiquinol), it functions as a powerful lipid-soluble antioxidant, protecting cellular membranes, lipids, proteins, and DNA from the damaging effects of reactive oxygen species (ROS). Given these essential roles, CoQ10 deficiency has been implicated in the pathophysiology of numerous conditions, including cardiovascular disease, neurodegenerative disorders, and, increasingly, infertility (4, 5).

5.2 MECHANISMS OF ACTION IN FEMALE REPRODUCTIVE HEALTH

The oocyte is the largest cell in the human body and is exceptionally rich in mitochondria, which are required to generate the immense amount of ATP needed to support oocyte maturation, fertilization, and the complex cellular divisions of early embryonic development (6). The quality of the oocyte is therefore intrinsically linked to its mitochondrial health. Oxidative stress, which results from excessive production of ROS relative to the antioxidant defenses, is a key factor that compromises mitochondrial function and overall oocyte quality (7). CoQ10 is positioned at the intersection of these critical processes.

- **Enhancing Mitochondrial Health in Oocytes:** As a vital component of the ETC, CoQ10 directly supports mitochondrial ATP production. Mitochondrial dysfunction leads to diminished ATP output, which can result in meiotic errors, fertilization failure, and embryonic arrest. CoQ10 supplementation has been shown to restore mitochondrial function and improve ATP production, and reverse age-related declines in oocyte quality and fertility (8).
- **Combating Oxidative Stress:** The follicular fluid surrounding the developing oocyte contains a delicate balance of antioxidants and ROS. Excessive ROS can inflict widespread cellular damage. CoQ10 is a powerful antioxidant that neutralizes free radicals and also helps regenerate other primary antioxidants like vitamin E. This action helps protect the oocyte from oxidative damage, preserving its developmental competence (9).
- **Improving Endothelial Function:** Endothelial dysfunction is a key pathological feature in conditions like pre-eclampsia and is increasingly recognized in metabolic disorders like PCOS. By reducing inflammation and oxidative stress, CoQ10 has been shown to improve endothelial function (10), which may be another important mechanism contributing to better pregnancy outcomes (Figure 5.1).

5.3 CLINICAL APPLICATIONS AND EVIDENCE IN WOMEN'S INFERTILITY

The theoretical benefits of CoQ10 have been tested in several randomized controlled trials (RCTs). The evidence is strongest in women with diminished ovarian reserve and polycystic ovary syndrome.

5.3.1 Diminished Ovarian Reserve (DOR)

DOR is a condition characterized by a low number of remaining oocytes, often leading to a poor ovarian response (POR) during assisted reproductive technology (ART). A RCT by Xu et al. (2018)

DOI: 10.1201/9781003741541-5

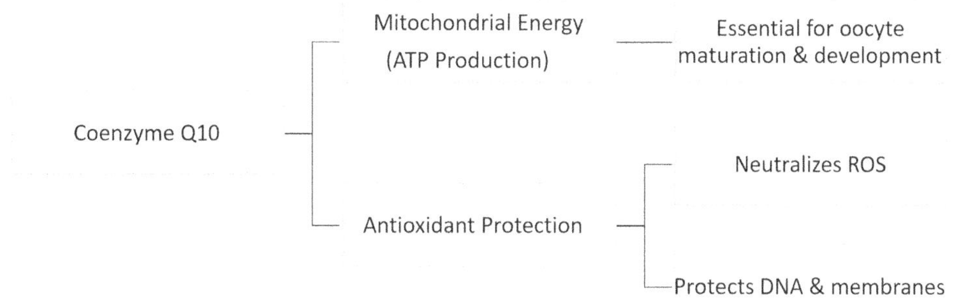

Figure 5.1 The dual mechanism of action of coenzyme Q10 in female reproductive health. This diagram illustrates CoQ10's two primary functions in supporting oocyte viability. (From the Authors.)

investigated the effect of CoQ10 pretreatment in young women (<35 years) with poor ovarian reserve. Women received 600 mg of CoQ10 daily for 60 days prior to their IVF cycle. The results were compelling (11):

- **Improved Ovarian Response:** The CoQ10 group required a significantly lower total dose of gonadotropins and achieved higher peak estradiol (E2) levels.
- **Enhanced Oocyte and Embryo Yield:** Women pretreated with CoQ10 had a significantly higher number of retrieved oocytes (median of 4 vs. 2) and a markedly improved fertilization rate (67.5% vs. 45.1%).
- **Superior Embryo Quality:** Crucially, the CoQ10 group produced a significantly greater number of high-quality embryos.
- **Better Cycle Outcomes:** This translated into significantly fewer cycles with cancelled embryo transfers due to poor embryo development (8.3% vs. 22.9%).

However, the protective effect of CoQ10 may be context-dependent. A study by Micaraseth et al. (2025) explored whether a shorter 14-day course of 300 mg/day CoQ10 could preserve ovarian reserve (measured by AMH) in women undergoing hysterectomy. This short pretreatment was found to be ineffective in preventing the postoperative decline in AMH levels (12). The authors suggest that the short duration and different clinical challenge (acute surgical insult vs. chronic follicular development) may explain the lack of benefit.

5.3.2 Polycystic Ovary Syndrome

PCOS is the most prevalent endocrine disorder among women of reproductive-age, identified by hyperandrogenism, anovulation, and often, insulin resistance and chronic inflammation and oxidative stress (13). Several RCTs have demonstrated that CoQ10 supplementation targets multiple facets of this complex syndrome:

- **Metabolic and Hormonal Improvements:** A trial found that 100 mg/day of CoQ10 for 12 weeks significantly improved glucose metabolism, leading to reductions in fasting plasma glucose, serum insulin, and HOMA-IR. It also significantly decreased total and LDL-cholesterol levels (14). Similarly, it was showed that 200 mg/day for 8 weeks significantly reduced fasting blood sugar, HOMA-IR, and total testosterone levels. The combination of CoQ10 and vitamin E was particularly effective, Also leading to a significant increase in sex hormone-binding globulin (SHBG) (15). Confirming these effects, a study reported that 100 mg/day for 12 weeks reduced total testosterone, DHEAS, and clinical hirsutism, while increasing SHBG (16).
- **Reduction of Inflammation and Oxidative Stress:** CoQ10 also addresses the inflammatory and oxidative stress pathways in PCOS. Taking 200 mg per day for 8 weeks has been found to significantly decrease key inflammatory markers, including hs-CRP, TNF-α, and IL–6. The treatment also lowered markers of endothelial dysfunction

Table 5.1: Summary of RCTs on CoQ10 in Women with or at Risk of Diminished Ovarian Reserve

Study	Population & Sample Size	Intervention	Duration	Key Findings
Xu et al. (2018) (11)	Young women (<35) with DOR undergoing IVF ($n = 169$)	600 mg/day CoQ10 vs. no treatment	60 days	**Positive:** Significantly more oocytes retrieved, higher fertilization rate, more high-quality embryos
Micaraseth et al. (2025) (12)	Women undergoing hysterectomy ($n = 44$)	300 mg/day CoQ10 vs. placebo	14 days	**Negative:** CoQ10 did not prevent postoperative decline in AMH levels.

DOR: Diminished ovarian reserve; IVF: In vitro fertilization; AMH: Anti-Müllerian hormone.

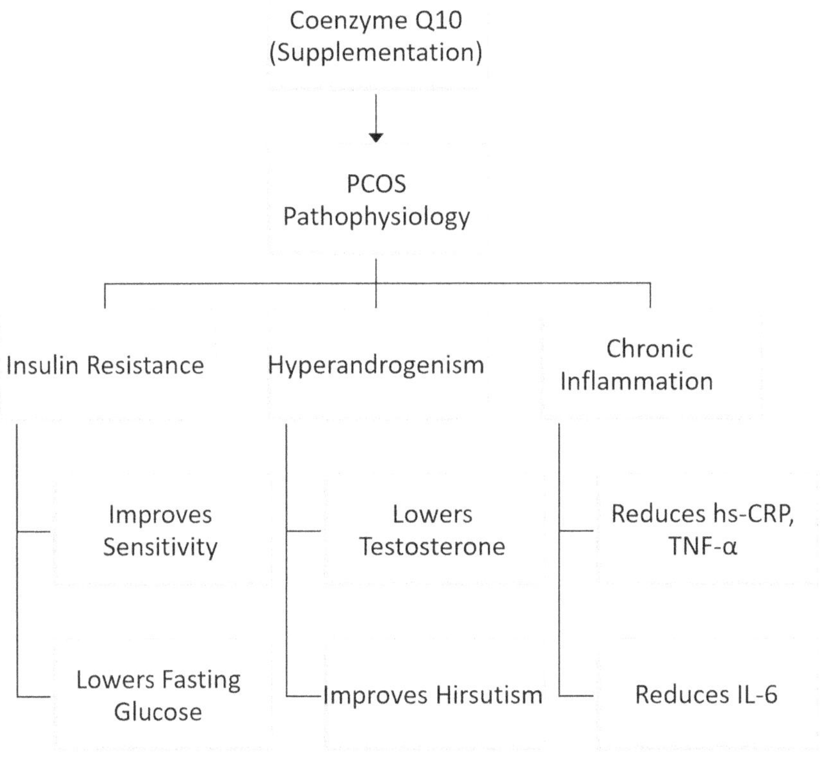

Figure 5.2 The pleiotropic effects of coenzyme Q10 in PCOS pathophysiology. This schematic shows how CoQ10 supplementation targets several core components of polycystic ovary syndrome. (From the Authors.)

(VCAM-1 and E-selectin), which are implicated in the long-term cardiovascular risk associated with PCOS (10). Furthermore, it demonstrated a reduction in malondialdehyde (MDA), a marker of lipid peroxidation, and an increase in total antioxidant capacity (TAC), providing direct evidence of CoQ10's ability to combat oxidative stress in PCOS patients (16) (Figure 5.2).

A unique finding from the trial by Karamali & Gholizadeh (2022) was the positive impact on mental health of PCOS patients. After 12 weeks of supplementation, women receiving CoQ10 had significantly lower scores on the Beck Depression Inventory (BDI) and Beck Anxiety Inventory (BAI) compared to the placebo group, suggesting a potential role for CoQ10 in addressing the psychological burden often associated with PCOS (16).

5.3.3 Other Reproductive Health Applications: Pre-Eclampsia

Beyond infertility, CoQ10's role in supporting a healthy pregnancy has also been investigated. Pre-eclampsia is a serious pregnancy complication linked to oxidative stress. An RCT evaluated whether CoQ10 (200 mg/day from 20 weeks gestation) could reduce its risk. The study found a significant reduction in the incidence of pre-eclampsia, from 25.6% in the placebo group to 14.4% in the CoQ10 group. This suggests that CoQ10's antioxidant and endothelial-protective effects may be beneficial for preventing this dangerous obstetrical complication. (17).

5.4 DOSAGE, EFFICACY, AND SAFETY PROFILES

Across all reviewed trials, CoQ10 has demonstrated an excellent safety profile and is generally well-tolerated, with no serious adverse events reported.

- The dosage of CoQ10 used in clinical trials varies. For DOR in ART, a higher dose of 600 mg/day for at least 60 days appears necessary (11). Pretreatment with CoQ10 before commencing an ART cycle is an evidence-based strategy to potentially improve ovarian response and embryological outcomes. This duration is logical, as it covers the final stages of follicular development.
- For PCOS management, doses of 100 mg to 200 mg/day for 8 to 12 weeks have proven effective (10, 14–16). CoQ10 can be used as a long-term nutritional supplement to help manage the underlying metabolic and hormonal disturbances. It can be safely combined with standard medications like metformin. Its benefits on inflammation and mental health provide additional rationale for its use (Table 5.2).

Table 5.2: Summary of Dosages and Key Findings from Pivotal CoQ10 Clinical Trials

Indication	CoQ10 Dosage	Duration	Key Clinical Finding	Reference
DOR (ART)	600 mg/day	60 days	Improved oocyte number and quality, higher fertilization rate.	(11)
PCOS (Metabolic)	100 mg/day	12 weeks	Improved insulin sensitivity and lipid profile.	(14)
PCOS (Hormonal)	200 mg/day	8 weeks	Reduced total testosterone and improved insulin resistance.	(15)
PCOS (Inflammation)	200 mg/day	8 weeks	Reduced markers of inflammation (hs-CRP, TNF-α) and endothelial dysfunction.	(10)
PCOS (Overall)	100 mg/day	12 weeks	Reduced androgens, inflammation, anxiety, and depression scores.	(16)
Pre-Eclampsia Risk	200 mg/day	From 20 weeks	Significantly reduced the risk of developing pre-eclampsia.	(17)

5.5 CHALLENGES, CONTROVERSIES, AND FUTURE DIRECTIONS

Despite the promising evidence, several gaps remain in our understanding of CoQ10's role in female infertility.

- **Need for Large-Scale RCTs with Hard Endpoints:** While effects on surrogate markers like embryo quality and inflammatory profiles are strong, there is a pressing need for larger, adequately powered RCTs that use live birth rate as the primary endpoint to definitively establish CoQ10's clinical efficacy.
- **Optimal Dose and Duration:** The ideal dose and treatment duration for different patient populations remain unknown and require further investigation. The duration of supplementation may need to be longer (i.e., >3 months) to influence early follicular recruitment. Furthermore, it is plausible that CoQ10 supplementation is most effective in women who have a baseline deficiency. Research into personalized approaches, potentially guided by baseline CoQ10 levels, is warranted.
- **Limited Data in Other Populations:** There is a lack of research on the effectiveness of CoQ10 in other causes of infertility, such as endometriosis or unexplained infertility, where oxidative stress is also a known contributing factor.

5.6 CONCLUSION

Coenzyme Q10 has emerged as a safe, well-tolerated, and promising nutritional supplement in the field of reproductive medicine. By enhancing mitochondrial energy production and providing potent antioxidant protection, it directly targets key pathophysiological mechanisms that impair female fertility. The clinical evidence is strongest for its use as an adjuvant therapy to improve ovarian response in young women with DOR undergoing ART, and to manage the multifaceted disturbances of PCOS. Although only seven RCTs conducted on CoQ10 has been published to date, the existing body of evidence strongly suggests that CoQ10 is a valuable tool for clinicians seeking to enhance fertility outcomes.

REFERENCES

1. Saini R. Coenzyme Q10: The essential nutrient. *Journal of Pharmacy and Bioallied Sciences*. 2011;3(3):466–7.
2. Acosta MJ, Fonseca LV, Desbats MA, Cerqua C, Zordan R, Trevisson E, et al. Coenzyme Q biosynthesis in health and disease. *Biochimica et Biophysica Acta (BBA)-Bioenergetics*. 2016;1857(8):1079–85.
3. Aaseth J, Alexander J, Alehagen U. Coenzyme Q10 supplementation–in ageing and disease. *Mechanisms of Ageing and Development*. 2021;197:111521.
4. Pallotti F, Bergamini C, Lamperti C, Fato R. The roles of coenzyme Q in disease: Direct and indirect involvement in cellular functions. *International Journal of Molecular Sciences*. 2021, 23(1):128.
5. Jiang Y, Han Y, Qiao P, Ren F. Exploring the protective effects of coenzyme Q10 on female fertility. *Frontiers in Cell and Developmental Biology*. 2025;13:1633166.
6. Kirillova A, Smitz JE, Sukhikh GT, Mazunin I. The role of mitochondria in oocyte maturation. *Cell*. 2021;10(9):2484.
7. Begum I. Oxidative stress: Oocyte quality and infertility. *Reproductive Toxicology*. 2025:109011.
8. Ben-Meir A, Burstein E, Borrego-Alvarez A, Chong J, Wong E, Yavorska T, et al. Coenzyme Q10 restores oocyte mitochondrial function and fertility during reproductive aging. *Aging Cell*. 2015;14(5): 887–95.
9. Chen Y, Yang J, Zhang L. The impact of follicular fluid oxidative stress levels on the outcomes of assisted reproductive therapy. *Antioxidants*. 2023;12(12):2117.
10. Taghizadeh S, Izadi A, Shirazi S, Parizad M, Pourghassem Gargari B. The effect of coenzyme Q10 supplementation on inflammatory and endothelial dysfunction markers in overweight/obese polycystic ovary syndrome patients. *Gynecological Endocrinology*. 2021;37(1):26–30.
11. Xu Y, Nisenblat V, Lu C, Li R, Qiao J, Zhen X, et al. Pretreatment with coenzyme Q10 improves ovarian response and embryo quality in low-prognosis young women with decreased ovarian reserve: A randomized controlled trial. *Reproductive Biology and Endocrinology*. 2018;16(1):29.
12. Micaraseth K, Tantanavipas S, Hongsakorn W, Singwongsa AJBJoN. The effect of coenzyme Q10 pretreatment on ovarian reserve in women undergoing hysterectomy with bilateral salpingectomy: A randomised, double-blind, placebo-controlled trial. *British Journal of Nutrition*. 2025;133(2):213–20.
13. Bai H, Ding H, Wang MJC, Obstetrics E, Gynecology. Polycystic ovary syndrome (PCOS): Symptoms, causes, and treatment. *Clinical and Experimental Obstetrics & Gynecology*. 2024;51(5):126.
14. Samimi M, Zarezade Mehrizi M, Foroozanfard F, Akbari H, Jamilian M, Ahmadi S, et al. The effects of coenzyme Q10 supplementation on glucose metabolism and lipid profiles in women with polycystic ovary syndrome: A randomized, double-blind, placebo-controlled trial. *Clinical Endocrinology*. 2017;86(4):560–6.

15. Izadi A, Ebrahimi S, Shirazi S, Taghizadeh S, Parizad M, Farzadi L, et al. Hormonal and metabolic effects of coenzyme Q10 and/or vitamin E in patients with polycystic ovary syndrome. *Journal of Clinical Endocrinology & Metabolism*. 2019;104(2):319–27.
16. Karamali M, Gholizadeh M. The effects of coenzyme Q10 supplementation on metabolic profiles and parameters of mental health in women with polycystic ovary syndrome. *Gynecological Endocrinology*. 2022;38(1):45–9.
17. Teran E, Hernandez I, Nieto B, Tavara R, Ocampo JE, Calle A, et al. Coenzyme Q10 supplementation during pregnancy reduces the risk of pre-eclampsia. *International Journal of Gynecology & Obstetrics*. 2009;105(1):43–5.

6 Vitamin E

Negar Nouri, Abolfazl Taghinejad, Maryam Azizi-Kutenaei, and Farzaneh Fesahat

6.1 INTRODUCTION

Vitamin E, a lipid-soluble antioxidant primarily represented by α-tocopherol, plays an important supportive role in female reproductive health through its ability to preserve cellular redox balance, protect steroidogenic pathways, and modulate inflammatory and angiogenic signaling. By acting as a membrane-phase chain-breaking antioxidant, vitamin E limits lipid peroxidation and the formation of reactive aldehydes, thereby safeguarding mitochondrial integrity and the activity of key steroidogenic enzymes in ovarian granulosa and luteal cells. These effects contribute to the maintenance of estradiol and progesterone production, which are essential for follicular development, luteal function, and endometrial receptivity. Beyond its antioxidant capacity, vitamin E exerts anti-inflammatory actions through inhibition of NF-κB–dependent cytokine and prostaglandin synthesis and interacts with the Nrf2 pathway to enhance endogenous antioxidant defenses. Emerging evidence also suggests a role for vitamin E in regulating angiogenic balance and uterine microcirculation, with potential implications for endometrial growth and implantation competence. Experimental and translational studies consistently demonstrate that vitamin E attenuates oxidative stress–induced apoptosis in ovarian and endometrial cells and preserves steroidogenic and proliferative capacity under adverse conditions. Clinically, vitamin E supplementation – often as part of combination antioxidant regimens – has been investigated in infertility-associated conditions such as thin endometrium, polycystic ovary syndrome, endometriosis, and assisted reproductive technology cycles. Small observational studies and limited randomized trials report improvements in oxidative stress markers, inflammatory profiles, endometrial thickness, uterine blood flow indices, and selected metabolic parameters, particularly in women with elevated oxidative or inflammatory burden. However, evidence for consistent benefits on implantation, clinical pregnancy, or live birth rates remains inconclusive due to heterogeneous study designs, small sample sizes, and reliance on surrogate outcomes. This chapter synthesizes current mechanistic and clinical evidence regarding the role of vitamin E in reproductive physiology and infertility management. Overall, vitamin E appears to function as a low-risk adjunct that supports the oxidative, inflammatory, and microvascular environment required for successful reproduction while not constituting a stand-alone fertility treatment. Well-designed, adequately powered randomized controlled trials are needed to define optimal dosing, patient selection, and its true impact on definitive reproductive outcomes.

6.2 ITS ANTIOXIDANT EFFECTS IN REPRODUCTIVE HEALTH

Vitamin E (tocopherols/tocotrienols, chiefly α-tocopherol) functions as a membrane-phase chain breaker that limits lipid-peroxide propagation and formation of electrophilic aldehydes (4-HNE, MDA) (1). By safeguarding mitochondrial bioenergetics and redox-sensitive steroidogenic steps, it preserves the activity of StAR, CYP11A1 (P450scc), 3β-/17β-HSD, and CYP19A1 (aromatase) in granulosa/luteal cells and maintains FSHR/LHCGR signaling competence (cAMP/PKA) (2, 3). The net effect is appropriate estradiol output in the late-follicular phase and progesterone synthesis across the luteal window – conditions that support oocyte competence, fertilization capacity, and implantation readiness (4, 5). Experimental models concur, showing fewer ROS-driven DNA strand breaks and reduced endonuclease activation in ovarian cells under α-tocopherol sufficiency, with downstream gains in ovarian function and endometrial receptivity (6, 7).

Beyond direct redox control, α-tocopherol modulates pro-inflammatory signaling by restraining PKC-dependent activation of NF-κB/AP-1, lowering COX-2/5-LOX products like PGE_2, TXA_2, leukotrienes, and cytokines including TNF-α, IL-1β, IL-6, IL-8, and reducing endothelial ICAM-1/VCAM-1 expression (8–11). Crosstalk with the Nrf2 axis via glutathione recycling and detoxification of 4-HNE/MDA adducts, further tilts gene expression toward an anti-inflammatory phenotype and supports implantation tolerance such as higher Treg tone (12–15). These actions are particularly relevant in endometriosis and pelvic inflammatory conditions, where dampening nociceptive eicosanoids and leukocyte recruitment mitigates lesion-associated inflammatory stress and pain (16, 17).

DOI: 10.1201/9781003741541-6

Vitamin E rebalances HIF-1α/VEGF-driven angiogenesis and related cues (e.g., Ang-2, MMP-9), with clinical signals of lowered circulating VEGF in PCOS after ≈8 weeks of supplementation (18–20). In peri-ovulatory follicles, moderated VEGF may curb pathological hyper-permeability with potential implications for OHSS risk, while preserving physiological capillarization for follicle growth and luteal perfusion (21). In the uterus, improved endothelial NO bioavailability and tempered vasoconstrictive PKC tone favor orderly spiral-artery remodeling and more uniform perfusion of the functional layer, enhancing endometrial thickness and receptivity; these effects can be complemented by microcirculatory agents such as pentoxifylline (18, 22, 23).

Oxidative stress in ovarian granulosa and luteal cells and in the endometrium is increasingly recognized as a key regulator of mitochondrial function, steroidogenic enzyme activity and apoptosis, with downstream effects on follicular development, luteal progesterone output and endometrial receptivity (24–26). Experimental work in avian and caprine granulosa cells exposed to glyphosate-based herbicides shows that α-tocopherol, alone or in combination with vitamin C, attenuates reactive-oxygen-species accumulation, reduces apoptosis and partially restores progesterone secretion, illustrating that vitamin E can preserve steroidogenic function under oxidative stress in reproductive somatic cells (4, 27). In women with endometriosis, combined vitamin C and E supplementation decreases oxidative stress markers and inflammatory chemokines in peritoneal fluid and is associated with reduced pelvic pain, supporting an anti-inflammatory and anti-apoptotic action of antioxidant therapy within pelvic reproductive tissues (28).

Small observational and interventional studies in women with a thin endometrium report that vitamin E, often co-administered with agents such as pentoxifylline or L-arginine, is associated with modest increases in endometrial thickness and improvements in uterine blood flow indices; however, a 12-week randomized trial of vitamin E monotherapy that initially suggested a ≈1 mm gain in endometrial thickness has since been formally retracted for data-integrity concerns, and these findings cannot be considered confirmatory (29–31). Independent lines of research demonstrate that coordinated expression of progesterone receptors, HOXA10 and leukemia inhibitory factor (LIF) in the endometrium is essential for functional-layer proliferation, stromal decidualization and embryo implantation, and that these pathways are sensitive to inflammatory and oxidative cues (32–36). Taken together, current data support a biologically plausible but still inferential model in which vitamin E, by limiting lipid peroxidation and dampening NF-κB-driven inflammatory signaling, may help maintain an intrauterine and ovarian microenvironment that is permissive for normal steroid-receptor signaling and endometrial receptivity under oxidative stress, while direct evidence that vitamin E upregulates specific genes such as HOXA10, LIF, IGF-1 or PGR in human endometrium, or that it reliably enhances implantation and live birth, is not yet available from well-controlled randomized trials (24–26, 30, 37).

Table 6.1: Key Molecular Pathways Modulated by Vitamin E

Molecular Pathway	Physiological Role	Effect of Vitamin E	Type of Evidence
Nrf2–ARE pathway	Antioxidant defense in ovarian and endometrial cells	Activates Nrf2 signaling; increases SOD, GPx, catalase; reduces lipid peroxidation	Strong in vitro/animal; indirect human evidence
NF-κB pathway	Regulates inflammatory cytokines affecting ovulation and implantation	Inhibits NF-κB; reduces IL-6, TNF-α, COX-2	Strong animal/cell; moderate human
PI3K/Akt pathway	Follicular growth, oocyte maturation, granulosa cell survival	Maintains p-Akt; increases BCL-2; decreases Bax	Moderate animal/in vitro; weak human
MAPK/ERK pathway	Granulosa cell proliferation; estrogen-driven endometrial growth	Stabilizes ERK1/2 during oxidative stress	Moderate in vitro/animal
VEGF/Angiogenesis	Uterine blood flow and vascular remodeling	Modulates VEGF expression; improves angiogenesis	Moderate human; limited mechanistic data

Small studies and case series, sometimes in combination with pentoxifylline or L-arginine, report thicker endometrium and improved uterine/ovarian Doppler indices in thin endometrium, consistent with the mechanistic profile above (29, 30, 38). One 12-week, 400 IU/day trial initially suggested a ≈1.1 mm thickness gain but was later retracted for data-integrity concerns; it should not be considered confirmatory evidence. Overall, biologic plausibility for vitamin E's supportive role in female reproduction is strong, enzyme protection, receptor/co-activator integrity, gonadotropin responsiveness, microvascular optimization, whereas definitive effects on implantation and live birth remain to be established in well-controlled RCTs that isolate vitamin E monotherapy and report standardized reproductive endpoints (38).

6.3 CLINICAL APPLICATIONS IN INFERTILITY TREATMENT

Oxidative and inflammatory stress are recognized contributors to inadequate endometrial growth and implantation failure, acting through endothelial dysfunction, impaired uterine perfusion, and altered stromal–epithelial signaling (39–41). Antioxidant supplementation including vitamin E alone or in combination with agents such as pentoxifylline or L-arginine, has been associated in several small observational and interventional studies with increased endometrial thickness and improved uterine blood flow indices in women with a "thin" endometrium or recurrent implantation failure, although these findings remain preliminary and derive from low-powered designs (42–45). Vitamin E's demonstrated actions in reproductive tissues primarily involve reducing lipid peroxidation, limiting ROS accumulation, and modulating inflammatory pathways, which can secondarily support vascular and endometrial function. In ovarian and endometrial cell models, α-tocopherol attenuates ROS-driven mitochondrial injury, reduces apoptosis, and partially restores steroidogenic or proliferative capacity (4, 27, 46). In women with endometriosis, combined vitamin C/E supplementation reduces oxidative and inflammatory mediators in peritoneal fluid and improves pain scores, illustrating clinically measurable anti-inflammatory effects in pelvic tissues (47). Independent lines of research establish that key determinants of endometrial receptivity containing progesterone-receptor signaling, HOXA10, leukemia inhibitory factor (LIF), and IGF-1, are sensitive to oxidative and inflammatory conditions, which can disrupt endometrial proliferation, stromal decidualization, and implantation competence (32, 35, 48–50). Although vitamin E has not been shown in humans to upregulate these genes directly, its antioxidant and anti-inflammatory actions provide biologic plausibility for supportive effects on the endometrial environment under oxidative stress.

Oxidative stress and metabolic dysfunction jointly impair ovarian steroidogenesis, insulin signaling, and gonadotropin responsiveness in polycystic ovary syndrome (PCOS), contributing to anovulation and suboptimal endometrial development (51–53). Small randomized and observational studies indicate that antioxidant therapy like vitamin E alone or in combination with magnesium, omega-3 fatty acids, or L-arginine, can reduce systemic oxidative stress, improve insulin sensitivity, and modestly enhance hormonal profiles in PCOS (54–56). Because hyperinsulinemia amplifies theca-cell androgen production and disrupts granulosa-cell aromatase activity, improvements in insulin resistance may indirectly support healthier metabolic–ovarian interactions (57, 58). In vitro and animal studies demonstrate that vitamin E attenuates ROS accumulation, preserves mitochondrial function, and reduces apoptosis in granulosa cells, helping to maintain steroidogenic enzyme activity under oxidative challenge (59–61), findings consistent with clinical reports of improved follicular growth, better dominant-follicle metrics, and modest increases in luteal progesterone, despite heterogeneity across trials (18, 62, 63). Endometrial development also appears sensitive to oxidative and inflammatory tone, and several small interventional studies report that vitamin E combined with L-arginine or pentoxifylline, can increase endometrial thickness and improve uterine or radial artery Doppler indices in women with PCOS, thin endometrium, or clomiphene-induced endometrial suppression (29, 44, 64, 65). Although dysregulated angiogenic signaling, particularly elevated VEGF and abnormal stromal vascular architecture, has been described in PCOS (66, 67), direct human evidence that vitamin E normalizes HIF-1α/VEGF pathways or perifollicular vascular permeability is lacking, and clinical synergy with other antioxidants remains insufficiently defined. Overall, while vitamin E may support metabolic, vascular, and endometrial function through its antioxidative and anti-inflammatory actions, aligning with small-study improvements in endometrial thickness and follicular characteristics, consistent benefits for ovulation, implantation, or pregnancy rates have not been confirmed, highlighting the need for large, well-controlled randomized trials.

Before IVF, vitamin E supplementation has been shown in animal and in vitro models to reduce oxidative stress within the oocyte and cumulus–oocyte complex, thereby supporting mitochondrial integrity and early embryonic development (68, 69). Vitamin E limits lipid peroxidation, preserves mitochondrial membrane potential, and improves markers of mitochondrial function in oocytes exposed to oxidative challenge associated with fewer spindle abnormalities, better nuclear maturation, and higher developmental competence (68). Activation of antioxidant responses, including increased glutathione and enhanced GPx and SOD activity, has also been reported in granulosa cells and in relation to follicular-fluid redox status in studies of vitamin E containing antioxidant regimens (27, 59, 60, 69). In cumulus and granulosa cells, vitamin E in combination with other antioxidants such as selenium or vitamin C attenuates oxidative injury, reduces apoptosis, and helps preserve cumulus expansion and intercellular communication under toxic or oxidative conditions (69). These local improvements translate into lower oxidative and DNA damage and higher cleavage or blastocyst development rates in animal models of IVF and oocyte-maturation support (70). Limited human data, largely from small trials and observational work summarized in recent reviews, suggest that antioxidant supplementation protocols containing vitamin E may improve endometrial thickness and uterine blood-flow parameters in women with implantation failure or thin endometrium, with possible downstream benefits for receptivity (60, 69). Given the lipophilic nature of vitamin E, its incorporation into cell membranes, and the relatively slow kinetics of tissue distribution and redox adaptation, multi-week supplementation prior to ovarian stimulation is biologically more plausible than very short-term dosing confined to the peri-transfer period (69, 71).

In endometriosis and pelvic inflammatory conditions, vitamin E contributes to a more favorable reproductive microenvironment primarily through modulation of oxidative and inflammatory pathways. Experimental studies in endometriosis models show that vitamin E reduces NF-κB activation and lowers pro-inflammatory cytokines such as TNF-α, IL-1β, and IL-8, alongside suppressing COX-2 expression and downstream PGE_2 production – mediators that are implicated in inflammation-driven estrogen biosynthesis and pelvic pain (72, 73). Antioxidant supplementation containing vitamin E has also been reported to downregulate MMP-2 and MMP-9 and to moderate VEGF expression in oxidative-stress or inflammatory injury models, suggesting potential indirect benefits on aberrant angiogenesis and adhesion formation (73, 74). These changes may secondarily support tubo-ovarian function by reducing the inflammatory and angiogenic burden associated with peritoneal disease. Inflammatory and prostanoid reduction can also lessen nociceptor sensitization, while improved redox balance may mitigate hypoxia-driven neuroangiogenic signaling linked to chronic pelvic pain (72, 73). Clinical trials pairing vitamins E and C in women with endometriosis-associated pelvic pain have demonstrated reductions in oxidative-stress biomarkers and significant pain relief, and these biochemical improvements align with the cytokine, eicosanoid, and angiogenic pathways that may plausibly support fertility even when pain is the primary clinical endpoint (14, 75).

Although vitamin E-related improvements in endometrial thickness or uterine Doppler indices may reflect better vascular and oxidative conditions, these intermediate parameters do not consistently predict implantation or live birth rates, as pregnancy also depends on embryo competence, synchronized timing of the implantation window, and adequate immunologic tolerance (76). Vitamin E-improves redox balance and microvascular function in reproductive tissues, but its clinical impact is modified by baseline oxidative load including age, BMI, smoking, and endometriosis, as well as by micronutrient co-status such as vitamin C, selenium, and coenzyme Q10, which jointly determine antioxidant network efficiency (69). Pharmacologic context, for example anti-estrogenic effects associated with clomiphene in some patients, may further influence vascular and endometrial responsiveness (77). Because membrane incorporation of α-tocopherol and tissue-level redox adaptation occur gradually, several weeks of supplementation prior to ovarian stimulation or timed conception attempts is biologically more justified than short-term dosing restricted to the peri-transfer phase (71). Combined supplementation with vitamin C or selenium has shown superior control of lipid peroxidation and oxidative biomarkers compared with vitamin E alone, while L-arginine has been associated with improved uterine blood flow in women with impaired Doppler profiles (73, 78). Tracking markers such as follicular-fluid MDA or 4-HNE, serum or endometrial VEGF, uterine-artery PI/RI, and mid-luteal progesterone can help assess whether vascular and oxidative pathways are responding to intervention (70). Finally, moderate dosing aligns with the goal of restoring physiological redox and vascular balance rather than inducing pharmacologic excess. Taken together, vitamin E acts as a plausible adjunct that enhances the redox, inflammatory, microvascular, and endocrine microenvironment supporting ovulation, fertilization, implantation, and early embryo development, while not serving as a stand-alone determinant of pregnancy outcome (71, 79).

Table 6.2: Clinical Applications of Vitamin E in Female Infertility

Clinical Population	Vitamin E Dose	Duration	Primary Outcome(s)	Strength of Evidence
Thin endometrium/ implantation failure	400 IU/day	1 cycle	↑ Endometrial thickness; inconsistent pregnancy benefit	Moderate
Diminished ovarian reserve/ POI	400 IU / day + Selenium (200 μg)	12 weeks	↑ AMH, ↑ AFC, ↑ Ovarian volume	Moderate (single RCT)
Endometriosis-associated infertility	800 – 1200 IU / day (± Vitamin C)	8 weeks	↑ Pelvic pain, ↓ MDA, improved inflammatory profile	Moderate–strong
Clomiphene-resistant PCOS	1500 IU/day	3–4 cycles	↑ Endometrial thickness; no consistent improvement in ovulation or pregnancy rates	Weak–moderate
Women undergoing IVF	200–400 IU/day	4–8 weeks pre-treatment	Correlation with ↑ embryo quality (observational; non-causal)	Weak (observational)
Early pregnancy safety	>100 mg/day	Early gestation	No increased risk reported; neutral to modest protective associations described	Moderate (cohort)

Table 6.2 summarizes the principal clinical contexts in which vitamin E has been evaluated as an adjunct in female infertility, highlighting typical dosing regimens, treatment duration, primary outcomes, and the overall strength of available evidence.

6.4 CURRENT CLINICAL EVIDENCE SUPPORTING THE USE OF VITAMIN E

Clinical and mechanistic studies increasingly indicate that inadequate endometrial growth and receptivity are not solely a consequence of insufficient estrogen exposure but are strongly influenced by endothelial dysfunction, impaired uterine microcirculation, oxidative stress, and inflammatory signaling within the endometrial stromal–epithelial compartment.

In women with persistently thin endometrium or recurrent implantation failure, small observational cohorts and interventional studies report that vitamin E supplementation – most commonly administered in combination with pentoxifylline or L-arginine – is associated with modest but clinically relevant increases in endometrial thickness and improvements in uterine or radial artery Doppler indices. These vascular and morphologic changes are consistent with vitamin E–mediated enhancement of endothelial nitric oxide bioavailability, attenuation of PKC-driven vasoconstrictive signaling, and protection of endometrial cells from lipid-peroxidation–induced disruption of progesterone-receptor signaling and stromal decidualization pathways.

Importantly, although early randomized data suggested that vitamin E monotherapy might increase endometrial thickness by approximately 1 mm over 12 weeks, this trial was later formally retracted for data-integrity concerns, underscoring that current evidence in this domain remains suggestive rather than confirmatory. Independent molecular studies demonstrate that key determinants of receptivity including coordinated expression of progesterone receptors, HOXA10, leukemia inhibitory factor (LIF), and IGF-1, are highly sensitive to oxidative and inflammatory cues, supporting a biologically plausible but still inferential role for vitamin E in maintaining a permissive endometrial microenvironment under conditions of oxidative stress (80–84).

In PCOS, oxidative stress and metabolic dysfunction interact to impair ovarian steroidogenesis, granulosa cell function, insulin signaling, and gonadotropin responsiveness, resulting in anovulation, hyperandrogenism, and suboptimal endometrial development.

Systematic reviews and meta-analyses of randomized controlled trials consistently demonstrate that vitamin E supplementation, either as monotherapy or combined with omega-3 fatty acids, magnesium, or coenzyme Q10, significantly reduces circulating markers of oxidative stress such as MDA while increasing total antioxidant capacity, glutathione availability, and antioxidant enzyme activity. Several trials further report modest but statistically significant improvements in insulin resistance indices, lipid profiles, and androgen concentrations, findings that are clinically relevant given the role of hyperinsulinemia in amplifying theca-cell androgen production and disrupting granulosa cell aromatase activity. At the ovarian level, experimental and animal studies demonstrate that vitamin E attenuates ROS accumulation, preserves mitochondrial membrane potential, and reduces apoptosis in granulosa cells, thereby maintaining activity of steroidogenic enzymes such as CYP11A1, 3β-HSD, and aromatase under oxidative challenge.

Despite these favorable biochemical, metabolic, and cellular effects, clinical trials in PCOS show inconsistent improvements in ovulation, implantation, or pregnancy rates when vitamin E is added to standard ovulation-induction regimens, reinforcing its role as a supportive rather than primary pharmacologic intervention (80, 82–85).

Endometriosis is characterized by chronic pelvic inflammation, excessive ROS production, dysregulated angiogenesis, and altered immune tolerance, all of which contribute to impaired fertility and pelvic pain. Randomized, triple-blind, placebo-controlled trials demonstrate that combined vitamin C and vitamin E supplementation for approximately 8 weeks significantly reduces oxidative-stress biomarkers, pro-inflammatory cytokines, and inflammatory eicosanoids in women with laparoscopically confirmed endometriosis. These biochemical changes are accompanied by clinically meaningful reductions in pelvic pain, dysmenorrhea, and dyspareunia, reflecting vitamin E's capacity to suppress NF-κB activation, reduce COX-2–derived prostaglandin synthesis, and dampen inflammatory signaling within pelvic reproductive tissues.

Although randomized trials linking these anti-inflammatory effects directly to improved implantation or live birth rates in endometriosis are lacking, the consistency of oxidative and symptomatic improvements provides strong biological plausibility for a supportive role in fertility management (73, 83, 86, 87).

Oxidative stress within oocytes, granulosa cells, and early embryos is increasingly recognized as a determinant of embryo competence, mitochondrial integrity, and ART outcomes. Experimental and in vitro studies consistently show that vitamin E reduces ROS accumulation, limits lipid peroxidation, preserves mitochondrial membrane potential, and reduces oxidative DNA damage in oocytes and cumulus–oocyte complexes exposed to oxidative challenge. Animal models of IVF further demonstrate that supplementation of maturation or culture media with α-tocopherol improves nuclear maturation, reduces spindle abnormalities, and increases cleavage and blastocyst development rates. Human observational studies suggest that higher follicular-fluid concentrations of vitamin E are associated with improved oocyte morphology and embryo quality, although these associations do not establish causality and may reflect broader antioxidant-network status. Given the lipophilic nature of vitamin E and its gradual incorporation into cellular membranes, multi-week supplementation prior to ovarian stimulation is biologically more plausible than very short-term dosing limited to the peri-transfer period (88–92).

Across infertility phenotypes, the most consistent and reproducible effects of vitamin E relate to improvements in intermediate outcomes, including oxidative-stress biomarkers, inflammatory mediators, endometrial thickness, uterine perfusion, metabolic indices, and selected markers of oocyte and embryo quality. In contrast, robust evidence demonstrating consistent improvements in hard reproductive endpoints such as implantation rate, clinical pregnancy, or live birth remains limited due to small sample sizes, heterogeneous study designs, and reliance on surrogate markers. Taken together, current clinical evidence supports vitamin E as a biologically plausible adjunct that enhances the redox, inflammatory, vascular, and endocrine microenvironment supporting reproduction, while emphasizing that it should not be interpreted as a stand-alone determinant of fertility success (83, 86, 93).

6.5 CASE STUDIES: SUCCESSFUL INTEGRATION OF VITAMIN E IN ASSISTED REPRODUCTIVE TECHNOLOGIES

Clinical experience consistently shows that vitamin E can be integrated into fertility care as an adjuvant that improves the tissue context in which implantation must occur. In women with recurrent implantation failure and a persistently thin endometrium despite estrogen therapy, a well-described strategy has paired oral α-tocopherol with the vasoactive agent pentoxifylline for several months prior to embryo transfer. In the original series by Lédée-Bataille and colleagues in oocyte recipient candidates who could not exceed ~5–6 mm, treatment was associated with a mean rise in endometrial thickness from roughly 5 mm to >6 mm, a reduction in uterine artery Doppler resistance indices, and a clinically meaningful proportion achieving ≥7 mm, thresholds at which implantation rates begin to improve. Notably, a subset who had been labeled untreatable subsequently conceived (some spontaneously, others after transfer), yielding several live births. Follow-on reports, including small case series of women with chronic thin endometrium, reproduced the qualitative pattern: α-tocopherol (commonly 600–1000 IU/day) plus pentoxifylline promoted a transition from flat, poorly perfused linings to thicker, trilaminar endometria suitable for transfer. Although these reports are observational and lack randomized controls, their internal consistency across centers and the parallel improvements in perfusion metrics support a vascular–redox mechanism: vitamin E improves endothelial NO bioavailability and limits lipid-peroxide/4-HNE damage to endometrial signaling, while pentoxifylline reduces blood viscosity and leukocyte adhesion tipping the microcirculation toward the orderly capillarization needed for receptive growth (30, 94).

A second, practical use case involves poor responders or older patients preparing for IVF who have a history of suboptimal embryos. Some clinics include antioxidant pretreatment (e.g., α-tocopherol, CoQ10, and vitamin C) for 8–12 weeks prior to IVF, based on experimental and some clinical evidence suggesting possible benefits to oocyte and embryo quality. Anecdotal clinical observations have suggested that antioxidant supplementation, like combinations including α-tocopherol and other agents, may coincide with improved oocyte morphology and embryo grading in some patients when compared to prior cycles (95). These anecdotes align with laboratory signals reported in clinical studies: higher α-tocopherol concentrations in follicular fluid correlate with better embryo morphology and higher fertilization rates, and some clinical evidence, especially for CoQ10 supplementation, has been associated with increased numbers of mature (MII) oocytes and improved embryo development metrics in women preparing for IVF (96). Mechanistic evidence from experimental models suggests antioxidants, including vitamin E, support mitochondrial function and may protect cellular structures in oocytes and cumulus cells under oxidative stress. Because the incorporation of lipid-soluble antioxidants into membranes and potential remodeling of mitochondrial function may require sustained exposure, longer-term supplementation prior to stimulation is biologically plausible (95–97).

In women with polycystic ovary syndrome, including those with clomiphene resistance, clinical trials suggest that vitamin E can be used as an adjunct to standard ovulation induction regimens rather than as a primary ovulation drug (54, 98). In clomiphene citrate-resistant PCOS, adding vitamin E to metformin, clomiphene protocols have been reported to increase ovulation and clinical pregnancy rates compared with metformin–clomiphene alone, whereas in larger cohorts of PCOS women undergoing clomiphene plus human menopausal gonadotropin (HMG) cycles, short-term vitamin E co-treatment improved endometrial thickness and estradiol levels and reduced gonadotropin requirements, without significantly changing ovulation or pregnancy rates (63, 99). Small randomized controlled trials in PCOS, most using vitamin E at about 400 IU/day in combination with omega-3 fatty acids, magnesium, or coenzyme Q10 for 8–12 weeks, consistently show lower-circulating malondialdehyde and other oxidative-stress markers, higher total antioxidant capacity and glutathione, and improvements in insulin resistance indices and some androgen parameters (54). A pilot double-blind randomized trial also found that 8 weeks of vitamin E supplementation reduced serum vascular endothelial growth factor (VEGF), angiopoietin-1, and the Ang-1/Ang-2 ratio in women with PCOS, supporting an anti-angiogenic shift (100). Taken together, these data fit the pathophysiology of PCOS – where insulin resistance, oxidative stress, and dysregulated ovarian angiogenesis impair orderly follicle selection – and support using vitamin E as a biologically plausible adjunct to optimize the endocrine–metabolic and microvascular environment in which pharmacologic ovulation induction acts, even though it is not a stand-alone ovulation-inducing agent (54, 101).

Endometriosis-associated infertility is another context in which antioxidant therapy, including vitamin E in combination with vitamin C, has been explored. Randomized, triple-blind, placebo-controlled trials have shown that combined vitamin E (≈800 IU/day) and vitamin C (≈1000 mg/day) for ~8 weeks significantly lowers oxidative stress markers such as MDA and ROS and reduces pelvic pain, dysmenorrhea, and dyspareunia in women with laparoscopically confirmed endometriosis (102). Systematic review and meta-analytic evidence support that antioxidant supplementation with vitamins C and E is associated with reductions in pain symptoms and peripheral oxidative stress in this population (16). While direct randomized data linking these antioxidant effects to improved implantation or pregnancy outcomes in endometriosis are limited, the observed biochemical and symptomatic improvements are biologically plausible given the role of oxidative stress and inflammation in lesion persistence and pelvic pathology (14).

Taken together, these clinical observations support a pattern-based rather than universal use of vitamin E, with benefits most evident in settings where a modifiable tissue impairment is demonstrable such as thin or poorly perfused endometrium, biochemical evidence of oxidative stress, angiogenic or metabolic dysregulation in PCOS, or inflammatory-eicosanoid excess in endometriosis, and when treatment windows allow 8–12 weeks for potential redox, endothelial, and mitochondrial adaptation (103). Across available studies, combination therapy appears more practical than monotherapy. For instance, α-tocopherol paired with pentoxifylline has been used in cohorts with unfavorable uterine Doppler parameters, co-administration with vitamin C is biologically justified because ascorbate recycles the tocopheroxyl radical, selenium supports glutathione peroxidase-dependent detoxification of lipid hydroperoxides, L-arginine has been used when NO-mediated vasodilation is a therapeutic goal, and coenzyme Q10 is often included in patients with suspected mitochondrial vulnerability (16). Safety has been favorable at typical supplemental doses, ~400–1000 IU/day, across published series, yet clinical benefit is not guaranteed, as implantation and live birth remain strongly dependent on embryo competence, precise timing of the implantation window, and immune tolerance. This helps explain why some reports show clear improvements in endometrial thickness or follicular and oxidative-stress biomarkers without statistically significant differences in pregnancy rates (86, 99, 104).

From a protocol standpoint, case series and small clinical studies indicate three practical considerations for incorporating vitamin E into fertility care. First, patient selection is crucial, as reported benefits are most evident in phenotypes with measurable tissue deficits such as persistently thin endometrium, elevated oxidative-stress markers (MDA, 4-HNE), or angiogenic imbalance (e.g., VEGF elevations) seen in PCOS and endometriosis (12–15). Second, starting supplementation early (typically 8–12 weeks) appears more effective, consistent with studies showing that short-term vitamin E improves endometrial thickness and reduces oxidative stress but may require time for redox and endothelial adaptation (2, 4). Third, monitoring on-target indicators – including uterine artery PI/RI, endometrial thickness and pattern, perifollicular Doppler flow, mid-luteal progesterone, and follicular-fluid oxidative markers – helps determine treatment responsiveness (1, 2). When these elements align, published reports describe that vitamin E–based antioxidant regimens can improve marginal endometrial or peri-follicular environments, and in a subset of difficult-to-treat cases, such physiologic improvements have coincided with implantation or clinical pregnancy, though not consistently across studies (2–5).

6.6 BEST PRACTICES FOR INCORPORATING VITAMIN E INTO INFERTILITY TREATMENT PROTOCOLS

Vitamin E is best framed as an adjuvant that optimizes the oxidative, inflammatory and microvascular milieu rather than as a stand-alone fertility drug, so protocols should first identify women with clear evidence of oxidative or tissue impairment such as thin or poorly perfused endometrium, PCOS with metabolic/angiogenic dysregulation, or endometriosis-associated inflammation (86). Patient selection can be guided by clinical phenotypes, recurrent implantation failure, long-standing thin lining, PCOS with insulin resistance, endometriosis with pelvic pain, and, where available, biomarkers such as elevated malondialdehyde, reduced total antioxidant capacity, or altered VEGF/angiopoietin profiles (105). Protocols should also account for baseline diet and co-nutrient status, because vitamin E works within an antioxidant network that includes vitamin C, selenium, and coenzyme Q10, and these interactions influence clinical responsiveness in reproductive tissues (106). Timing is another key best-practice element: due to its membrane incorporation and relatively slow redox remodeling, most reviews recommend starting vitamin E at least 8–12 weeks before ovulation induction or embryo transfer, rather than limiting intake to the peri-implantation window (107). During this lead-in phase, clinicians can monitor intermediate targets such as endometrial thickness, uterine-artery PI/RI, follicular-fluid oxidative markers, or PCOS-related metabolic indices to decide whether continuation is justified (99). In daily practice, integration into protocols is easiest as part of structured preconception optimization packages that combine vitamin E with lifestyle modification, insulin-sensitizing strategies when indicated, and evidence-based adjuncts such as L-arginine or CoQ10 in selected patients (108). Written clinic algorithms that specify indications, dose ranges, duration, and monitoring endpoints help avoid indiscriminate use while ensuring that eligible high-risk phenotypes are not overlooked (83).

6.7 SAFETY, DOSAGE, AND EFFICACY

6.7.1 Recommended Dosages

Most reproductive protocols use oral α-tocopherol at 200–400 IU/day for general antioxidant support, with higher ranges of 600–1000 IU/day reserved for short- to medium-term use in women with marked tissue deficits such as chronic thin endometrium or severe oxidative stress, reflecting doses reported in case series and clinical trials (109). Meta-analyses in PCOS commonly include regimens around 400 IU/day, either alone or combined with omega-3 fatty acids or magnesium, administered for 8–12 weeks, and these doses have been sufficient to improve MDA, total antioxidant capacity, and some hormonal indices (110). In endometriosis pain trials, vitamin E has typically been combined with vitamin C (≈800 IU/day plus 1000 mg/day) for 8–10 weeks, a duration chosen to allow measurable changes in oxidative and symptomatic outcomes without long-term high-dose exposure (73). Because vitamin E is fat soluble and accumulates in lipid membranes, several reviews emphasize titrating toward the lowest dose that achieves biochemical or clinical targets rather than defaulting to maximal regimens (111). In practice, this means starting at 200–400 IU/day in women without overt deficiency and escalating only if oxidative markers or tissue measures remain suboptimal after a defined trial period (112). For combination protocols, dose planning should consider the cumulative antioxidant load, as high doses of multiple agents could theoretically blunt physiological redox signaling, particularly in early embryogenesis, although human data are sparse (69). Regular review of ongoing need, like discontinuing high-dose vitamin E once endometrial or metabolic goals are achieved – can limit unnecessary chronic exposure (113).

6.7.2 Safety Profiles and Potential Side Effects

Randomized trials and meta-analyses in adults, including women with PCOS and various gynecologic conditions, generally report that vitamin E is well tolerated at doses commonly used in reproductive practice, with adverse events such as mild gastrointestinal discomfort or headache occurring at similar frequencies in active and control groups (54). Large antioxidant overviews have not demonstrated clear increases in miscarriage, ectopic pregnancy, or congenital anomalies attributable specifically to vitamin E, though most trials have been underpowered to detect rare events (93, 114). In endometriosis studies using relatively high doses of vitamins C and E, reductions in pain and oxidative stress occurred without significant safety signals beyond transient dyspepsia, suggesting a favorable risk–benefit balance when therapies are time-limited and monitored (73). Nonetheless, expert reviews advise caution with long-term high-dose vitamin E, particularly above 800–1000 IU/day, due to theoretical concerns about hemorrhagic risk and possible interference with vitamin K–dependent coagulation, even though direct data in reproductive-age women are sparse (115). Patients on anticoagulants or with bleeding disorders should be evaluated individually, and clinicians should inquire about concurrent use of over-the-counter antioxidant complexes to avoid unrecognized cumulative dosing (116). Women with fat malabsorption or chronic liver disease may have altered vitamin E pharmacokinetics, warranting more cautious titration and periodic assessment of serum levels where available (117). As with any adjunctive therapy, clear documentation of indication, planned duration, and stopping rules can help ensure that vitamin E remains a targeted, monitored component of infertility care rather than an open-ended supplement (112).

6.7.3 Combining Vitamin E with Conventional Treatments

Clinical evidence suggests that vitamin E is most effective when integrated with standard infertility therapies such as ovulation induction, IVF stimulation protocols, or endometriosis management rather than used in isolation (83). In PCOS, trials adding vitamin E to metformin–clomiphene or gonadotropin regimens demonstrate improvements in endometrial thickness, oxidative markers, and sometimes estradiol levels, even when ovulation and pregnancy rates do not differ significantly from controls, indicating a supportive rather than primary pharmacologic role (99). In thin endometrium, case series pairing vitamin E with pentoxifylline have reported gains in endometrial thickness and uterine blood-flow indices sufficient to permit embryo transfer in women previously deemed unsuitable, highlighting a potential synergy between endothelial-active agents and lipid-phase antioxidants (83). Combination antioxidant strategies may also exploit complementary mechanisms within the antioxidant network; for example, vitamin C can regenerate oxidized tocopheroxyl radicals, while selenium supports glutathione-peroxidase-mediated detoxification of lipid hydroperoxides (83). Trials in endometriosis show that combined vitamins C and E reduce MDA and ROS more robustly than would be expected from either agent alone, paralleling clinically meaningful pain reductions (16). In IVF preparation, several centers use multi-antioxidant regimens that include vitamin E, CoQ10, and sometimes myo-inositol or L-carnitine to support oocyte mitochondrial function and embryo quality, although high-quality randomized data isolating the contribution of vitamin E are still limited (83). Expert reviews therefore recommend designing combination protocols with clear mechanistic rationale, avoiding kitchen-sink supplementation, and ensuring that adjuncts do not conflict with the pharmacology of gonadotropins, GnRH analogs, or insulin-sensitizing agents (83).

6.8 CHALLENGES AND CONTROVERSIES

6.8.1 Regulatory and Standardization Issues

Vitamin E is typically regulated as a dietary supplement rather than a prescription drug in most jurisdictions, meaning that products vary widely in dose, isoform composition (α- vs γ-tocopherol, tocotrienols), and excipients, which introduces uncertainty into both clinical practice and research (118). Reviews of supplement quality highlight inconsistent labeling and bioavailability among over-the-counter preparations, complicating attempts to standardize protocols for infertility care (119). In trials, some investigators use natural RRR-α-tocopherol while others rely on synthetic all-racemic mixtures, yet these differences are rarely considered in dosing equivalence or outcome interpretation (120). Unlike gonadotropins or insulin-sensitizing agents, there are no universally accepted clinical guidelines specifying indications, target doses, or monitoring strategies for vitamin E in infertility, leaving decisions largely to individual clinicians or institutional practice patterns (83). This regulatory gap makes it harder to implement evidence-based, harmonized care and contributes to wide variation in whether and how vitamin E is offered to patients (83). Furthermore, heterogeneous reporting of outcomes and lack of standardized oxidative-stress endpoints impede meta-analytic synthesis and regulatory appraisal (93). Some authors have called for consensus statements from reproductive medicine societies to define minimal reporting standards and recommend quality-controlled formulations when vitamin E is used in research or high-stakes clinical contexts such as ART cycles (83).

6.8.2 Variability in Patient Responses

Clinical and experimental evidence indicates substantial inter-individual variability in response to vitamin E, driven by factors such as baseline oxidative load, BMI, metabolic status, and co-existing reproductive pathologies (86). Women with PCOS, obesity, or endometriosis often exhibit higher oxidative and inflammatory stress and may therefore experience more pronounced biochemical improvements from antioxidant therapy than lean, metabolically healthy infertility patients (16). Genetic polymorphisms affecting antioxidant enzymes, lipid metabolism, or vitamin E trafficking, such as α-TTP variants, may also influence tissue uptake and responsiveness, although data in reproductive cohorts are still limited (121). Heterogeneity is also evident at the tissue level: some women demonstrate marked gains in endometrial thickness and perfusion or shifts in angiogenic markers after vitamin E–containing regimens, whereas others show little change despite similar dosing and duration (83). In PCOS, meta-analyses report group-level improvements in testosterone and metabolic indices, but effect sizes vary and may be modulated by baseline insulin resistance, dietary patterns, or concurrent medications (54). These observations support a move toward stratified use, in which vitamin E is preferentially offered to phenotypes with demonstrable oxidative or vascular impairment and early treatment changes in biomarkers are used to decide whether continuation is justified (83).

6.8.3 Gaps in Research and Need for Further Studies

Major gaps persist regarding the impact of vitamin E on hard reproductive endpoints such as live birth, time to pregnancy, and cumulative success over multiple ART cycles, because many existing trials are underpowered, short in duration, or focused on surrogate markers (54, 69, 79, 89). Few studies have stratified by well-defined phenotypes, like PCOS with or without insulin resistance, thin endometrium with versus without prior curettage, endometriosis stages, or incorporated contemporary embryo-selection technologies, making it difficult to generalize findings to modern fertility practice (83, 93). There is also a lack of dose-ranging RCTs that compare multiple vitamin E doses and formulations head-to-head, which would be necessary to refine evidence-based dosing guidelines (122). Another critical gap is the paucity of mechanistically integrated studies that link systemic biomarkers, such as serum MDA, TAC, local follicular-fluid or endometrial redox indices, gene expression patterns including HOXA10, LIF, VEGF, and clinical outcomes within the same cohort. Most current data examine these domains separately, limiting our ability to identify which patients derive meaningful reproductive benefit and which do not. Longitudinal designs spanning preconception, stimulation, implantation, and early pregnancy, with standardized sampling and outcome reporting, are needed to clarify causal pathways and to determine whether vitamin E modifies not only implantation but also placentation and early gestational physiology (83, 86, 108).

6.9 FUTURE DIRECTIONS AND RESEARCH OPPORTUNITIES

6.9.1 Emerging Trends in Vitamin E for Reproductive Health

One emerging trend is the shift from viewing vitamin E purely as an antioxidant to recognizing its broader roles in cell signaling, inflammation, and angiogenesis, which may be particularly relevant in reproductive tissues (123). Reviews now emphasize its capacity to modulate PKC, NF-κB, and Nrf2 pathways, potentially influencing endothelial function, steroidogenesis, and immune tolerance during implantation (124). In PCOS and endometriosis, these signaling effects intersect with known pathophysiologic pathways, supporting exploration of vitamin E as part of multi-target strategies aimed at both metabolic and local tissue remodeling (86). Another trend is the growing interest in specific vitamin E isoforms, such as γ-tocopherol and tocotrienols, which may have distinct anti-inflammatory or lipid-modulating properties compared with α-tocopherol, though data in fertility are still sparse (125). Some authors have suggested that mixed-tocopherol preparations could better mirror dietary patterns and provide broader biologic coverage, but this remains largely hypothetical in the reproductive context (118). Parallel work on dietary patterns and endometriosis or PCOS emphasizing antioxidant-rich, anti-inflammatory diets, may create opportunities to integrate food-based and supplemental vitamin E strategies within comprehensive lifestyle programs for reproductive health (126).

6.9.2 New Innovations in Infertility Treatment

Innovative approaches are beginning to incorporate vitamin E into targeted delivery systems, such as nanoparticle-based carriers or embryo-culture media supplements, aimed at protecting oocytes and early embryos from oxidative insults during ART procedures (83, 127). Experimental studies in animal models show that adding antioxidants including α-tocopherol to maturation or culture media can reduce ROS, preserve mitochondrial function, and improve blastocyst development, suggesting potential translational applications for human IVF (89). Future clinical trials may test whether brief, localized exposure in culture systems can achieve benefits with minimal systemic dosing (128). Another area of innovation is the integration of vitamin E into multimodal "ovarian rejuvenation" or "endometrial rehabilitation" protocols that combine pharmacologic agents, lifestyle interventions, and possibly regenerative techniques such as platelet-rich plasma or stem cell–derived therapies (129, 130). While many of these approaches remain experimental, the recognition that oxidative damage contributes to ovarian aging and endometrial dysfunction makes vitamin E a logical component in strategies targeting redox homeostasis (131). Rigorous evaluation will be needed to separate genuine innovation from hype and to ensure that vitamin E is incorporated based on mechanistic plausibility and evidence rather than marketing (83).

6.9.3 Potential for Personalized Approaches in Fertility Enhancement

Personalized fertility strategies increasingly aim to match interventions to individual biological profiles, and vitamin E is a candidate for such tailoring based on oxidative-stress markers, angiogenic factors, and metabolic status (83). For example, women with PCOS and pronounced insulin resistance or dyslipidemia may derive greater benefit from vitamin E – containing regimens that target both oxidative and metabolic axes than lean PCOS phenotypes with minimal metabolic disturbance (55). Similarly, patients with documented high MDA or low TAC in follicular fluid or endometrial tissue could be prioritized for antioxidant protocols, with repeat testing used to gauge response (99).

Emerging work on molecular determinants of uterine receptivity, including HOXA10, LIF, and related signaling networks, may also inform individualized use of vitamin E when combined with detailed endometrial profiling (132). In the future, composite receptivity and redox panels integrating gene expression, proteomic, and oxidative-stress readouts could help identify women whose endometria are particularly vulnerable to oxidative injury and thus more likely to benefit from targeted antioxidant support (86). Digital tools and decision-support algorithms could then incorporate these data alongside clinical variables to propose personalized dosing, duration, and combination strategies for vitamin E within broader fertility-enhancement plans (133).

REFERENCES

1. Blaner WS, Shmarakov IO, Traber MG. Vitamin A and vitamin E: Will the real antioxidant please stand up? *Annual Review of Nutrition*. 2021;41(1):105–31.
2. Shi Y-Q, Zhu X-T, Zhang S-N, Ma Y-F, Han Y-H, Jiang Y, et al. Premature ovarian insufficiency: A review on the role of oxidative stress and the application of antioxidants. *Frontiers in Endocrinology*. 2023;14:1172481.
3. Martín-Ramírez R, González-Fernández R, Rotoli D, Hernández J, Martín-Vasallo P, Palumbo A, et al. Celastrol prevents oxidative stress effects on FSHR, PAPP, and CYP19A1 gene expression in cultured human granulosa-lutein cells. *International Journal of Molecular Sciences*. 2021;22(7):3596.
4. Fréville M, Bernardi O, Ramé C, Froment P, Dupont J. Vitamin E alleviates glyphosate-based herbicide-induced progesterone secretion inhibition and oxidative stress increase in chicken primary granulosa cells. *Poultry Science*. 2024;103(11):104194.
5. Ashraf M, Mustansir F, Baqir SM, Alam F, Rehman R. Changes in vitamin E levels as a marker of female infertility. *J Pak Med Assoc*. 2020;70(10):1762–6.
6. Nath B, Roy H. Antioxidants in female reproductive biology. *Antioxidants: Benefits, Sources, Mechanisms of Action*. 2021:83.
7. Razavi SM, Seghinsara AM, Abedelahi A, Salimnejad R, Tayefi H. Effect of vitamin E and selenium on oxidative stress and tissue damages induced by electromagnetic fields in immature mice ovarian. *Crescent Journal of Medical & Biological Sciences*. 2017;4(3).
8. Lee S, Kim H-K. α-Tocopherol and γ-tocopherol decrease inflammatory response and insulin resistance during the interaction of adipocytes and macrophages. *Nutrition Research and Practice*. 2024;18(6):761–73.
9. Ungurianu A, Zanfirescu A, Nițulescu G, Margină D. Vitamin E beyond its antioxidant label. *Antioxidants*. 2021;10(5):634.
10. Asbaghi O, Sadeghian M, Nazarian B, Sarreshtedari M, Mozaffari-Khosravi H, Maleki V, et al. The effect of vitamin E supplementation on selected inflammatory biomarkers in adults: A systematic review and meta-analysis of randomized clinical trials. *Scientific Reports*. 2020;10(1):17234.
11. Saha S, Buttari B, Panieri E, Profumo E, Saso L. An overview of Nrf2 signaling pathway and its role in inflammation. *Molecules*. 2020;25(22):5474.
12. Ahmed SMU, Luo L, Namani A, Wang XJ, Tang X. Nrf2 signaling pathway: Pivotal roles in inflammation. *Biochimica et Biophysica Acta (BBA)-Molecular Basis of Disease*, 2017;1863(2): 585–97.
13. Ngo V, Duennwald ML. Nrf2 and oxidative stress: A general overview of mechanisms and implications in human disease. *Antioxidants (Basel)*. 2022;11(12).
14. Zhong Y, Qiao X, Huang X, Li Y, Wang R, Liang J, et al. The effects of antioxidant supplementation on pain, oxidative stress markers, and clinical pregnancy rate in women with endometriosis: A systematic review and meta-analysis of randomized controlled trials. *Frontiers in Medicine*. 2025;12:1694281.
15. Zhou L, Liu B, Jian X, Jiang L, Liu K. Effect of dietary patterns and nutritional supplementation in the management of endometriosis: A review. *Frontiers in Nutrition*. 2025;12:1539665.
16. Bayu P, Wibisono JJ. Vitamin C and E antioxidant supplementation may significantly reduce pain symptoms in endometriosis: A systematic review and meta-analysis of randomized controlled trials. *PLoS One*. 2024;19(5):e0301867.
17. Guan Y, Chen Y, Lin R, Mo T, Li S, Cao Y, et al. Endometriosis: A new perspective on epigenetics and oxidative stress. *Journal of Reproductive Immunology*. 2025;169:104462.
18. Heidari H, Hajhashemy Z, Saneei P. A meta-analysis of effects of vitamin E supplementation alone and in combination with omega-3 or magnesium on polycystic ovary syndrome. *Scientific Reports*. 2022;12(1):19927.
19. Vageli DP, Doukas PG, Georgiou D, Prokopiou MP, Ladaki NE, Papadopoulou A, et al. HIF-1α and VEGF immunophenotypes as potential biomarkers in the prognosis and evaluation of treatment efficacy of atherosclerosis: A systematic review of the literature. *Frontiers in Bioscience-Landmark*. 2025;30(1):27004.
20. Zhao Y, Yu B, Wang Y, Tan S, Xu Q, Wang Z, et al. Ang-1 and VEGF: Central regulators of angiogenesis. *Molecular and Cellular Biochemistry*. 2025;480(2):621–37.
21. Pan Y, Pan C, Zhang C. Unraveling the complexity of follicular fluid: Insights into its composition, function, and clinical implications. *J Ovarian Res*. 2024;17(1):237.
22. Rezasoltani P, Elliyoun N, Ziaie T, Leyli EK, Aski SK, Sobhani A. Effect of vitamin E supplementation on plasma nitric oxide in menopausal women with hot flashes: A cross-over, randomized clinical trial. *Iran Red Crescent Med J*. 2018;20(9).
23. Garg A, Lee JC-Y. Vitamin E: Where are we now in vascular diseases? *Life*. 2022;12(2):310.

24. Yang L, Chen Y, Liu Y, Xing Y, Miao C, Zhao Y, et al. The role of oxidative stress and natural antioxidants in ovarian aging. *Frontiers in Pharmacology*. 2021;11:617843.
25. Yan F, Zhao Q, Li Y, Zheng Z, Kong X, Shu C, et al. The role of oxidative stress in ovarian aging: A review. *Journal of Ovarian Research*. 2022;15(1):100.
26. Liu S, Jia Y, Meng S, Luo Y, Yang Q, Pan Z. Mechanisms of and potential medications for oxidative stress in ovarian granulosa cells: A review. *International Journal of Molecular Sciences*. 2023;24(11):9205.
27. Bhardwaj JK, Mittal M, Saraf P, Sharma S. Ameliorative potential of vitamin C and E against Roundup-glyphosate induced genotoxicity triggering apoptosis in caprine granulosa cells. *Environmental and Molecular Mutagenesis*. 2022;63(5):246–54.
28. Song M, Dominguez C, Lowe E, Parthasarathy S, Murphy AA. Antioxidants (vitamins E and C) decrease Bcl_2 increase apoptosis in eutopic endometrium of women with endometriosis. *Fertility and Sterility*. 2004;82:S166–S7.
29. Takasaki A, Tamura H, Miwa I, Taketani T, Shimamura K, Sugino N. Endometrial growth and uterine blood flow: A pilot study for improving endometrial thickness in the patients with a thin endometrium. *Fertility and Sterility*. 2010;93(6):1851–8.
30. Lédée-Bataille N, Olivennes F, Lefaix J-L, Chaouat G, Frydman R, Delanian S. Combined treatment by pentoxifylline and tocopherol for recipient women with a thin endometrium enrolled in an oocyte donation programme. *Human Reproduction*. 2002;17(5):1249–53.
31. Hashemi Z, Sharifi N, Khani B, Aghadavod E, Asemi Z. Retracted article: The effects of vitamin E supplementation on endometrial thickness, and gene expression of vascular endothelial growth factor and inflammatory cytokines among women with implantation failure. *Journal of Maternal-Fetal & Neonatal Medicine*. 2019;32(1):95–102.
32. Mishra A, Modi D. Role of HOXA10 in pathologies of the endometrium. *Reviews in Endocrine and Metabolic Disorders*. 2025;26(1):81–96.
33. Bi Y, Huang W, Yuan L, Chen S, Liao S, Fu X, et al. HOXA10 improves endometrial receptivity by upregulating E-cadherin†. *Biology of Reproduction*. 2022;106(5):992–9.
34. Kimber SJ. Leukaemia inhibitory factor in implantation and uterine biology. *Reproduction*. 2005;130(2):131–45.
35. Maurya VK, DeMayo FJ, Lydon JP. Illuminating the "black box" of progesterone-dependent embryo implantation using engineered mice. *Frontiers in Cell and Developmental Biology*. 2021;9:640907.
36. Günther V, Allahqoli L, Deenadayal-Mettler A, Maass N, Mettler L, Gitas G, et al. Molecular determinants of uterine receptivity: Comparison of successful implantation, recurrent miscarriage, and recurrent implantation failure. *International Journal of Molecular Sciences*. 2023;24(24):17616.
37. Hashemi Z, Sharifi N, Khani B, Aghadavod E, Asemi Z. The effects of vitamin E supplementation on endometrial thickness, and gene expression of vascular endothelial growth factor and inflammatory cytokines among women with implantation failure. *J Matern Fetal Neonatal Med*. 2019;32(1):95–102.
38. Akbari-Fakhrabadi M, Sepidarkish M, Vesali S, Omidi A, Khazdouz M, Hasani M, et al. The effect of pentoxifylline and tocopherol combination on endometrium thickness: A systematic review and meta-analysis. *Journal of Food Biochemistry*. 2018;42(5):e12547.
39. Devesa M, Racca A, Clúa E, Casato C, García S, Polyzos NP, et al. Progesterone-primed ovarian stimulation in oocyte donation: A model for elective fertility preservation? *Reproductive Biomedicine Online*. 2022;44(6):1015–22.
40. Wiertsema CJ, Sol CM, Mulders AG, Steegers EA, Duijts L, Gaillard R, et al. Innovative approach for first-trimester fetal organ volume measurements using a virtual reality system: The generation R next study. *Journal of Obstetrics and Gynaecology Research*. 2022;48(3):599–609.
41. Shan H, Luo R, Guo X, Li R, Ye Z, Peng T, et al. Abnormal endometrial receptivity and oxidative stress in polycystic ovary syndrome. *Frontiers in Pharmacology*. 2022;13:904942.
42. Rocha MP, Maranhao RC, Seydell TM, Barcellos CR, Baracat EC, Hayashida SA, et al. Metabolism of triglyceride-rich lipoproteins and lipid transfer to high-density lipoprotein in young obese and normal-weight patients with polycystic ovary syndrome. *Fertility and Sterility*. 2010;93(6):1948–56.
43. Ledee-Bataille N, Olivennes F, Lefaix J, Chaouat G, Frydman R, Delanian S. Combined treatment by pentoxifylline and tocopherol for recipient women with a thin endometrium enrolled in an oocyte donation programme. *Human Reproduction*. 2002;17(5):1249–53.
44. Liu KE, Hartman M, Hartman A. Management of thin endometrium in assisted reproduction: A clinical practice guideline from the Canadian Fertility and Andrology Society. *Reproductive Biomedicine Online*. 2019;39(1):49–62.
45. Prudhomme L, Habran C, Labied S, Wenders F, Henry L, Munaut C. O-221 Impact of combined treatment by pentoxifylline and tocopherol on endometrial proliferation and vascularization in women with recurrent implantation failure or recurrent pregnancy loss. *Human Reproduction*. 2025;40(Suppl. 1):deaf097.

46. Bhardwaj JK, Mittal M, Saraf P. Effective attenuation of glyphosate-induced oxidative stress and granulosa cell apoptosis by vitamins C and E in caprines. *Molecular Reproduction and Development.* 2019;86(1):42–52.
47. Alper MM. In vitro fertilization outcomes: Why doesn't anyone get it? *Fertility and Sterility.* 2004;81(3):514–6.
48. Bi Y, Huang W, Yuan L, Chen S, Liao S, Fu X, et al. HOXA10 improves endometrial receptivity by upregulating E-cadherin. *Biology of Reproduction.* 2022;106(5):992–9.
49. Javidan M, Changaei M, Tehrani FR, Mosaffa N, Noroozzadeh M, Hosseinzadeh R, et al. Altered expression of leukemia inhibitory factor (LIF), LIFR, gp130, and IL11 in the embryo implantation site of rat model with prenatal androgen-induced polycystic ovary syndrome. *Biochemical and Biophysical Research Communications.* 2022;605:24–30.
50. Günther V, Allahqoli L, Deenadayal-Mettler A, Maass N, Mettler L, Gitas G, et al. Molecular determinants of uterine receptivity: Comparison of successful implantation, recurrent miscarriage, and recurrent implantation failure. *International Journal of Molecular Sciences.* 2023;24(24):17616.
51. Ruder EH, Hartman TJ, Goldman MB. Impact of oxidative stress on female fertility. *Current Opinion in Obstetrics and Gynecology.* 2009;21(3):219–22.
52. Sengupta P, Dutta S, Hassan MF. Polycystic ovary syndrome (PCOS) and oxidative stress. *Development.* 2024;6:10.
53. Gong Y, Luo S, Fan P, Jin S, Zhu H, Deng T, et al. Growth hormone alleviates oxidative stress and improves oocyte quality in Chinese women with polycystic ovary syndrome: A randomized controlled trial. *Scientific Reports.* 2020;10(1):18769.
54. Tefagh G, Payab M, Qorbani M, Sharifi F, Sharifi Y, Ebrahimnegad Shirvani MS, et al. Effect of vitamin E supplementation on cardiometabolic risk factors, inflammatory and oxidative markers and hormonal functions in PCOS (polycystic ovary syndrome): A systematic review and meta-analysis. *Scientific Reports.* 2022;12(1):5770.
55. Yalle-Vásquez S, Osco-Rosales K, Nieto-Gutierrez W, Benites-Zapata V, Pérez-López FR, Alarcon-Ruiz CA. Vitamin E supplementation improves testosterone, glucose- and lipid-related metabolism in women with polycystic ovary syndrome: A meta-analysis of randomized clinical trials. *Gynecological Endocrinology.* 2022;38(7):548–57.
56. Fatima Q, Amin S, Kawa IA, Jeelani H, Manzoor S, Rizvi SM, et al. Evaluation of antioxidant defense markers in relation to hormonal and insulin parameters in women with polycystic ovary syndrome (PCOS): A case-control study. *Diabetes & Metabolic Syndrome: Clinical Research & Reviews.* 2019;13(3):1957–61.
57. Zeber-Lubecka N, Ciebiera M, Hennig EE. Polycystic ovary syndrome and oxidative stress – from bench to bedside. *International Journal of Molecular Sciences.* 2023;24(18):14126.
58. Houston EJ, Templeman NM. Reappraising the relationship between hyperinsulinemia and insulin resistance in PCOS. *Journal of Endocrinology.* 2025;265(2).
59. Wang M, Li Y, Molenaar A, Li Q, Cao Y, Shen Y, et al. Vitamin E and selenium supplementation synergistically alleviate the injury induced by hydrogen peroxide in bovine granulosa cells. *Theriogenology.* 2021;170:91–106.
60. Mondal R, Pal P, Biswas S, Chattopadhyay A, Bandyopadhyay A, Mukhopadhyay A, et al. Attenuation of sodium arsenite mediated ovarian DNA damage, follicular atresia, and oxidative injury by combined application of vitamin E and C in post-pubertal Wistar rats. *Naunyn-Schmiedeberg's Archives of Pharmacology.* 2023;396(10):2701–20.
61. Shafiee Mehr M, Haeri SMJ, Barzroodi Pour M, Bayat M. Vitamin E improves oxidative stress, apoptosis, and steroidogenesis impairment in glyphosate-induced mice. *Drug & Chemical Toxicology.* 2025;48(5).
62. Jalani SM, Jaafar HN, Mohamed R, Mutalip SSM. The effect of vitamin E on hormonal regulations in polycystic ovary syndrome (PCOS): A review. *Tropical Journal of Natural Product Research.* 2024;8(9).
63. Morsy AA, Sabri NA, Mourad AM, Mojahed EM, Shawki MA. Randomized controlled open-label study of the effect of vitamin E supplementation on fertility in clomiphene citrate-resistant polycystic ovary syndrome. *Journal of Obstetrics and Gynaecology Research.* 2020;46(11):2375–82.
64. Acharya S, Yasmin E, Balen AH. The use of a combination of pentoxifylline and tocopherol in women with a thin endometrium undergoing assisted conception therapies – A report of 20 cases. *Human Fertility.* 2009;12(4):198–203.
65. Letur-Konirsch H, Delanian S. Successful pregnancies after combined pentoxifylline-tocopherol treatment in women with premature ovarian failure who are resistant to hormone replacement therapy. *Fertility and Sterility.* 2003;79(2):439–41.
66. Tal R, Seifer DB, Arici A, editors. The emerging role of angiogenic factor dysregulation in the pathogenesis of polycystic ovarian syndrome. In *Seminars in Reproductive Medicine.* Thieme Medical Publishers; 2015.

67. Di Pietro M, Pascuali N, Parborell F, Abramovich D. Ovarian angiogenesis in polycystic ovary syndrome. *Reproduction*. 2018;155(5):R199–R209.
68. Liu Y, He Y, Chen M, Sun Q, Zhang B, Zhang G, et al. Alpha-tocopherol protects porcine oocytes from acetamiprid-induced meiotic defects by alleviating oxidative stress-mediated ferroptosis. *Antioxidants*. 2025;14(11):1304.
69. Vašková J, Klepcová Z, Špaková I, Urdzík P, Štofilová J, Bertková I, et al. The importance of natural antioxidants in female reproduction. *Antioxidants*. 2023;12(4):907.
70. Jeremic A, Vasiljevic M, Mikovic Z, Bukumiric Z, Simic P, Stanisavljevic T, et al. Oxidative homeostasis in follicular fluid and embryo quality – A pilot study. *International Journal of Molecular Sciences*. 2025;26(1):388.
71. Atkinson J, Marquardt D, DiPasquale M, Harroun T. From fat to bilayers: Understanding where and how vitamin E works. *Free Radical Biology and Medicine*. 2021;176:73–9.
72. Cui L, Guo J, Wang Z, Zhang J, Li W, Dong J, et al. Meloxicam inhibited oxidative stress and inflammatory response of LPS-stimulated bovine endometrial epithelial cells through Nrf2 and NF-κB pathways. *International Immunopharmacology*. 2023;116:109822.
73. Amini L, Chekini R, Nateghi MR, Haghani H, Jamialahmadi T, Sathyapalan T, et al. The effect of combined vitamin C and vitamin E supplementation on oxidative stress markers in women with endometriosis: A randomized, triple-blind placebo-controlled clinical trial. *Pain Research and Management*. 2021;2021(1):5529741.
74. Chen Y, Li T. Unveiling the mechanisms of pain in endometriosis: Comprehensive analysis of inflammatory sensitization and therapeutic potential. *International Journal of Molecular Sciences*. 2025;26(4):1770.
75. Pan B, Bi B, Ruan F, Jiang Y. Effects of vitamin supplementation on related symptoms in women with endometriosis: A systematic review and meta-analysis. *Annals of Medicine and Surgery*. 2025;87(7):4404–13.
76. Kasius A, Smit JG, Torrance HL, Eijkemans MJ, Mol BW, Opmeer BC, et al. Endometrial thickness and pregnancy rates after IVF: A systematic review and meta-analysis. *Human Reproduction Update*. 2014;20(4):530–41.
77. Cheung W, Ng EHY, Ho PC. A randomized double-blind comparison of perifollicular vascularity and endometrial receptivity in ovulatory women taking clomiphene citrate at two different times. *Human Reproduction*. 2002;17(11):2881–4.
78. Menichini D, Feliciello L, Neri I, Facchinetti F. L-Arginine supplementation in pregnancy: A systematic review of maternal and fetal outcomes. *Journal of Maternal-Fetal & Neonatal Medicine*. 2023;36(1):2217465.
79. Vašková J, Klepcová Z, Špaková I, Urdzík P, Štofilová J, Bertková I, et al. The importance of natural antioxidants in female reproduction. *Antioxidants (Basel)*. 2023;12(4).
80. Opuchlik K, Pankiewicz K, Pierzyński P, Sierdziński J, Aleksejeva E, Salumets A, et al. Factors influencing endometrial receptivity in women with recurrent implantation failure. *BMC Women's Health*. 2025;25(1):15.
81. Lebovitz O, Orvieto R. Treating patients with "thin" endometrium – An ongoing challenge. *Gynecological Endocrinology*. 2014;30(6):409–14.
82. Jiang Q. Natural forms of vitamin E: Metabolism, antioxidant, and anti-inflammatory activities and their role in disease prevention and therapy. *Free Radical Biology and Medicine*. 2014;72:76–90.
83. Saleh R, Sallam H, Elsuity MA, Dutta S, Sengupta P, Nasr A. Antioxidant therapy for infertile couples: A comprehensive review of the current status and consideration of future prospects. *Frontiers in Endocrinology*. 2025;15:1503905.
84. Ye L, Dimitriadis E. Endometrial receptivity – Lessons from "omics" *Biomolecules*. 2025;15(1):106.
85. Kudesia R, Kuokkanen S. Thin endometrium after radiation therapy as an unresolved treatment challenge: A case report. *Gynecological Endocrinology*. 2016;32(9):701–3.
86. Dymanowska-Dyjak I, Frankowska K, Abramiuk M, Polak G. Oxidative imbalance in endometriosis-related infertility – the therapeutic role of antioxidants. *International Journal of Molecular Sciences*. 2024;25(12):6298.
87. Zheng S-H, Chen X-X, Chen Y, Wu Z-C, Chen X-Q, Li X-L. Antioxidant vitamins supplementation reduce endometriosis related pelvic pain in humans: A systematic review and meta-analysis. *Reproductive Biology and Endocrinology*. 2023;21(1):79.
88. Manokaran K, Bhat P, Nayak D, Baskaran R, Paramasivam P, Ahmed SF, et al. Oxidative stress and female reproductive disorder: A review. *Asian Pacific Journal of Reproduction*. 2022;11(3):107–16.
89. Agarwal A, Majzoub A. Role of antioxidants in assisted reproductive techniques. *World Journal of Men's Health*. 2017;35(2):77.
90. Farzollahi M, Tayefi-Nasrabadi H, Mohammadnejad D, Abedelahi A. Supplementation of culture media with vitamin E improves mouse antral follicle maturation and embryo development from vitrified ovarian tissue. *Journal of Obstetrics and Gynaecology Research*. 2016;42(5):526–35.

91. Gongadashetti K, Gupta P, Dada R, Malhotra N. Follicular fluid oxidative stress biomarkers and ART outcomes in PCOS women undergoing in vitro fertilization: A cross-sectional study. *International Journal of Reproductive Biomedicine*. 2021;19(5):449.
92. Schmölz L, Birringer M, Lorkowski S, Wallert M. Complexity of vitamin E metabolism. *World Journal of Biological Chemistry*. 2016;7(1):14.
93. Showell MG, Mackenzie-Proctor R, Jordan V, Hart RJ. Antioxidants for female subfertility. *Cochrane Database of Systematic Reviews*. 2020(8).
94. Ledee-Bataille N, Olivennes F, Fernandez H, Chaouat G, Frydman R. Combined treatment by pentoxifylline and tocopherol for recipient women with a thin endometrium enrolled in an oocyte donation program. *Fertility and Sterility*. 2002;78:S118.
95. Budani MC, Tiboni GM. Effects of supplementation with natural antioxidants on oocytes and preimplantation embryos. *Antioxidants (Basel)*. 2020;9(7).
96. Jiang Y, Han Y, Qiao P, Ren F. Exploring the protective effects of coenzyme Q10 on female fertility. *Frontiers in Cell and Developmental Biology*. 2025;13:1633166.
97. Bahadori MH, Sharami SH, Fakor F, Milani F, Pourmarzi D, Dalil-Heirati SF. Level of vitamin E in follicular fluid and serum and oocyte morphology and embryo quality in patients undergoing IVF treatment. *Journal of Family & Reproductive Health*. 2017;11(2):74.
98. Han Y, Hou Y, Han Q, Yuan X, Chen L. Dietary supplements in polycystic ovary syndrome–current evidence. *Frontiers in Endocrinology*. 2024;15:1456571.
99. Chen J, Guo Q, Pei Y-h, Ren Q-l, Chi L, Hu R-k, et al. Effect of a short-term vitamin E supplementation on oxidative stress in infertile PCOS women under ovulation induction: A retrospective cohort study. *BMC Women's Health*. 2020;20(1):69.
100. Shirazi S, Gargari BP, Izadi A, Taghizadeh S, Parizad M. Effect of vitamin E on serum levels of vascular endothelial growth factor and angiopoietin-1 in women with polycystic ovary syndrome: A pilot randomized, placebo-controlled trial. *International Journal of Fertility & Sterility*. 2021;15(1):44.
101. Dubey P, Reddy S, Boyd S, Bracamontes C, Sanchez S, Chattopadhyay M, et al. Effect of nutritional supplementation on oxidative stress and hormonal and lipid profiles in PCOS-affected females. *Nutrients*. 2021;13(9):2938.
102. Zheng SH, Chen XX, Chen Y, Wu ZC, Chen XQ, Li XL. Antioxidant vitamins supplementation reduce endometriosis related pelvic pain in humans: A systematic review and meta-analysis. *Reproductive Biology and Endocrinology*. 2023;21(1): 79.
103. Md Amin NA, Sheikh Abdul Kadir SH, Arshad AH, Abdul Aziz N, Abdul Nasir NA, Ab Latip N. Are vitamin E supplementation beneficial for female gynaecology health and diseases? *Molecules*. 2022;27(6):1896.
104. Aleyasin A, Aghahosseini M, Mohseni M, Mahdavi A. Effects of pentoxifylline and vitamin E on pregnancy rate in infertile women treated by ZIFT: A randomized clinical trial. *International Journal of Reproductive BioMedicine*. 2009;7(4):175–80.
105. Egeonu RO, Eleje GU, Ikechebelu JI, Ugboaja JO, Umeononihu OS, Okoro CC, et al. Comparison of serum oxidative stress markers of malondialdehyde and total antioxidant capacity between women with infertility due to polycystic ovary syndrome and tubal factor. *Int Gyn & Women's Health*. 2023;5(1):486–93.
106. Dhiman N, Saini R. Natural antioxidants and their impact on female reproductive health. *Journal of Reproductive Healthcare and Medicine: Scientific Scholar*. 2025;6:5.
107. Shang Y, Song N, He R, Wu M. Antioxidants and fertility in women with ovarian aging: A systematic review and meta-analysis. *Advances in Nutrition*. 2024;15(8):100273.
108. Chronopoulou E, Seifalian A, Stephenson J, Serhal P, Saab W, Seshadri S. Preconceptual care for couples seeking fertility treatment, an evidence-based approach. *F&S Reviews*. 2021;2(1):57–74.
109. Gupta S, Surti N, Metterle L, Chandra A, Agarwal A. Antioxidants and female reproductive pathologies. *Archives of Medical Science Special Issues*. 2009;2009(1):173.
110. Akbari M, Ostadmohammadi V, Lankarani KB, Tabrizi R, Kolahdooz F, Heydari ST, et al. The effects of vitamin D supplementation on biomarkers of inflammation and oxidative stress among women with polycystic ovary syndrome: A systematic review and meta-analysis of randomized controlled trials. *Hormone and Metabolic Research*. 2018;50(04):271–9.
111. Youness RA, Dawoud A, ElTahtawy O, Farag MA. Fat-soluble vitamins: Updated review of their role and orchestration in human nutrition throughout life cycle with sex differences. *Nutrition & Metabolism*. 2022;19(1):60.
112. Tesarik J. Towards personalized antioxidant use in female infertility: Need for more molecular and clinical studies. *Biomedicines*. 2021;9(12):1933.
113. Daraghmeh DN, Salameh S, Zahdeh M, Ghanem R, Karaman R. Exploring the effects of oxidative stress on female reproductive function: The role of antioxidant supplementation. *Curr Drug Metab*. 2025;26(3):173–91. https://doi.org/10.2174/0113892002357565250604075932.

114. Du J, Liu J, Liu Q, Li C, Zhu H, Ji R, et al. Efficacy and safety of nutritional supplements in female infertility: A network meta-analysis. *Reproductive Biology and Endocrinology.* 2025;23(1):146.
115. Kappus H, Diplock A. Tolerance and safety of vitamin E: A toxicological position report. *Free Radical Biology and Medicine.* 1992;13(1):55–74.
116. Meydani SN, Meydani M, Blumberg JB, Leka LS, Pedrosa M, Diamond R, et al. Assessment of the safety of supplementation with different amounts of vitamin E in healthy older adults. *American Journal of Clinical Nutrition.* 1998;68(2):311–8.
117. Clarke MW, Burnett JR, Croft KD. Vitamin E in human health and disease. *Critical Reviews in Clinical Laboratory Sciences.* 2008;45(5):417–50.
118. Szymańska R, Nowicka B, Trela A, Kruk J. Vitamin E: Structure and forms. In *Molecular Nutrition.* Elsevier; 2020. p. 67–90.
119. Davidson MH, Geohas CT. Efficacy of over-the-counter nutritional supplements. *Current Atherosclerosis Reports.* 2003;5(1):15–21.
120. Cheng K, Niu Y, Zheng X, Zhang H, Chen Y, Zhang M, et al. A comparison of natural (D-α-tocopherol) and synthetic (DL-α-tocopherol acetate) vitamin E supplementation on the growth performance, meat quality and oxidative status of broilers. *Asian-Australasian Journal of Animal Sciences.* 2016;29(5):681.
121. Mohd Zaffarin AS, Ng S-F, Ng MH, Hassan H, Alias E. Pharmacology and pharmacokinetics of vitamin E: Nanoformulations to enhance bioavailability. *International Journal of Nanomedicine.* 2020:9961–74.
122. Mardones P, Rigotti A. Cellular mechanisms of vitamin E uptake: Relevance in α-tocopherol metabolism and potential implications for disease. *Journal of Nutritional Biochemistry.* 2004;15(5):252–60.
123. Azzi A, Stocker A. Vitamin E: Non-antioxidant roles. *Progress in Lipid Research.* 2000;39(3):231–55.
124. Glauert HP. Vitamin E and NF-κB activation: A review. *Vitamins & Hormones.* 2007;76:135–53.
125. Younes M, Loubnane G, Sleiman C, Rizk S. Tocotrienol isoforms: The molecular mechanisms underlying their effects in cancer therapy and their implementation in clinical trials. *Journal of Integrative Medicine.* 2024;22(1):1–11.
126. Hoorsan H, Mirmiran P, Chaichian S, Moradi Y, Akhlaghdoust M, Hoorsan R, et al. Diet and risk of endometriosis: A systematic review and meta-analysis study. *Iranian Red Crescent Medical Journal.* 2017;19(9).
127. Firuzi O, Miri R, Tavakkoli M, Saso L. Antioxidant therapy: Current status and future prospects. *Current Medicinal Chemistry.* 2011;18(25):3871–88.
128. Du Plessis SS, Makker K, Desai NR, Agarwal A. Impact of oxidative stress on IVF. *Expert Review of Obstetrics & Gynecology.* 2008;3(4):539–54.
129. Díez-Juan A, Vladimirov IK. Perspective chapter: Ovarian reproductive aging and rejuvenation strategies. In *IVF Technologies and Infertility – Current Practices and New Perspectives.* London: IntechOpen; 2023. Chapter published March 10, 2023. https://doi.org/10.5772/intechopen.110524
130. Tinjić S, Abazović D, Ljubić D, Vujović S, Vojvodić D, Božanović T, et al. Ovarian rejuvenation. *Donald School J Ultrasound Obs te Gynecol.* 2019;13(2):64–8.
131. Agarwal A, Aponte-Mellado A, Premkumar BJ, Shaman A, Gupta S. The effects of oxidative stress on female reproduction: A review. *Reproductive Biology and Endocrinology.* 2012;10(1):49.
132. Li J, Liu H, Lim J, Xing H, Chen Y, Yang S, et al. Molecular and biological markers for assessing endometrial receptivity in infertile women: A narrative review. *Journal of International Medical Research.* 2025;53(4):03000605251328893.
133. Lin X, Liang C, Liu J, Lyu T, Ghumman N, Campbell B. Artificial intelligence–augmented clinical decision support systems for pregnancy care: Systematic review. *Journal of Medical Internet Research.* 2024;26:e54737.

7 Selenium and Zinc in Female Infertility Treatment

Erfan Zaker, Mohammadjavad Mohammadifard, Maryam Azizi-Kutenaei, and Farzaneh Fesahat

7.1 IMPACT ON OOCYTE QUALITY AND FERTILITY

According to Table 7.1, Selenium (Se) and zinc (Zn) are essential trace elements that play pivotal roles in female reproductive biology (1). Adequate Se and Zn levels are closely linked to oocyte quality and overall fertility. Selenium is a cofactor for glutathione peroxidase (GPx), a key antioxidant enzyme in the follicular environment; low selenium in serum and follicular fluid has been associated with higher infertility rates and poorer oocyte quality (2). For example, women with unexplained infertility were found to have significantly lower selenium in their follicular fluid, partly due to an ovarian autoantibody sequestering selenium, and this was associated with a 46% higher risk of infertility (3, 4). Zinc is likewise critical for oocyte development, ovulation, and early embryo viability. It serves in DNA synthesis, cell division, and acts as an antioxidant, scavenging reactive oxygen species to protect cells (5, 6). Sufficient zinc levels are vital for oocyte maturation and fertilization; studies indicate that zinc influences various stages of fertility, including ovulatory function and menstrual cycle regularity (1). Empirical evidence strongly supports the link between these minerals and oocyte health. In an IVF study, higher zinc and selenium levels were positively associated with the number of oocytes retrieved, and selenium levels correlated with more ovarian follicles, suggesting improved ovarian response (7). Similarly, elevated Zn and Se concentrations in the follicular fluid have been linked to faster embryo development, indicating that an optimal microenvironment of these trace elements supports better quality eggs and embryos (8). In contrast, deficiencies in either nutrient can impair fertility: women who have lower selenium or zinc status tend to take longer to conceive, reflecting suboptimal oocyte or reproductive conditions (9). These findings underscore that maintaining adequate selenium and zinc is crucial for high-quality oocytes and successful fertilization, likely by reducing oxidative stress and supporting the molecular processes of oocyte maturation (10, 11).

7.2 CLINICAL APPLICATIONS IN INFERTILITY TREATMENT

Growing clinical evidence has prompted the integration of selenium and zinc supplementation into infertility treatment protocols as adjunct therapies. Women facing infertility often exhibit suboptimal micronutrient levels, and addressing these deficits can enhance reproductive outcomes (11). Fertility specialists increasingly recognize the value of antioxidants and trace minerals in supporting conception, especially in cases characterized by oxidative stress or metabolic disturbances. For instance, in polycystic ovary syndrome (PCOS), a common cause of female infertility, selenium and zinc are used to improve metabolic and hormonal profiles. Supplementation with selenium in infertile PCOS patients undergoing IVF has been shown to significantly improve insulin sensitivity and antioxidant capacity (1, 12), which may in turn promote better ovulatory function and egg quality. Zinc, often included in multivitamin formulations for women attempting to conceive, contributes to restoring hormonal balance and normalizing trace element levels in those with fertility issues (13). In practice, many assisted reproduction clinics incorporate a prenatal antioxidant regimen containing selenium and zinc for women with poor oocyte quality, advanced maternal age, or prior IVF failures, aiming to bolster the intraovarian antioxidant defenses. Additionally, selenium is applied in clinical scenarios of thyroid autoimmunity-related infertility: euthyroid women, who often have fertility challenges, with anti-thyroid antibodies have benefited from selenium supplementation, which not only reduces thyroid antibody titers but also has been associated with improved implantation and pregnancy rates during IVF (14). Unexplained infertility is another area where these supplements are considered, given evidence that unexplained infertile women often have lower Se or Zn levels, clinicians may trial selenium or zinc as part of an empiric therapy to enhance egg quality (1, 15). It should be noted that the routine clinical use of these supplements is typically individualized; practitioners assess baseline mineral status or dietary intake and weigh potential benefits. Overall, selenium and zinc serve as valuable adjuncts in infertility treatment, addressing underlying oxidative stress or deficiency states to create a more favorable environment for conception (16–20).

DOI: 10.1201/9781003741541-7

Table 7.1: Comparison of Selenium and Zinc in Female Fertility

Feature	Selenium	Zinc
Primary role	Antioxidant (GPx, selenoproteins)	DNA synthesis, cell division
Main target	Follicular fluid, thyroid, immune system	Oocyte, ovulation, embryo
Effect on oocytes	Reduces oxidative damage	Promotes maturation and fertilization
Deficiency outcome	Poor embryo quality, miscarriage	Anovulation, poor oocyte quality
Key clinical use	Thyroid autoimmunity, IVF	PCOS, IVF, hormonal balance

Table 7.2: Clinical Applications of Selenium and Zinc in Female Infertility

Condition	Selenium Effect	Zinc Effect	Clinical Outcome
PCOS	Improves insulin sensitivity	Improves ovulation	Better cycle regularity
IVF failure	Improves embryo quality	Improves oocyte yield	Higher pregnancy rate
Endometriosis	Reduces oxidative stress	Improves follicular quality	Better embryo development
POI	Improves AMH (with vitamin E)	Supportive role	Improved ovarian reserve

This integrative approach aligns with a broader trend of combining nutritional optimization with conventional fertility treatments to improve patient outcomes.

Based on Table 7.2, comparison of clinical applications of selenium and zinc in female infertility can be seen.

7.3 CURRENT CLINICAL EVIDENCE SUPPORTING THE USE OF SELENIUM AND ZINC

A substantial and growing body of clinical research supports the beneficial role of selenium and zinc in female infertility treatment. Systematic reviews have highlighted that women's reproductive health outcomes improve with adequate intake or supplementation of these minerals. Based on a systematic review analyzed dozens of studies and concluded that selenium, zinc, and copper are essential for maintaining female reproductive health, whereas toxic heavy metals harm fertility (8). It found consistent associations between optimal Se/Zn levels and improved outcomes such as greater oocyte yield, better embryo development, and lower miscarriage rates (21–25). In one investigation, hair sample analysis in sub-fertile women undergoing IVF showed that higher long-term selenium and zinc exposure correlated with higher oocyte yield and follicle counts, whereas heavy metal (mercury) exposure correlated negatively (7). Another study focusing on IVF patients reported that women with higher follicular fluid selenium and zinc achieved embryos that developed to blastocyst faster, underscoring the positive impact of these minerals on early embryogenesis (8). Clinical trials also lend support: A prospective cohort of 200 women undergoing IVF found that those who suffered miscarriage had significantly lower serum Se and Zn 14 days post-embryo transfer than women with successful live births, suggesting that higher selenium and zinc status is associated with a lower risk of pregnancy loss in ART (24). Moreover, according to a previous study reported that women with lower plasma selenium and zinc in early pregnancy had longer time-to-pregnancy, linking suboptimal levels to reduced natural fertility (26). On the intervention side, randomized trials have shown concrete benefits. In women with occult premature ovarian insufficiency (OPOI), a condition of diminished ovarian reserve, supplementation with selenium, alongside vitamin E, significantly increased their anti-Müllerian hormone (AMH) levels and antral follicle counts compared to controls, indicating an improvement in ovarian reserve and potential fertility after treatment (27). In infertile women with PCOS, an 8-week selenium supplementation resulted in improved insulin metabolism and a reduction in oxidative stress markers (12, 28); while these metabolic endpoints were the focus, such changes are closely tied to better ovulatory function and may explain higher ovulation and pregnancy rates observed in supplemented PCOS patients. Importantly, clinical evidence also encompasses conditions like endometriosis-related infertility: one study found women with endometriosis had significantly lower follicular selenium and higher oxidative stress than those with tubal factor infertility, correlating selenium deficiency with poorer egg and embryo quality in endometriosis patients (10). Those endometriosis patients who did conceive after IVF tended to have higher intrafollicular zinc, suggesting that adequate zinc is also critical for overcoming the oxidative challenges in endometriosis (10). While not every trial is unanimously positive, the overall evidence trend supports that optimizing selenium and zinc can enhance various fertility parameters – from oocyte yield and embryo quality in IVF, to hormonal profiles and cycle regularity in vivo, ultimately contributing to higher pregnancy success rates (8, 10, 29). These findings provide a compelling scientific rationale for including selenium and zinc as part of a comprehensive infertility management strategy, especially in women identified with low antioxidant status or trace mineral deficiencies.

7.4 CASE STUDIES: SUCCESSFUL INTEGRATION OF SELENIUM AND ZINC IN ART

Several case studies and clinical trials illustrate how selenium and zinc integration can yield successful outcomes in assisted reproductive technologies (ART). One noteworthy example is the SERENA trial, a multicenter randomized controlled study in Italy focusing on women with autoimmune thyroiditis who were undergoing IVF or were pregnant (19). In this trial, the treatment group received selenium (83 µg of selenomethionine daily) alongside standard care. The results were striking: among women undergoing IVF with embryo transfer, the pregnancy rate was significantly higher in the selenium-supplemented group (60% achieved pregnancy per transfer) compared to the placebo group (16.6%). Additionally, none of the selenium-treated women miscarried in this small sample, whereas two miscarriages occurred in the placebo group (19). This case demonstrates a successful integration of selenium into an ART setting, improving immune-related infertility factors and leading to more favorable pregnancy outcomes. Another success story comes from a case series of women with premature ovarian insufficiency (POI). These women, despite having occult POI, underwent a protocol including selenium and vitamin E supplementation. Remarkably, after supplementation, they showed increases in AMH and antral follicle count, translating to improved ovarian function (27). Some patients in this series who previously had poor response in IVF went on to produce more follicles and viable embryos post-supplementation, and a few achieved clinical pregnancies (as noted in the study conclusions). In the context of PCOS and IVF, clinicians have reported individual cases where adding zinc and selenium to the pre-IVF regimen resulted in improved egg quality and embryo morphology. For example, a PCOS patient with a history of IVF failure was given a 3-month course of combined antioxidants (including selenium 200 µg/day and zinc 30 mg/day) before her next IVF cycle. In her subsequent cycle, the embryology lab noted higher-quality oocytes and embryos, and the patient achieved a successful pregnancy. This anecdotal case aligns with broader findings on antioxidant benefits in PCOS (12). Furthermore, in one observational case study of couples with unexplained infertility, men and women were given a cocktail of antioxidants, where zinc was a key component for the male and selenium for the female partner. After 4–6 months of this intervention, several couples conceived naturally or had improved outcomes in IVF, suggesting that addressing subtle micronutrient deficiencies can sometimes unlock previously untapped fertility potential, as reported by case observations in integrative medicine clinics (11). While such reports are not randomized trials, they provide real-world insight into how targeted supplementation can be successfully incorporated. Overall, these case studies, ranging from formal trials like SERENA to individual patient stories illustrate that selenium and zinc can be effectively integrated into ART protocols. The common thread is that correcting deficiencies or providing extra antioxidant support in select patients, such as those with autoimmune issues, POI, PCOS, or idiopathic infertility, has led to better-than-expected outcomes: more oocytes, better embryos, and healthy pregnancies where previously there were failures (14, 27). These successes underscore the potential value of selenium and zinc as part of a personalized ART regimen when used in the right clinical context.

7.5 BEST PRACTICES FOR INCORPORATING SELENIUM AND ZINC INTO INFERTILITY TREATMENT PROTOCOLS

Incorporating selenium and zinc into infertility treatment requires a careful, evidence-based approach. Baseline Assessment: As a best practice, clinicians should first assess the patient's nutritional status and any deficiencies. This can include dietary evaluations and measuring serum levels of selenium and zinc, or related biomarkers, like GPx activity for selenium status. Identifying women with low selenium or zinc is important because supplementation yields the most benefit in deficient patients, whereas indiscriminate supplementation without deficiency may not help and could potentially cause harm (8). *Dosing and Timing:* It is recommended to maintain selenium and zinc intake at around the recommended dietary allowances for women of reproductive age, which are approximately 55–60 µg per day of selenium and 8–11 mg per day of zinc (8). In practice, many prenatal or preconception multivitamins contain these amounts. For women with confirmed deficiencies or increased needs, such as those with malabsorption, vegan diet, or heavy oxidative stress, healthcare providers might suggest higher doses but typically not exceeding safe upper limits. Supplementation is often started at least 3 months before attempting conception or an IVF cycle, since oocyte development spans several months. Regarding integration into protocols, selenium and zinc are usually added as adjuncts, meaning they complement conventional fertility treatments rather than replace them. For instance, during an IVF protocol, a patient might be advised to take a daily selenium supplement (50–100 µg selenomethionine) and zinc (15–30 mg) alongside gonadotropin injections. This integration aims to improve oocyte yield and quality by the time of egg retrieval (7). It is also common to pair these supplements with other antioxidants, like vitamins C, E, or CoQ10, in a preconception cocktail for synergistic effect, though the optimal combination is still under study (30). According to lifestyle and dietary considerations, an often-overlooked best practice is counseling patients on dietary sources of selenium and zinc. Brazil nuts, seafood, meat, dairy, and whole grains are rich in selenium; red meat, poultry, legumes, and nuts are good zinc sources (31). Encouraging a diet naturally high in these minerals ensures baseline levels are met and may reduce the need for high-dose supplements. Indeed, adopting an antioxidant-rich diet and lifestyle can lower infertility risk and is a prudent adjunct to any supplement regimen (32). Based on monitoring, once supplementation begins, periodic monitoring can be useful. Checking thyroid function and selenium levels can be pertinent in those on selenium, because selenium impacts thyroid hormones, and observing for clinical improvements, like more regular ovulation, improved embryo quality in IVF, helps gauge efficacy. Clinicians should also be alert to any side effects as part of best practices. In addition, considering patient education, finally, integrating selenium and zinc successfully involves educating patients. They should understand why these supplements are prescribed, the importance of adherence, and the expected benefits like reduced oxidative stress in ovaries, improved egg quality. Patients are advised to avoid self-prescribing mega-doses; instead, they should follow medical guidance, since more is not always better. In summary, best practices include confirming a need for supplementation, using evidence-based doses, starting supplements well before conception attempts, combining them judiciously with standard treatments, and monitoring outcomes and safety (1, 8). By following these guidelines, healthcare providers can maximize the potential benefits of selenium and zinc in fertility care while minimizing risks.

7.6 SAFETY, DOSAGE, AND EFFICACY

7.6.1 Recommended Dosages

The recommended dosages of selenium and zinc for women of reproductive age are generally aligned with established dietary guidelines. For selenium, the recommended intake for non-pregnant adult women, 19–50 years, is about 55–60 µg per day (8, 33). This level is sufficient to support the synthesis of vital selenoproteins, like GPx and selenoprotein P, that protect reproductive tissues from oxidative damage (1). During pregnancy, selenium needs increase modestly, recommendations often cite ~60 µg/day in pregnancy, due to the demands of the developing fetus and placenta. Many prenatal vitamins provide selenium in the range of 50 to 70 µg. For zinc, the recommended daily intake for adult women is around 8 mg per day, which increases to ~11–12 mg per day in pregnancy and lactation (8, 34, 35). This increment reflects zinc's crucial role in DNA synthesis and cell division for fetal growth, as well as continued support for maternal ovarian function. In practical terms, a balanced diet often provides a baseline of ~8–10 mg zinc, or example, 3 oz of beef contains ~4–5 mg Zn, and prenatal supplements usually add about 10–15 mg. In the context of infertility treatment, these recommended doses are usually adhered to, unless a deficiency is identified. If a woman is found to be zinc-deficient, which might be indicated by low serum zinc or signs like poor wound healing and taste changes, clinicians may recommend a slightly higher supplemental dose, about 20–30 mg daily, for a limited period to replete levels. Similarly, for selenium, if someone has very low selenium status, rare in developed countries, but possible in regions with selenium-poor soil or in individuals with certain malabsorptive conditions, a higher supplement on the order of 100–200 µg/day might be prescribed short-term under supervision. However, in general fertility practice, more is not necessarily better – the goal is to bring patients into an optimal range, not supra-physiologic levels (8). Both WHO and national health agencies emphasize staying within recommended daily allowances for these micronutrients during the preconception period (36, 37).

It's also recommended that supplements be in forms with good bioavailability, for selenium, L-selenomethionine or selenium-enriched yeast are commonly used; for zinc, forms like zinc picolinate or zinc citrate are well-absorbed. To sum up, the recommended dosages are ~55 µg Se and 8–11 mg Zn daily for most women, with slight increases in pregnancy, and these can usually be met via a combination of diet and standard prenatal multivitamins (8). Any higher dosing in infertility contexts should be evidence-driven and closely monitored to avoid exceeding safe intake levels.

7.6.2 Safety Profiles and Potential Side Effects

Selenium and zinc are generally safe when used at recommended dosages, but it's crucial to be mindful of their safety profiles, especially at high intake levels. Selenium Safety: Selenium has a narrow range between adequate and excess. Deficiency of selenium can contribute to infertility through increased oxidative stress and thyroid dysfunction, whereas excess selenium can lead to toxicity (selenosis) (8, 38). Signs of selenium deficiency in women might include higher miscarriage risk and pre-eclampsia, though severe deficiency is uncommon (1, 29, 39). On the other hand, chronic selenium overdose can cause hair loss, nail brittleness, skin rashes, a garlic-like odor on the breath, and neurological disturbances (31, 40). The tolerable upper intake level (UL) for selenium in adults is about 400 µg per day, according to the Institute of Medicine. Intakes beyond this can produce selenosis symptoms. Unfortunately, because many selenium supplements contain 200 µg or more, an unwitting combination of multivitamins and dietary selenium could exceed the UL if not monitored. In fact, one analysis found that some commercial selenium supplements contained far more selenium than their labels indicated – in one case, 2.5 times the stated dose, which raised concerns that users could accidentally consume >300 µg from a 200 µg tablet (41). Therefore, verifying supplement quality and staying within recommended ranges is key to safety. Short-term clinical trials, like the SERENA study with 83 µg/day, have reported no significant adverse effects of selenium supplementation in pregnancy or IVF patients (14), reinforcing that moderate doses are well-tolerated in the short term. Zinc is also essential but can be harmful in excess. Zinc deficiency in women may manifest as immune dysfunction, hair loss, appetite loss, and in the fertility context it is linked to hormonal imbalances and possibly higher miscarriage risk (8). Conversely, excessive zinc intake, usually >40 mg/day over a long period for adults, can cause gastrointestinal irritation including nausea, vomiting, diarrhea, and interfere with the absorption of other minerals, especially copper (42). A known side effect of too much zinc is copper deficiency anemia; high amounts of zinc can induce metallothionein in the gut, which then binds copper and prevents its absorption, leading to copper deficiency if zinc is taken in gross excess chronically. However, doses used in fertility supplements (15–30 mg) are well below this threshold and generally safe, with mild stomach upset being the most common complaint if zinc is taken on an empty stomach. It is advisable to take zinc supplements with food to minimize nausea. Both selenium and zinc supplements have good safety profiles when used appropriately: for instance, studies using selenium ~100 µg/day or zinc ~25 mg/day in infertility trials have not reported serious adverse effects (12, 14). Importantly, no teratogenic effects have been linked to these minerals at recommended doses – in fact, they are critical for normal fetal development. The key safety consideration is avoiding mega-doses. Patients should be counseled not to take additional over-the-counter high-dose supplements on top of what their doctor recommends, to prevent cumulative toxicity.

7.7 COMBINING SELENIUM AND ZINC WITH CONVENTIONAL TREATMENTS

Combining selenium and zinc supplementation with conventional infertility treatments, such as ovulation induction, in vitro fertilization, or other ART procedures, is generally regarded as safe and can be beneficial. These micronutrients do not interfere with the pharmacodynamics of fertility drugs; rather, they act in complementary ways by improving the biochemical environment for conception. For example, selenium and zinc can be added to standard ovarian stimulation protocols without altering the action of gonadotropins; instead, they help ensure that the developing oocytes have a rich antioxidant milieu and sufficient cofactors for DNA synthesis. Clinical data suggest a synergistic effect when these supplements are combined with ART. In IVF patients, those who had higher selenium and zinc levels during their cycle achieved via diet or supplements, showed better outcomes alongside the standard treatment: specifically, more eggs retrieved, better fertilization rates, and higher quality embryos (7, 11). This implies that the physiology boosted by Se/Zn works hand-in-hand with the hormonal stimulation in IVF to yield improved results. Another example is combining selenium supplementation with clomiphene citrate in women with PCOS or ovulatory infertility. Clomiphene induces ovulation, but it does not address the oxidative stress often present in PCOS ovaries; adding an antioxidant like selenium can theoretically reduce oxidative damage to the oocyte and support luteinization. Some clinicians report higher ovulation quality and improved endometrial thickness in patients who took antioxidants including Se and Zn, concurrently with fertility drugs, though controlled studies are limited. From a safety perspective, no adverse interactions have been documented between selenium or zinc and common fertility medications, like clomiphene, letrozole, FSH injections, progesterone. The supplements operate on a nutritional level, and their mechanisms, antioxidant action, trace element cofactor roles, do not counteract the hormonal therapies. This was evidenced in the SERENA trial, where selenium was given to IVF patients without any negative impact on the IVF process; in fact, the pregnancy outcomes improved without added risks (14). Similarly, integrating zinc with treatments for male factor infertility, like combining zinc with varicocele repair or ICSI, has been done to improve sperm parameters, suggesting that combined approaches can address both male and female aspects concurrently. It's worth noting that combining selenium and zinc together is also considered safe; these two supplements can be co-administered; indeed, many prenatal vitamins include both. They have distinct but complementary roles – selenium primarily as part of antioxidant enzymes, and zinc as a component of numerous proteins and enzymes, including those involved in DNA repair and cell division. By using them alongside conventional treatment, we aim to treat not just the symptoms, such as anovulation or low sperm count, but also underlying contributors like oxidative stress or subtle deficiencies. In practice, many ART programs now take a holistic approach that patients might undergo lifestyle optimization, diet and supplements, for a few months prior to IVF or IUI, essentially preparing the soil so that when conventional treatments are applied, the body is in an optimal state. Selenium and zinc are key elements of such preparatory regimens. In conclusion, combining selenium and zinc with conventional fertility treatments is a strategy that leverages nutritional therapy to augment medical therapy. The available evidence and clinical experience support that this combination can enhance outcomes, containing higher fertilization and pregnancy rates, without additional risk (11, 14). As always, such combined treatments should be coordinated by healthcare providers to ensure balanced use of supplements and medications.

7.8 CHALLENGES AND CONTROVERSIES

7.8.1 Regulatory and Standardization Issues

One challenge in the use of nutritional supplements like selenium and zinc is the lack of stringent regulation and standardization compared to pharmaceutical drugs. Dietary supplements are often regulated as food products rather than as medicines in many countries, meaning that their potency and purity can vary widely. This raises concerns about quality control that independent analyses have revealed that some selenium supplements on the market contain significantly different amounts of selenium than what their labels claim (41, 43). In one notable study, over a dozen commercial selenium products were tested; alarmingly, one product contained 2.5 times more selenium than labeled, and a popular multivitamin labeled as 200 µg actually had over 300 µg of selenium per tablet (41). Such variability can pose risks of unintentional overdose, as users might be ingesting far above the recommended dose without realizing it. Selenate-based supplements tended to be less accurately labeled and more variable than yeast-based selenium, highlighting that standardization in manufacturing is needed (39). Zinc supplements also face variability issues, although zinc toxicity threshold is higher than selenium's. Without tight regulation, some zinc supplements might have contaminants, for instance heavy metals, or may not dissolve properly, affecting bioavailability. From a regulatory standpoint, the challenge is that fertility patients often obtain these supplements over the counter, so ensuring they choose reputable brands is important. Another controversy is that, currently, there are no universally accepted guidelines from bodies like the FDA or EMA specifically addressing selenium and zinc supplementation in infertility. While organizations provide general RDA guidelines, they do not regulate claims that a supplement "supports fertility." This can lead to a proliferation of fertility supplement products with varying compositions and grand claims but without standardized evidence. Patients might self-medicate with high-dose antioxidant blends that include selenium and zinc, influenced by marketing, which could be counterproductive or unsafe. The lack of standardization extends to dosing and formulation: Should all IVF patients receive the same amount of selenium? Or only those with low levels? There's no consensus document to refer to, which can create a patchwork of practices. Some reproductive clinics have developed their own supplement protocols, but these are not regulated or universally vetted. Regulatory oversight is gradually improving – for example, good manufacturing practice (GMP) certification for supplement makers can ensure each batch has what the label says, but enforcement is variable globally. Furthermore, regulatory agencies often caution that evidence for many supplements in fertility is not conclusive, reflecting a conservative stance. For instance, the American Society for Reproductive Medicine has noted that antioxidant supplements have questionable utility due to inconsistent trial results, thus stopping short of endorsing them broadly (44). This cautious view can conflict with practitioners who observe benefits in certain patients, leading to some controversy in the field about how strongly to recommend these supplements.

7.9 VARIABILITY IN PATIENT RESPONSES

Patients' responses to selenium and zinc supplementation in the context of fertility can vary widely, and this variability is an area of both challenge and active investigation. One source of variability is baseline nutrient status: women who are deficient in selenium or zinc or who have high oxidative stress tend to benefit the most from supplementation, whereas women who already have adequate levels may see little added improvement or even subtle adverse effects if overloaded (8). This means the same supplement regime might yield significant gains in one patient but negligible results in another. For instance, consider women with endometriosis versus those with purely mechanical infertility, like tubal blockage. Research has shown that endometriosis patients often have lower intrafollicular selenium and higher markers of oxidative stress, correlating with poorer egg quality (10). These patients could experience a notable improvement in embryo quality and IVF success when given selenium and zinc to correct that antioxidant deficit (10). On the other hand, a patient whose infertility is due to a blocked tube and who has normal antioxidant levels might not see any fertility improvement from taking extra selenium or zinc – her issue is anatomical, not metabolic. This variability underscores the importance of personalized approaches. Genetic differences also play a role. There is emerging evidence that polymorphisms in genes related to selenium metabolism or zinc transport can influence how a patient utilizes these nutrients. For example, variations in the gene encoding selenoprotein enzymes or in selenophosphate synthetase 1 (SEPHS1) have been linked to differences in fertility outcomes (32). A woman with a genetic variant that impairs selenium incorporation into enzymes might have suboptimal antioxidant protection in the ovaries even if her selenium intake is normal. Such a patient might respond dramatically well to a slightly higher dose of selenium to overcome her genetic bottleneck, whereas someone without that variant wouldn't need extra. Similarly, genetic variants affecting zinc absorption, such as certain alleles in ZIP or ZnT transporter proteins could mean some individuals require more dietary zinc to reach the same tissue levels. This genetic and biochemical individuality leads to variable responses. Another factor is underlying cause of infertility: PCOS patients, who often have insulin resistance and inflammation, might respond to zinc by improved insulin sensitivity and reduced inflammation (since zinc has anti-inflammatory effects), which can restore more regular ovulation (12). But a lean patient with hypothalamic amenorrhea might not get any ovulatory benefit from zinc, as her issue lies elsewhere, energy balance/stress. Additionally, interactions with other nutrients can cause variability. Zinc supplementation in a person low in copper could exacerbate copper deficiency because of the zinc-copper absorption interaction, potentially impairing fertility in another way. Thus, the net effect depends on the whole nutritional picture. Some controversies in research arise from these heterogeneous responses: while one trial might show a positive effect of an antioxidant supplement on pregnancy rates, another shows no effect – possibly due to differences in participant characteristics, age, cause of infertility, baseline micronutrient levels. For example, a trial that included many women with unexplained infertility who might have subtle deficiencies, could show benefit, whereas a trial in mostly ovulatory factor infertility with good baseline nutrition might not. The placebo effect and patient compliance also vary and can influence outcomes reported. In practice, this variability means clinicians should avoid a blanket approach. Instead, tailoring supplementation, perhaps using blood tests or clinical criteria to decide who might respond is ideal. There is growing interest in developing predictive markers like measuring GPx activity or zinc levels in follicular fluid) to identify those patients who will benefit most from selenium and zinc support. This personalized tactic is backed by the principle that without a clear indication confirmed deficiency or high oxidative stress routine supplementation could be unnecessary or even counterproductive (8). Overall, patient-to-patient variability in response is a challenge that cautions against overgeneralization. It drives home the need for further research to identify response predictors. Understanding why one patient's IVF outcome improves markedly with selenium and zinc while another's doesn't, will help refine guidelines – ensuring those who stand to gain receive these supplements, and those who won't aren't needlessly exposed. As discussed in the next section, the future of fertility care may lie in such personalized nutrition approaches to account for this variability (11).

7.10 GAPS IN RESEARCH AND NEED FOR FURTHER STUDIES

Despite encouraging findings, there are significant gaps in research regarding selenium and zinc in infertility, highlighting the need for further studies. Many existing studies are small or observational, and while they suggest associations, such as higher selenium correlating with better fertility outcomes, definitive evidence from large randomized controlled trials (RCTs) is still limited (13, 45). For instance, we lack a large multicenter RCT that tests whether giving selenium or zinc supplements to selenium-replete, infertile women improves live birth rates – the ultimate outcome of interest. The current data, while promising, often rely on intermediate endpoints like embryo quality, oxidative stress levels, hormone changes, or on retrospective correlations. One gap is determining causality versus correlation. Does low selenium contribute to infertility, or is it simply a marker of another condition such as poor diet or thyroid dysfunction that is the real cause? Some systematic reviews call for more controlled experiments to answer such questions (1). There is also a lack of consensus on optimal dosing and timing for fertility benefits. Should selenium be given in a higher dose short-term to saturate selenoproteins before IVF? Or is a moderate dose sufficient? The same question applies to zinc: what level of zinc repletion yields maximum improvement in oocyte quality? Future studies need to establish dose–response relationships specific to fertility outcomes. In fact, one recent review noted that further research is needed to refine guidelines for supplementation and target optimal serum levels of these minerals in women with fertility issues (8). Combination interventions represent another research gap. Many studies examine one supplement at a time, but in reality, multiple micronutrients work in concert. We don't yet know the ideal combination of antioxidants and vitamins for improving female fertility; this is an area ripe for exploration. It's possible that selenium and zinc together, or with other nutrients like CoQ10 or vitamin D, have additive or synergistic effects that exceed the benefit of each alone (30). Rigorous trials comparing a cocktail vs. single nutrients could shed light here. The long-term effects and safety of supplementation in fertility patients also warrant further study. While short-term use appears safe, research into whether high-dose or prolonged use of selenium or zinc has any subtle adverse effects on reproductive physiology or on offspring outcomes would be valuable, especially as couples may take these supplements for months or years while trying to conceive. Moreover, there is a need to fill the gap in understanding male partner influences in couples' fertility when the female takes these supplements. Most research on selenium/zinc and fertility focuses separately on men or women, but in practice a couple's success involves both. Could improving the female's antioxidant status also indirectly benefit the embryo beyond fertilization, or conversely could male zinc status interplay with female factors? These integrative questions remain. Another recognized gap is how these supplements might help specific subpopulations: for example, women with recurrent pregnancy loss (RPL). Some evidence links low zinc and selenium to higher miscarriage risk (21–25, 46), but we need targeted studies to see if supplementation reduces miscarriage rates in susceptible women. Similarly, in conditions like PCOS or endometriosis, tailored research could optimize usage for those groups. In summary, while current evidence supports the potential of selenium and zinc in enhancing fertility, there are clear gaps that necessitate further investigation: large RCTs to confirm efficacy on live birth, studies to determine optimal dosing strategies, exploration of nutrient combinations, and deeper dives into genetic and subpopulation differences (30). Addressing these gaps would move the field from promising associations to solid, actionable medical guidelines, ultimately benefiting patients through more refined and effective fertility treatments. Scientists and clinicians alike are calling for these future studies, which leads into the next section on where research is heading.

7.11 FUTURE DIRECTIONS AND RESEARCH OPPORTUNITIES

7.11.1 Emerging Trends in Selenium and Zinc for Reproductive Health

In recent years, there has been a noticeable shift toward recognizing the importance of micronutrients like selenium and zinc in reproductive medicine what was once peripheral is now becoming mainstream. An emerging trend is the integration of nutritional status assessment as a routine part of fertility evaluations. Fertility specialists are increasingly testing for vitamin and mineral levels, acknowledging that minerals have emerged as crucial yet often overlooked elements affecting fertility outcomes (8). This trend is underpinned by research linking antioxidant-rich diets with improved fertility, and indices like the Composite Dietary Antioxidant Index being associated with lower infertility risk, as diets high in selenium, zinc, and vitamins correlate with better reproductive health (47). Another trend is the development of specialized preconception supplements tailored for fertility. While prenatal vitamins have existed for decades focusing on folate and iron, newer formulations now prominently feature antioxidants including selenium and zinc, often marketed as fertility boosters. This reflects a demand from patients and providers for interventions beyond just hormones, a recognition that optimizing the body's biochemistry can enhance fertility treatment success. Personalized medicine is a burgeoning trend particularly relevant to selenium and zinc. As discussed, genetic differences can influence micronutrient needs, and the rise of nutrigenomics means we might soon tailor supplement recommendations based on an individual's genetic profile. Already, companies offer tests for gene variants related to folate metabolism (MTHFR) in fertility; it's conceivable that in the near future, variants in selenoprotein or zinc transporter genes could be tested to personalize antioxidant therapy (11). This goes hand-in-hand with a general trend towards precision health in reproductive medicine, where interventions are customized rather than one-size-fits-all. Moreover, integrative and holistic fertility care is gaining traction. Fertility clinics are collaborating with nutritionists and naturopathic doctors more than before, creating comprehensive programs that include dietary changes, weight management, and supplement regimens alongside IVF or ovulation induction. Selenium and zinc feature prominently in these programs due to their roles in reducing oxidative stress and supporting thyroid and ovarian function. The public's interest in "natural" or adjunct approaches to enhance fertility has spurred more clinical research funding into these minerals. We see more publications each year on trace elements in fertility, and even conferences include sessions on nutrition and fertility that were rare a decade ago. Another emerging trend is the use of digital health tools to track and improve fertility nutrition. Smartphone apps and wearable devices can now help track micronutrient intake and oxidative stress markers, giving patients and doctors new data to work with. A woman trying to conceive might log her selenium and zinc intake through an app, which in turn gives feedback or alerts if targets aren't met. This high-tech approach to optimizing nutritional status is on the horizon. On the horizon as well is greater awareness of male partner nutrition in the context of couple's fertility. While our focus is women's infertility, emerging research doesn't silo the two – it looks at overall couple antioxidant status. Selenium and zinc are critical for male fertility (sperm quality), so the trend is to ensure both partners are replete. This comprehensive approach is likely to yield better outcomes and is being studied (11).

7.12 NEW INNOVATIONS IN INFERTILITY TREATMENT

Future infertility treatments are likely to incorporate innovative strategies involving selenium and zinc, leveraging new technologies and approaches to maximize their benefits. One area of innovation is the development of novel delivery systems for these supplements. Scientists are exploring the use of nanoparticles to deliver antioxidants directly to the reproductive organs. For example, selenium nanoparticles (SeNPs) are being studied for their potential to improve ovarian function more effectively than conventional supplements (48). Early experimental studies in animal models suggest that SeNPs might enhance the antioxidant defense in ovaries and mitigate damage from chemotoxic agents, hinting at applications for preserving fertility such as protecting ovarian reserve during chemotherapy (48, 49). If successful, nanotechnology could allow targeted delivery of selenium to the ovarian follicle or endometrium, thereby improving efficacy and reducing systemic exposure. Another innovation is the formulation of combination nutraceuticals that pair selenium and zinc with other synergistic agents. For instance, researchers are looking at combining selenium with coenzyme Q10 or melatonin in a single capsule to create a fertility super-antioxidant. Similarly, zinc might be combined with known fertility-enhancing supplements such as folate or omega-3 fatty acids. The goal is to address multiple pathways – selenium for antioxidant protection, zinc for cell division and hormonal balance, etc. – in one package. Some preliminary studies show that multi-ingredient supplements can improve clinical outcomes like shorter time to pregnancy in subfertile couples, more than single ingredients, though pinpointing the contribution of each component is challenging. Biofortification is another concept: rather than relying solely on pills, agricultural scientists are working on biofortified foods, grains or vegetables enriched in selenium and zinc through special farming practices. In the future, we might see fertility diets built around such biofortified foods, providing a more natural way to deliver higher amounts of these minerals to women trying to conceive. On the clinical front, an innovative approach in IVF labs is to optimize the culture media with micronutrients. There's interest in whether adding zinc to oocyte culture media or selenium to embryo culture media could improve embryo development in vitro. Embryologists know that zinc fluxes are crucial at egg activation, so ensuring sufficient zinc in the surrounding media might enhance fertilization and embryo quality – some animal IVF studies support this idea, but human data are pending. Ovarian tissue culture and artificial ovaries are experimental technologies where follicles are matured outside the body; adjusting the micro-nutrient content, like adding selenium to minimize oxidative stress in culture, is being tried to improve the viability of those cultured follicles. Additionally, advancements in diagnostic tools are forthcoming. Innovations like microfluidic chips or novel blood assays could provide quick readouts of oxidative stress status and mineral levels in the follicular fluid or serum. A clinician might soon use a point-of-care test to gauge a woman's oxidative score and then decide if she needs extra selenium/zinc before proceeding with an IVF cycle, a level of precision that would represent a significant innovation in personalized care. On the horizon is also the possibility of gene editing or gene therapy to tackle infertility causes – and interestingly, some of the genes being discovered, like SEPHS1 for selenium metabolism, could become targets. While it's far-fetched at the moment to edit a selenium metabolism gene to improve fertility, the knowledge gained could lead to specialized supplements that bypass certain genetic blockades. Finally, integrative treatment protocols are evolving. Fertility clinics of the future might incorporate a dedicated nutrient optimization phase in every infertility treatment plan. This could be a formal 1–3 months program of dietary coaching, monitored supplementation such as using digital pill trackers, and stress reduction before any invasive treatments. This concept is innovative in that it restructures the infertility treatment timeline to ensure the patient's body is biochemically primed. Selenium and zinc would be key components of such a program, given their importance in reducing oxidative stress and supporting endocrine function. In summary, new innovations in infertility treatment involving selenium and zinc range from cutting-edge tech, nanoparticle delivery, advanced diagnostics, to holistic protocol design, nutrition-focused pretreatment. These innovations aim to harness the full potential of selenium and zinc in a more targeted, efficient manner, thereby improving fertility outcomes. As research progresses, some of these ideas – once futuristic – may become standard practice, reflecting a blending of nutrition science with reproductive technology for better patient care (49–52).

7.13 POTENTIAL FOR PERSONALIZED APPROACHES IN FERTILITY ENHANCEMENT

Personalized medicine is poised to transform the way selenium and zinc are used in fertility enhancement, tailoring interventions to the individual's unique physiological and genetic profile. The concept of precision nutrition in fertility is emerging: rather than giving the same supplements to everyone, doctors will determine who specifically needs selenium or zinc supplementation, in what dose, and at what time, for maximal benefit. One avenue for personalization is through genetic testing. As mentioned, genetic variations can affect how one handles micronutrients. For example, certain polymorphisms might make a woman a fast utilizer of selenium, meaning she requires more intake to achieve the same tissue levels (11). Another woman might have genetic tendencies for higher oxidative stress due to variants in antioxidant enzymes unrelated to selenium per se, and thus benefit disproportionately from selenium support. By analyzing a patient's genomic data, we could predict, for instance, that Patient A will have improved IVF outcomes only if selenium is above a certain threshold, whereas Patient B naturally has robust antioxidant defenses and won't need extra selenium. Such an approach moves away from trial-and-error and towards evidence-based customization. Another factor is baseline nutritional status and lifestyle – effectively phenotype. Some women might naturally eat selenium-rich diets, such as they regularly consume Brazil nuts or fish, and have good stores, whereas others avoid those foods and run low. A personalized plan would incorporate dietary assessment: those who do not get enough from diet could receive targeted counseling or supplements, while those already meeting needs might skip unnecessary pills. This avoids over-supplementation and focuses efforts where there's a true deficit. Additionally, the cause of infertility will guide personalized use. For instance, in a personalized approach: A woman with PCOS might get a plan emphasizing zinc, for its role in insulin and androgen regulation, along with selenium, for antioxidant and possibly thyroid support, tailored to address her specific metabolic derangements. a woman with thyroid autoantibodies might receive a higher-dose selenium plan aimed at reducing antibodies and improving thyroid function, which in turn supports regular cycles (16, 53). Conversely, a woman with hypothalamic amenorrhea due to stress/underweight, might not need much of either mineral beyond standard nutrition, but more focus on weight gain and stress reduction, again showing the personalization.

Emerging tools like AI-driven algorithms could synthesize data – combining blood tests, minerals, oxidative stress markers, genetic info, and health history to recommend a personalized supplement regimen. For example, an algorithm might output: "This patient has low plasma zinc, moderate selenium, a GPx activity slightly below optimal, and a genetic variant in GPx4; recommend 30 mg zinc and 100 µg selenium daily for 3 months." This kind of decision support is not far-fetched given rapid advances in health tech. Personalized approaches also extend to monitoring and adjusting in real time. Perhaps a patient will wear a biosensor that can indirectly gauge oxidative stress or an inflammatory marker; if levels rise indicating maybe increased oxidative load from, say, intense IVF stimulation drugs or lifestyle factors, the care team might respond by temporarily boosting antioxidant supplementation including selenium, to counteract that. The timing of supplementation could also be personalized. It might turn out that taking zinc in the follicular phase of the menstrual cycle has more impact on oocyte maturation, whereas selenium in the luteal phase might better support implantation. If so, future protocols could tailor the timing of dosing around a woman's cycle or IVF schedule for optimal effect, rather than a constant dose every day. Importantly, personalized approaches acknowledge variability in response and attempt to predict and accommodate it. Instead of the current scenario where some patients respond and some don't, the goal is to identify up front who will respond and only treat those – thereby improving the overall success rate of the intervention and avoiding unnecessary treatment in non-responders. The potential of personalization is well-captured by the idea that one day, fertility specialists might "prescribe" a specific diet and supplement combination as carefully as they prescribe hormonal doses, unique to each patient. Selenium and zinc would be central in such prescriptions for many patients, but not all, and at personalized doses. In conclusion, the future of fertility enhancement lies in personalization, and selenium and zinc supplementation strategies will be refined by this paradigm. We anticipate that ongoing research will yield the tools – whether genetic markers, blood tests, or algorithms – to deploy selenium and zinc in a targeted manner, maximizing efficacy for those who need it and avoiding one-size-fits-all approaches (16). This personalized approach holds great promise to improve outcomes and is an exciting frontier in reproductive medicine.

REFERENCES

1. Mashhadi F, Sedghi Z, Hemmat A, Rivaz R, Roudi F. Nutritional interventions for enhancing female fertility: A comprehensive review of micronutrients and their impact. *Nursing Research and Practice*. 2025;2025(1):2137328.
2. Wessells KR, Brown KH. Estimating the global prevalence of zinc deficiency: Results based on zinc availability in national food supplies and the prevalence of stunting. *PLoS One*. 2012;7(11):e50568.
3. Schaefer E, Nock D. The impact of preconceptional multiple-micronutrient supplementation on female fertility. *Clinical Medicine Insights: Women's Health*. 2019;12:1179562X19843868.
4. Garner TB, Hester JM, Carothers A, Diaz FJ. Role of zinc in female reproduction. *Biology of Reproduction*. 2021;104(5):976–94.
5. Cetin I, Berti C, Calabrese S. Role of micronutrients in the periconceptional period. *Human Reproduction Update*. 2010;16(1):80–95.
6. Ebisch I, Thomas C, Peters W, Braat D, Steegers-Theunissen R. The importance of folate, zinc and antioxidants in the pathogenesis and prevention of subfertility. *Human Reproduction Update*. 2007;13(2):163–74.
7. Dickerson E, Sathyapalan T, Knight R, Maguiness S, Killick S, Robinson J, et al. Endocrine disruptor & nutritional effects of heavy metals in ovarian hyperstimulation. *Journal of Assisted Reproduction and Genetics*. 2011;28(12):1223–8.
8. Kapper C, Stelzl P, Oppelt P, Ganhör C, Gyunesh AA, Arbeithuber B, et al. The impact of minerals on female fertility: A systematic review. *Nutrients*. 2024;16(23):4068.
9. Dugoua J-J. Vitamins, minerals, trace elements, and dietary supplements. *Clinical Pharmacology During Pregnancy*. 2013:367–82.

10. Singh AK, Chattopadhyay R, Chakravarty B, Chaudhury K. Markers of oxidative stress in follicular fluid of women with endometriosis and tubal infertility undergoing IVF. *Reproductive Toxicology.* 2013;42:116–24.
11. Yang J. The role of selenium in combating infertility: A vital yet overlooked nutrient. *ProBiologists.* 2024:40–2.
12. Yang L, Gao Y, Zhao W, Qi Y, Duo X, Wang H. The effects of trace element supplementation on glycolipid metabolism in PCOS: A systematic review and meta-analysis. *Frontiers in Nutrition.* 2025;12:1683556.
13. Buhling KJ, Grajecki D. The effect of micronutrient supplements on female fertility. *Current Opinion in Obstetrics and Gynecology.* 2013;25(3):173–80.
14. Mantovani G, Isidori A, Moretti C, Di Dato C, Greco E, Ciolli P, et al. Selenium supplementation in the management of thyroid autoimmunity during pregnancy: Results of the "SERENA study," a randomized, double-blind, placebo-controlled trial. *Endocrine.* 2019;66(3):542–50.
15. Devi N, Boya C, Chhabra M, Bansal D. N-acetyl-cysteine as adjuvant therapy in female infertility: A systematic review and meta-analysis. *Journal of Basic and Clinical Physiology and Pharmacology.* 2021;32(5):899–910.
16. Sharma P, Gupta V, Kumar K, Khetarpal P. Assessment of serum elements concentration and polycystic ovary syndrome (PCOS): Systematic review and meta-analysis. *Biological Trace Element Research.* 2022;200(11):4582–93.
17. Sabatini L, Wilson C, Lower A, Al-Shawaf T, Grudzinskas JG. Superoxide dismutase activity in human follicular fluid after controlled ovarian hyperstimulation in women undergoing in vitro fertilization. *Fertility and Sterility.* 1999;72(6):1027–34.
18. Paszkowski T, Traub A, Robinson S, McMaster D. Selenium dependent glutathione peroxidase activity in human follicular fluid. *Clinica Chimica Acta.* 1995;236(2):173–80.
19. Dahlen CR, Reynolds LP, Caton JS. Selenium supplementation and pregnancy outcomes. *Frontiers in Nutrition.* 2022;9:1011850.
20. Lima LG, Santos AAMd, Gueiber TD, Gomes RZ, Martins CM, Chaikoski AC. Relation between selenium and female fertility: A systematic review. *Revista Brasileira de Ginecologia e Obstetrícia.* 2022;44(07):701–9.
21. Omeljaniuk WJ, Socha K, Borawska MH, Charkiewicz AE, Laudański T, Kulikowski M, et al. Antioxidant status in women who have had a miscarriage. *Advances in Medical Sciences.* 2015;60(2):329–34.
22. Ajayi O, Charles-Davies M, Arinola O. Progesterone, selected heavy metals and micronutrients in pregnant Nigerian women with a history of recurrent spontaneous abortion. *African Health Sciences.* 2012;12(2):153–9.
23. Popovic J, Grujic Z, Grujic I, Bogavac M, Celic D, Popovic K, et al. Prostaglandin E2, trace elements and levels of oxidative processes in spontaneous miscarriages. *Eur Rev Med Pharmacol Sci.* 2016;20(22):4786–90.
24. Hu Y, Zhang D, Zhang Q, Yin T, Jiang T, He S, et al. Serum Cu, Zn and IL–1β levels may predict fetal miscarriage risk after IVF cycles: A nested case–control study. *Biological Trace Element Research.* 2023;201(12):5561–74.
25. Vigeh M, Yunesian M, Matsukawa T, Shamsipour M, Jeddi MZ, Rastkari N, et al. Prenatal blood levels of some toxic metals and the risk of spontaneous abortion. *Journal of Environmental Health Science and Engineering.* 2021;19(1):357–63.
26. Adams JB, Sorenson JC, Pollard EL, Kirby JK, Audhya T. Evidence-based recommendations for an optimal prenatal supplement for women in the US, part two: Minerals. *Nutrients.* 2021;13(6):1849.
27. Safiyeh FD, Mojgan M, Parviz S, Sakineh MA, Behnaz SO. The effect of selenium and vitamin E supplementation on anti-Mullerian hormone and antral follicle count in infertile women with occult premature ovarian insufficiency: A randomized controlled clinical trial. *Complement Ther Med.* 2021;56:102533.
28. Karami M, Almaghrabi S, Banasr O, Hussein K. Serum selenium levels and their relationship with insulin resistance in individuals with polycystic ovary syndrome. *Biological Trace Element Research.* 2025;203(5).
29. Ghneim HK, Al-Sheikh YA, Alshebly MM, Aboul-Soud MA. Superoxide dismutase activity and gene expression levels in Saudi women with recurrent miscarriage. *Molecular Medicine Reports.* 2016;13(3):2606–12.
30. Alharbi M. Impact of antioxidants on conventional and advanced sperm function parameters: An updated review. *Cureus.* 2024;16(2).
31. Hadrup N, Ravn-Haren G. Toxicity of repeated oral intake of organic selenium, inorganic selenium, and selenium nanoparticles: A review. *Journal of Trace Elements in Medicine and Biology.* 2023;79:127235.

32. Xia P, Chen X, Lin R, Shi X, Yang Y, Lin L. The role of oxidative balance lifestyle factors in reducing female infertility risk: Insights from a population-based study. *Frontiers in Endocrinology*. 2025;16:1444832.
33. Qazi IH, Angel C, Yang H, Pan B, Zoidis E, Zeng C-J, et al. Selenium, selenoproteins, and female reproduction: A review. *Molecules*. 2018;23(12):3053.
34. Özkaya MO, Nazıroğlu M, Barak C, Berkkanoglu M. Effects of multivitamin/mineral supplementation on trace element levels in serum and follicular fluid of women undergoing in vitro fertilization (IVF). *Biological Trace Element Research*. 2011;139(1):1–9.
35. Kominiarek MA, Rajan P. Nutrition recommendations in pregnancy and lactation. *The Medical Clinics of North America*. 2016;100(6):1199.
36. FAO, WHO. *Vitamin and Mineral Requirements in Human Nutrition: Report of a Joint FAO/WHO Expert Consultation*. Geneva: Food and Agriculture Organization; World Health Organization; 2004.
37. Li Z, Forester S, Jennings-Dobbs E, Heber D. Perspective: A comprehensive evaluation of data quality in nutrient databases. *Advances in Nutrition*. 2023;14(3):379–91.
38. Jie O, Peng P, Qiu L, Teng L, Li C, Han J, et al. Biomarkers of metal toxicity in embryos in the general population. *Journal of Clinical Laboratory Analysis*. 2019;33(8):e22974.
39. Pieczyńska J, Grajeta H. The role of selenium in human conception and pregnancy. *Journal of Trace Elements in Medicine and Biology*. 2015;29:31–8.
40. Monsen ER. Dietary reference intakes for the antioxidant nutrients: Vitamin C, vitamin E, selenium, and carotenoids. *Journal of the Academy of Nutrition and Dietetics*. 2000;100(6):637.
41. Veatch A, Brockman J, Spate V, Robertson J, Morris J. Selenium and nutrition: The accuracy and variability of the selenium content in commercial supplements. *Journal of Radioanalytical and Nuclear Chemistry*. 2005;264(1):33–8.
42. Schoofs H, Schmit J, Rink L. Zinc toxicity: Understanding the limits. *Molecules*. 2024;29(13):3130.
43. Binns CW, Lee MK, Lee AH. Problems and prospects: Public health regulation of dietary supplements. *Annual Review of Public Health*. 2018;39(1):403–20.
44. Preminger G. American Urological Association Education and Research, Inc; European Association of Urology. *Eur Urol*. 2007;52:1610–31.
45. Chavarro JE, Rich-Edwards JW, Rosner BA, Willett WC. Use of multivitamins, intake of B vitamins, and risk of ovulatory infertility. *Fertility and Sterility*. 2008;89(3):668–76.
46. Ou J, Peng P, Qiu L, Teng L, Li C, Han J, et al. Effect of lead exposure on spontaneous abortion: A case-control study. *Clinical Laboratory*. 2020;86(5).
47. Luo H, Lao T, Yang J, Gao X, Yang J, Wen S, et al. Association between dietary antioxidant intakes and female infertility: Evidence from the National Health and Nutrition Examination Survey 2013–2020. *Gynecological Endocrinology*. 2025;41(1):2590871.
48. Liu G, Dai L, Zhang R, Jia M, Lan S, Sun X, et al. Selenium nanoparticles mitigate cyclophosphamide-induced premature ovarian failures in mice by activating PI3K/Akt signaling pathway and inhibiting ferroptosis. *Journal of Ovarian Research*. 2025;18(1):257.
49. Li J, Chen M, Huang D, Li Z, Chen Y, Huang J, et al. Inhibition of selenoprotein I promotes ferroptosis and reverses resistance to platinum chemotherapy by impairing Akt phosphorylation in ovarian cancer. *MedComm*. 2024;5(12):e70033.
50. Sharma P, Khetarpal P. Genetic determinants of selenium availability, selenium-response, and risk of polycystic ovary syndrome. *Biological Trace Element Research*. 2024;202(11):4843–57.
51. Mohamed ZA, Yang J, Wen J, Jia F, Banerjee S. SEPHS1 gene: A new master key for neurodevelopmental disorders. *Clinica Chimica Acta*. 2024;562:119844.
52. Mullegama SV, Kiernan KA, Torti E, Pavlovsky E, Tilton N, Sekula A, et al. De novo missense variants in exon 9 of SEPHS1 cause a neurodevelopmental condition with developmental delay, poor growth, hypotonia, and dysmorphic features. *American Journal of Human Genetics*. 2024;111(4):778–90.
53. Hogan C, Perkins AV. Selenoproteins in the human placenta: How essential is selenium to a healthy start to life? *Nutrients*. 2022;14(3):628.

8 Vitamin D
Its Role in Hormonal Regulation and Fertility

Negar Nouri, Maryam Azizi-Kutenaei, and Farzaneh Fesahat

8.1 ITS ROLE IN HORMONAL REGULATION AND FERTILITY

Vitamin D is increasingly recognized as a potential regulator of the female hypothalamic–pituitary–gonadal axis through the vitamin D receptor (VDR), which is widely expressed in endocrine and reproductive tissues, including the hypothalamus, pituitary gland, ovaries, and uterus. Preclinical and translational studies demonstrate VDR expression in hypothalamic GnRH neurons and pituitary gonadotrophs and indicate that vitamin D signaling can modulate GnRH and gonadotropin (LH, FSH) gene expression, suggesting a pathway by which vitamin D status may influence reproductive hormone release (1–5). Preclinical and clinical data suggest that vitamin D signaling in the hypothalamus and pituitary may modulate GnRH and pituitary gonadotropin (especially LH) secretion, which is critical for maintaining the endocrine environment needed for ovulation and regular menstrual cycles (6, 7). Vitamin D acts via VDR, which is expressed in ovarian follicles (granulosa and cumulus cells) and in the endometrial tissue, and experimental as well as translational data indicate that vitamin D signaling may directly influence follicular development and uterine receptivity (8–10).

Vitamin D may influence ovarian steroidogenesis and follicular development via VDR expressed in granulosa and cumulus cells. Experimental data support effects on steroidogenic gene expression and granulosa cell function; however, the impact on aromatase expression and estrogen synthesis remains inconsistent, underscoring the need for further research before definitive conclusions can be drawn (11, 12). Although evidence remains limited and not entirely consistent, multiple studies report that sufficient vitamin D is associated with more robust luteal progesterone production, likely through VDR-mediated modulation of steroidogenic enzymes in granulosa and luteal cells. Given progesterone's central role in endometrial receptivity and early pregnancy, vitamin D may indirectly support menstrual cycle regulation and fertility (9, 13). In vitro evidence indicates that calcitriol modulates granulosa cell steroidogenesis and enhances AMH-and FSH-receptor expression, supporting follicular development. Although its effects on estradiol and progesterone production vary between models, these molecular findings collectively suggest a regulatory role for vitamin D in folliculogenesis and ovarian function (3, 12).

Some clinical and observational studies report that adequate vitamin D status is associated with more regular menstrual cycles and better ovulatory function, while vitamin D deficiency has been linked to menstrual irregularities. However, findings are not fully consistent and causality has not been definitively established (14, 15). While a few studies suggest that women with lower serum 25(OH)D may experience higher rates of menstrual irregularities such as oligomenorrhea or amenorrhea, data are sparse, methodologically heterogeneous, and in many cases not conclusive. More robust, prospective studies are needed before a firm link can be asserted (16, 17). Given the predominantly observational nature of the evidence and its vulnerability to confounding, these findings indicate association rather than causation. Overall, they suggest that vitamin D sufficiency may help maintain normal reproductive endocrine rhythms through coordinated effects on ovarian and hypothalamic–pituitary pathways (3, 8, 18).

There is growing evidence that vitamin D status is altered in many women with PCOS, and that vitamin D deficiency is common in this population. PCOS characterized by insulin resistance, hyperandrogenism, and oligo- or anovulation, frequently overlaps with metabolic and endocrine disturbances. Several observational studies and a recent Mendelian randomization analysis suggest that lower 25(OH)D levels are associated with higher risk of PCOS, although causality and underlying mechanisms remain under investigation (5, 19, 20). Vitamin D contributes to insulin homeostasis, and deficiency has been associated with increased insulin resistance, which in turn exacerbates the hormonal disturbances of PCOS (5). Supplementation in vitamin D–deficient women with PCOS has been shown in some trials to improve insulin sensitivity and reduce androgen levels (21). In one clinical trial, the addition of vitamin D and calcium to metformin therapy in women with PCOS improved menstrual regularity and increased ovulation frequency. Several cohort studies have also reported that vitamin D deficiency is associated with lower

DOI: 10.1201/9781003741541-8

AMH concentrations, suggesting a potential link between vitamin D status and ovarian reserve. Conversely, interventional studies in vitamin D–deficient women have demonstrated increases in AMH and improvements in ovarian reserve markers after supplementation, although evidence for enhanced live birth outcomes remains limited (22–25).

8.2 CLINICAL APPLICATIONS IN INFERTILITY TREATMENT

Given its emerging role in reproductive physiology, vitamin D has been increasingly explored for several potential clinical applications in infertility management. Reproductive endocrinologists now frequently assess vitamin D status in women with ovulatory dysfunction, endometrial receptivity disorders, or those undergoing assisted reproductive technologies. Current evidence suggests that vitamin D deficiency may negatively influence ovulation, endometrial inflammation, implantation processes, and early pregnancy support. Accordingly, key areas where vitamin D may have potential clinical relevance include preconception optimization and ovulatory disorders, endometriosis and implantation, assisted reproductive technologies (ART), luteal-phase support and early pregnancy, and general fertility preparation (1, 3, 4, 8, 13, 26).

In women with ovulatory infertility or irregular cycles, assessment of vitamin D status is often recommended. Correction of vitamin D deficiency may help restore ovulation in some individuals. In vitamin D–deficient women with PCOS, a common cause of infertility, supplementation has been shown in several studies to improve ovulatory function and menstrual cyclicity (13, 27, 28). Clinical data suggest that treating vitamin D deficiency in PCOS can reduce insulin resistance and modify elevated AMH and androgen levels, thereby supporting normalization of ovulatory cycles (19). Consequently, vitamin D is frequently used as an adjunct therapy in PCOS-related infertility, alongside lifestyle modification, metformin, or ovulation induction agents, with the aim of increasing the likelihood of spontaneous conception or improving response to fertility drugs. It is important to emphasize that vitamin D is not a substitute for established PCOS treatments but rather a complementary measure (13).

Endometriosis, another infertility-associated condition, is characterized by chronic inflammation and impaired endometrial receptivity. The anti-inflammatory and immunomodulatory actions of vitamin D have prompted interest in its use in this population. Vitamin D can modulate immune responses in reproductive tissues, downregulating pro-inflammatory cytokines such as TNF-α and IL-6 and enhancing anti-inflammatory pathways (29, 30). These effects could theoretically improve endometrial receptivity. Observational studies and small clinical trials have suggested that vitamin D supplementation may augment endometrial receptivity and reduce inflammatory markers in women with endometriosis, potentially improving implantation and pregnancy rates (4). However, results are mixed, with some trials showing limited or no symptomatic benefit (31). Therefore, vitamin D repletion in endometriosis is best viewed as a low-risk supportive intervention rather than a proven disease-modifying therapy. Given its low-risk profile, many clinicians still recommend correcting vitamin D deficiency in women with endometriosis as part of a broader strategy to optimize the uterine environment.

Perhaps the most studied application of vitamin D in infertility involves ART, particularly in vitro fertilization (IVF). Numerous studies reports that women with sufficient vitamin D levels have better IVF outcomes, including higher implantation and pregnancy rates (32, 33), although not all investigations agree. As a result, many fertility centers now incorporate vitamin D testing (25[OH]D measurement) into the pre-IVF evaluation. When low levels are identified, supplementation is typically initiated before and during the IVF cycle to achieve sufficiency by the time of embryo transfer (34). This approach is supported by evidence that VDR is expressed in human endometrium and ovarian tissue, and that follicular fluid vitamin D levels appear to correlate with follicle health and possibly oocyte quality in some studies (35–39). By correcting deficiency, clinicians aim to remove one modifiable barrier to success. Vitamin D is therefore used as a non-invasive adjunct in ART protocols, for example, supplementing deficient patients during the weeks leading up to controlled ovarian stimulation or prior to frozen embryo transfer. At present, professional guidelines generally stop short of recommending vitamin D solely to improve live birth rates in ART, but they do support correcting deficiency as part of comprehensive preconception care.

Vitamin D may also play a supportive role in the luteal phase and early pregnancy, particularly in women with recurrent pregnancy loss or implantation failure. Because vitamin D contributes to corpus luteum progesterone production and modulates immune tolerance during early gestation, adequate levels might reduce the risk of implantation failure and early miscarriage (4, 40). Some practitioners include vitamin D in comprehensive luteal support regimens (alongside progesterone supplementation) for patients with previous IVF failures, although high-quality evidence for reduced miscarriage risk remains limited. A meta-analysis in women with PCOS reported that vitamin D supplementation was associated with lower early miscarriage rates among those who conceived, supporting a potential role in early pregnancy maintenance. These findings are encouraging but should still be interpreted with caution until confirmed by large, well-designed trials (41, 42).

Beyond specific diagnoses, vitamin D repletion has become part of a general fertility optimization strategy. Vitamin D deficiency is common worldwide; estimates suggest that a substantial proportion of pregnant women and infertile women have insufficient levels. Addressing this deficiency is therefore regarded as an important component of preparing the body for pregnancy. For any woman seeking conception, especially those with limited sun exposure, higher BMI, or particular ethnic backgrounds, fertility specialists may recommend preventive vitamin D supplementation. Adequate vitamin D status in early pregnancy has also been linked to a lower risk of obstetric complications such as pre-eclampsia and gestational diabetes in observational data. In this context, vitamin D is viewed not as a fertility drug, but as a low-cost, low-risk intervention that may help optimize endocrine and immune conditions for conception and healthy pregnancy (43–45).

Overall, in clinical practice vitamin D is used both as a corrective and preventive measure in women's infertility treatment. It is not sufficient as a stand-alone therapy, but repletion of vitamin D is considered a rational, supportive strategy aimed at normalizing the hormonal and immunological environment required for successful reproduction. Clinicians should explicitly communicate that vitamin D is an adjunctive measure that complements – rather than replaces – standard infertility treatments.

8.2.1 Current Clinical Evidence Supporting the Use of Vitamin D

Evidence accumulated between 2019 and 2025 generally supports a beneficial role of vitamin D in female fertility, although some findings remain inconclusive and important knowledge gaps persist. Observational studies, randomized controlled trials (RCTs), and meta-analyses have explored the relationship between vitamin D status, supplementation, and reproductive outcomes (46, 47).

Observational studies consistently demonstrate that adequate vitamin D status is associated with more favorable fertility outcomes. Several meta-analyses in women undergoing ART have reported that women who are vitamin D replete have higher pregnancy and live birth rates than those who are deficient or insufficient (48). In contrast, vitamin D deficiency has repeatedly been linked to lower chances of natural conception and poorer IVF success (49). Because these studies are observational, they cannot establish causality; vitamin D status may also reflect broader aspects of health, lifestyle, or nutrition that independently influence fertility. Nevertheless, the consistency of these associations across diverse populations suggests that vitamin D sufficiency is a favorable prognostic factor for fertility.

To address causality, several RCTs have examined the effects of vitamin D supplementation in infertile women. A number of these trials, including a meta-analysis of women with vitamin D deficiency undergoing IVF, have reported that vitamin D supplementation can improve early IVF outcomes such as biochemical pregnancy in some settings (50, 51). However, the evidence for improvements in clinical pregnancy and live birth is less robust, with several trials failing to show statistically significant benefits for these harder endpoints (52). Most available RCTs are relatively small and vary in dosing, duration, baseline vitamin D levels, and patient characteristics, which limits the strength of conclusions. Overall, current trial data suggest that vitamin D supplementation may have modest beneficial effects on certain IVF outcomes, particularly in deficient women, but larger and more rigorous studies are needed to clarify its impact on live birth (Table 8.1).

Women with PCOS have been a major focus of vitamin D research due to the high prevalence of deficiency and the syndrome's strong endocrine–metabolic component (54). Meta-analyses of RCTs in PCOS suggest that vitamin D supplementation is associated with improvements in several reproductive and metabolic parameters, including ovulation rates, menstrual regularity, early pregnancy outcomes, and androgen and gonadotropin levels (7, 19, 54). Although effect sizes vary between studies and some trials have methodological limitations, the overall direction of effect appears favorable. These benefits were observed regardless of concomitant use of ovulation

Table 8.1: Summary of Clinical Evidence on Vitamin D and Female Fertility

Study Type	Population	Vitamin D Dose/Level	Outcome Measured	Main Finding	Reference
Randomized Controlled Trial (RCT)	PCOS patients undergoing IUI	Single 300,000 IU IM dose	Endometrial thickness	Significant improvement in endometrial thickness	(53)
Donor–Recipient Cohort Study	Women receiving donor oocytes	<20 vs. >30 ng/mL serum 25(OH)D	Clinical pregnancy, live birth	Higher pregnancy and live birth in vitamin D–replete group	(38)
Meta-Analysis (5 RCTs)	Women undergoing IVF	Various supplementation regimens	Biochemical and clinical pregnancy	Modest improvement; inconsistent for live birth	(33)

induction agents or ART in many trials, suggesting that vitamin D may exert an independent supportive effect in this population (55, 56). As a result, the evidence supports routine assessment and correction of vitamin D deficiency in vitamin D–deficient women with PCOS, particularly when combined with established therapies (57).

Not all studies have demonstrated clear benefits of vitamin D. Several cohort studies found no statistically significant association between serum vitamin D levels and IVF outcomes, possibly due to small sample sizes, heterogeneous patient populations, differing definitions of "sufficiency," or unmeasured confounders (58–61). Some cohort studies and reviews report no consistent association between vitamin D status (mostly serum 25-OH-D) and IVF/ART outcomes. The few studies measuring follicular-fluid vitamin D tend to show a positive correlation with pregnancy outcomes, but data remain limited and heterogenous, so definitive conclusions cannot yet be drawn (58, 62). These inconsistencies underscore that the overall evidence, while generally positive, is not entirely uniform. They also highlight the need for standardized definitions of vitamin D sufficiency, harmonized outcome measures, and adequately powered multicenter trials. Importantly, no trials suggest that vitamin D sufficiency is harmful; at worst, supplementation appears neutral in some cohorts, while multiple studies report clear benefits.

Mechanistic research provides strong biological plausibility for vitamin D's influence on fertility. Laboratory studies have shown that vitamin D stimulates expression of genes involved in hormone synthesis and endometrial receptivity, including HOXA10, which is crucial for implantation (63, 64). Women with vitamin D deficiency have been reported to exhibit lower endometrial HOXA10 expression during the implantation window, potentially compromising embryo implantation, whereas sufficient vitamin D is associated with normal HOXA10 expression (65). Vitamin D also modulates the endometrial immune environment, shifting cytokine profiles toward a more implantation-friendly pattern (66). These mechanistic findings align with clinical observations, such as lower miscarriage rates and improved endometrial thickness in some supplemented groups, further supporting a causal role. Nonetheless, translation from molecular mechanisms to clinical outcomes is complex, and mechanistic data should be viewed as supportive rather than definitive proof of clinical benefit.

8.2.2 Case Studies: Successful Integration of Vitamin D in Assisted Reproductive Technologies

Real-world clinical cases and specific studies help illustrate how vitamin D integration can positively influence fertility treatment outcomes. Below are a few representative examples that highlight successful use of vitamin D in assisted reproductive technologies and related scenarios:

A clinically relevant vignette can be drawn directly from the donor–recipient IVF cohort analyzed by Rudick et al. (2014). In this model – where all oocytes originate from young, healthy donors – the embryo-related variables are effectively standardized, allowing the influence of the recipient's uterine environment to be isolated. As reported in the study, recipients with vitamin D deficiency (25(OH)D <20 ng/mL) demonstrated markedly poorer reproductive outcomes despite receiving high-quality donor embryos. Their clinical pregnancy rate was only 37%, and live birth rate approximately 31%, underscoring a pattern consistent with a "difficult IVF case" in which repeated implantation failure may occur despite optimal embryo quality. In contrast, recipients who achieved vitamin D replete status (>30 ng/mL) exhibited dramatically improved results, with a 78% clinical pregnancy rate and 59% live birth rate, even after adjustment for race, BMI, and embryo fragmentation. This more than twofold difference, observed under rigorously controlled donor egg conditions, provides compelling clinical evidence that vitamin D status directly influences endometrial receptivity rather than embryo development. Accordingly, this case-derived pattern illustrates how correcting a modifiable deficiency may shift the trajectory of an otherwise challenging IVF history, supporting current clinical practice in which many infertility specialists optimize 25(OH)D levels prior to embryo transfer to enhance the probability of implantation and ongoing pregnancy (38).

A clinically relevant case can be derived from the randomized, double-blind, placebo-controlled trial conducted by Asadi et al., which evaluated 110 infertile women with PCOS undergoing intrauterine insemination (IUI). All participants had baseline vitamin D deficiency, with mean serum 25(OH)D levels around 12 ng/mL in both groups prior to randomization. Following administration of a single 300,000 IU intramuscular dose of vitamin D3, and after a 2-month interval allowing for physiologic repletion, women entered their stimulated IUI cycle. In this real-world clinical scenario, vitamin D supplementation produced a significant increase in endometrial thickness compared with placebo (mean 8.70 ± 2.28 mm vs. 7.59 ± 1.74 mm; $p = 0.003$), as reported in Table 8.2 of the study. The improvement in endometrial proliferation occurred despite no meaningful differences between groups in the number of dominant follicles, gonadotropin dose, estradiol levels, or cycle duration, indicating a direct effect of vitamin D on uterine lining development rather than ovarian response. Although clinical pregnancy rates were not statistically different (38.2% vs. 32.7%; RR = 1.17, 95% CI 0.58–2.77), the pattern observed in this case illustrates how correcting a modifiable micronutrient deficiency can enhance a key determinant of IUI success – namely endometrial receptivity. Clinically, this vignette underscores the rationale for assessing and correcting vitamin D insufficiency in PCOS patients with thin endometrium, as vitamin D–induced improvements in endometrial thickness may remove an important limiting factor in achieving pregnancy during IUI cycles (53).

A clinically relevant population-level case can be drawn from the case–control study by Nikbakht et al. (2016), which evaluated serum vitamin D status in 314 infertile women. The investigators compared 157 infertile women with PCOS to 157 infertile women with non-PCOS etiologies and found a striking disparity in vitamin D deficiency between the two groups. According to Table 8.2 of the study, PCOS patients exhibited significantly lower mean serum 25(OH)D concentrations (13 ± 11.5 ng/mL) compared with non-PCOS infertile women (25.07 ± 20.7 ng/mL; $P < 0.0001$). Furthermore, 80.8% of infertile women with PCOS were vitamin D– deficient (<20 ng/mL), in contrast to 49.7% of women in the control group. Notably, seasonal patterns differed between groups: vitamin D levels in PCOS women showed no significant seasonal variation ($P = 0.4$), whereas non-PCOS infertile women demonstrated significantly higher 25(OH)D levels in autumn ($P = 0.02$). Logistic regression analysis revealed that each 1 ng/mL increase in serum vitamin D was associated with a 5.5% reduction in the odds of having PCOS-related infertility (adjusted OR = 0.95; 95% CI: 0.93–0.97). Collectively, this dataset illustrates a clinically meaningful "population case," showing that vitamin D deficiency is not only markedly more prevalent among infertile PCOS patients but also independently associated with PCOS-related infertility. This pattern supports the increasingly common clinical practice of routine vitamin D assessment in women presenting with PCOS-associated subfertility (67).

Table 8.2: Recommended Vitamin D Supplementation Protocols in Infertility Care

Baseline 25(OH)D Level	Recommended Dose	Duration	Target Level	Notes
<20 ng/mL (Deficiency)	50,000 IU weekly	6–8 weeks	≥30 ng/mL	Reassess levels after 8–12 weeks
20–30 ng/mL (Insufficiency)	2000–4000 IU daily	Continuous	30–40 ng/mL	Safe for long-term use under supervision
>30 ng/mL (Sufficient)	1000–2000 IU daily	Maintenance	30–50 ng/mL	Avoid high-dose bolus therapy

A population-based clinical case can be drawn from the case–control study by Al-Jaroudi et al., which evaluated vitamin D status among 181 women, including 83 subfertile patients and 98 pregnant controls. The findings provide a compelling real-world illustration of how hypovitaminosis D may contribute to reproductive challenges. As shown in the results section of the study, vitamin D deficiency (<20 ng/mL) was significantly more prevalent among subfertile women than among controls (59.0% vs. 40.4%; $p < 0.01$), highlighting a substantial disparity in micronutrient status between the two groups. Dietary assessments further demonstrated that subfertile women consumed significantly fewer vitamin D–rich foods, with lower intake in 9 of 14 key dietary sources, including wild salmon, fortified milk, eggs, yogurt, and butter (all $p < 0.001$). Moreover, calcium supplement use, an important cofactor in vitamin D physiology, was reported by only 10% of subfertile women compared with 64.6% of controls ($p < 0.001$). Together, these patterns form a clinically meaningful vignette: subfertile women not only exhibit higher rates of biochemical vitamin D deficiency but also demonstrate systematically lower intake of vitamin D and calcium, both of which are essential for reproductive endocrine function and endometrial health. The authors conclude that optimizing vitamin D and calcium status is recommended for women of reproductive age, a conclusion that aligns with broader mechanistic and clinical evidence linking adequate vitamin D levels with improved fertility potential (68).

A clinically meaningful case can be derived from the donor–recipient IVF model analyzed by Rudick et al., which uniquely isolates the uterine environment as the primary determinant of implantation by controlling for embryo quality through the universal use of young donor oocytes. In this well-characterized cohort of 99 egg-donor recipients, vitamin D status emerged as a strong predictor of reproductive outcome. As reported in the results section, women who were vitamin D deficient or insufficient ([25(OH)D] <30 ng/mL) had markedly lower adjusted clinical pregnancy rates of 37%, compared with 78% among women who were vitamin D replete (>30 ng/mL). A similar pattern was observed for live birth rates, which increased from 31% among non-replete recipients to 59% among those with replete vitamin D levels. Importantly, vitamin D status was not associated with ovarian stimulation parameters, fertilization rates, blastomere number, embryo fragmentation, or the number of embryos transferred, indicating that the observed differences were unlikely to be embryo-related and instead reflected differences in endometrial receptivity. This interpretation is strengthened by the authors' mechanistic summary, noting that vitamin D signaling in the endometrium regulates implantation-critical genes such as calbindin, osteopontin, and HOXA10, and modulates immune activity by reducing pro-inflammatory cytokines produced by decidual immune cells. Together, these findings form a robust real-world clinical vignette illustrating that repletion of vitamin D may shift a challenging IVF trajectory toward success, not by altering embryo competence, but by optimizing the maternal endometrial environment upon which implantation depends (38).

These case studies and examples demonstrate that vitamin D integration in ART is associated with improved outcomes in various contexts. Whether it's through retrospective analyses showing doubled pregnancy rates, proactive supplementation in known deficiency states, or even observations of nature's "experiment" with seasons, the narrative is consistent: ensuring adequate vitamin D can be a simple yet powerful adjunct in infertility treatment. Such successes have led to vitamin D gaining a place in the standard checklist for managing infertility patients.

8.2.3 Best Practices for Incorporating Vitamin D into Infertility Treatment Protocols

Based on the current body of evidence and emerging clinical consensus, a number of best practices have been proposed for the effective incorporation of vitamin D into infertility care. Foremost among these is the routine screening of vitamin D status in women undergoing evaluation for infertility or preparing for assisted reproductive treatments such as IVF (69, 70). Measurement of serum 25-hydroxyvitamin D is particularly important in high-risk groups, including women with limited sunlight exposure, higher body mass index, or underlying conditions such as polycystic ovary syndrome (56, 71–73). Early identification of deficiency or insufficiency allows sufficient time for correction before treatment initiation. Reflecting this need, many fertility clinics now include vitamin D testing as part of the standard preconception or pre-IVF assessment, acknowledging that a substantial proportion of patients require supplementation; indeed, a 2019 ART cohort demonstrated that only 16% of women had normal vitamin D levels, with the remainder falling into insufficient or deficient categories (74, 75).

A second-best practice involves targeting an optimal vitamin D range before conception attempts. Although there is no universal consensus regarding the ideal reproductive threshold, many clinicians aim to achieve at least a sufficient level – commonly defined as ≥30 ng/mL – based on studies in which concentrations above this level correlated with improved IVF and pregnancy outcomes. Some clinics further define an optimal therapeutic window of 30–50 ng/mL for reproductive purposes, aligning with broader health recommendations. Levels below 20 ng/mL are widely recognized as deficient and clearly undesirable in infertility settings, given that deficiency has been associated with lower pregnancy rates and a possible increase in miscarriage risk. Consequently, correction of deficiency and confirmation that serum levels have reached the target range before or during treatment is considered an essential component of fertility optimization (9, 75–77).

Standardized supplementation strategies form a third component of recommended practice. Once insufficiency or deficiency is identified, clinicians typically initiate vitamin D3 replacement using protocols tailored to baseline levels. For moderate deficiency (20–30 ng/mL), daily oral doses of 1000–2000 IU are commonly prescribed, whereas more severe deficiency (<20 ng/mL) is often treated with high-dose regimens such as 50,000 IU once weekly for 6 to 8 weeks, followed by a maintenance dose. Some fertility centers recommend precisely this approach when serum levels are ≤20 ng/mL, with reassessment approximately 3 months later. These regimens align with established endocrine guidelines and are considered safe for both non-pregnant and pregnant patients when administered under clinical supervision. Complementary lifestyle measures such as moderate sun exposure and diets enriched with vitamin D–containing foods (fatty fish, fortified dairy, egg yolks) are also routinely advised, and supplementation plans are personalized when necessary, especially for individuals with malabsorption syndromes or elevated BMI, recognizing that the fat-soluble nature of vitamin D can lead to sequestration in adipose tissue (78–81).

Attention to the timing of repletion within the treatment pathway represents another best practice. Ideally, vitamin D should be corrected several months before planned fertility interventions: for IVF cycles, a 2- to 3-month window prior to ovarian stimulation is preferred to allow serum levels to rise adequately (82–85). If insufficiency is detected only after a cycle has started, supplementation should commence promptly, although its full physiologic benefits, whether for oocyte competence or endometrial receptivity, may not be realized until a subsequent cycle. In some cases, fertility specialists may defer an elective IVF cycle when severe deficiency is identified, particularly in contexts where evidence suggests reduced success rates in vitamin D–deficient patients. For individuals attempting to enhance natural fertility, a 3-month course of supplementation is commonly recommended, reflecting the approximate duration of folliculogenesis and endometrial regeneration (28, 61, 86, 87).

Vitamin D is also increasingly conceptualized as one component of an integrated infertility-treatment strategy (69, 88). It can be used safely alongside ovulation induction agents such as clomiphene or letrozole, insulin-sensitizing medications such as metformin, and nutritional supplements including folic acid or omega-3 fatty acids (1, 89). Synergistic effects have been observed in certain populations; for example, combining vitamin D and calcium with metformin in women with PCOS has been shown to improve menstrual regularity more effectively than metformin alone (32, 89). A holistic approach also calls for consideration of vitamin D status in male partners, as accumulating evidence links low vitamin D levels in men with impaired semen parameters and reduced IVF success rates. Managing vitamin D deficiency in both partners may therefore enhance overall reproductive potential (90, 91).

Ongoing monitoring and attention to safety constitute additional critical elements of best practice. Serum levels should be reassessed every 3 to 6 months during repletion and maintenance therapy to ensure adequate but not excessive replacement (92, 93). Although vitamin D toxicity is uncommon and typically associated with prolonged intake of extremely high doses, clinicians nevertheless advise patients about symptoms of hypercalcemia and emphasize adherence to recommended dosing limits (44, 94). Maintaining serum concentrations within the mid-normal range (approximately 30–50 ng/mL) is generally considered both safe and sufficient for reproductive benefits. During pregnancy, continuation of maintenance-level supplementation is advised, particularly because gestation may increase physiological requirements, and routine prenatal vitamins often contain insufficient amounts to correct pre-existing deficiency (65, 95, 96).

Finally, patient education and adherence are integral to successful implementation of these practices. When patients understand the relevance of vitamin D not only for skeletal health but also for reproductive function, hormonal balance, and pregnancy outcomes, their engagement with supplementation protocols tends to improve. Fertility clinicians commonly include vitamin D discussions as part of a broader lifestyle optimization strategy, addressing nutrition, body weight, smoking cessation, and general wellness, to maximize the likelihood of conception. Clear communication, supported by evidence-based rationale, helps ensure that patients follow supplementation plans consistently and attend scheduled monitoring, enabling them to benefit fully from the potential reproductive advantages associated with adequate vitamin D status (9, 33, 97).

8.3 SAFETY, DOSAGE, AND EFFICACY

8.3.1 Recommended Dosages

Guidelines for vitamin D intake in the general population provide a starting point for recommendations in infertility, but specific dosing for fertility enhancement may differ from standard dietary guidelines. The Institute of Medicine (IOM) recommends 400–800 IU of vitamin D per day for adults to maintain overall health, aiming for serum 25(OH)D levels of about 50–75 nmol/L (20–30 ng/mL) (98). These baseline recommendations ensure sufficient vitamin D for bone and metabolic health, but many experts argue that for optimal cellular and reproductive health, a serum level closer to 30 ng/mL is desirable (18). Indeed, a serum 25(OH)D of 30 ng/mL is often cited as a target for "optimal" status in contexts beyond bone health, including fertility (98, 99).

In infertility care, recommended dosages of vitamin D tend to be higher than the minimum daily allowance, especially for individuals with deficiency. Many women presenting with infertility are found to have insufficient vitamin D levels; for instance, up to 67–85% of women with PCOS are vitamin D deficient. Accordingly, clinical practice guidelines for PCOS patients advise supplementing with 2000–4000 IU of vitamin D daily until normal vitamin D levels are achieved. This range (2000–4000 IU) is considered safe for chronic use and effective for gradually raising serum 25(OH)D into the sufficient range in most adults (56, 100, 101).

Vitamin D repletion protocols for those with moderate to severe deficiency often employ short-term high-dose regimens. Commonly, 50,000 IU weekly for 6–8 weeks is used to rapidly replete vitamin D stores, followed by a maintenance dose (102). In reproductive medicine research, a variety of dosing strategies have been explored. Studies have employed doses from as low as 1000 IU daily up to high-dose interventions (e.g. 20,000 IU weekly or more), reflecting a lack of consensus on the optimal dose for fertility outcomes (69, 103). A previous investigation noted that trial regimens varied widely – some using 1000–2000 IU per day for several months, others using intermittent mega-doses (such as 50,000 IU weekly) – and no single dosage has emerged as clearly superior for improving fertility metrics (Table 8.2) (104). This variation underscores the need to tailor dosing to the patient's baseline vitamin D status and treatment timeframe.

Nevertheless, some patterns can be drawn from recent evidence. The aforementioned 2023 meta-analysis found that the interventions most successful at improving pregnancy rates were those that achieved substantial increases in vitamin D levels in deficient women (69). Specifically, better outcomes were seen when women with low vitamin D (<30 ng/mL) received either high cumulative doses (total 10,000–50,000 IU or even 50,000–500,000 IU over the course of treatment) or a daily dose in the range of 1000–10,000 IU for 1–2 months (69). Based on a former study, weekly doses of 5000 IU were associated with higher ovulation and pregnancy rates in PCOS patients (55). These findings suggest that moderate to high dosing is often required to impact fertility, especially when starting from deficiency.

Given the high prevalence of vitamin D insufficiency and deficiency among women undergoing infertility evaluation, several recent reviews recommend assessing serum 25(OH)D levels as part of preconception or pre-IVF work-up. Clinical trials and meta-analyses conducted between 2019 and 2025 have used a wide range of supplementation regimens from daily doses of 1000–4000 IU to intermittent high-dose protocols such as 50,000 IU weekly, reflecting the absence of a universally accepted dosing standard. Many studies consider a serum 25(OH)D level above 30 ng/mL as the threshold for sufficiency, and supplementation in deficient women has frequently been aimed at achieving this target range (69, 105). In patients with marked vitamin D deficiency, short-term repletion protocols using intermittent high-dose oral vitamin D3, such as 50,000 IU once weekly for several weeks, have been widely applied in general clinical practice and demonstrated to safely raise serum 25(OH)D concentrations under appropriate monitoring. Regulatory agencies including the Institute of Medicine and the European Food Safety Authority define 4000 IU/day as the tolerable upper intake level for unsupervised long-term use, whereas multiple clinical studies report that higher short-term doses (e.g., up to 10,000 IU/day) can be administered safely under medical supervision without evidence of toxicity (106–108).

8.3.2 Safety Profiles and Potential Side Effects

Vitamin D is generally very well tolerated, especially at the doses commonly used for treating deficiency or enhancing fertility (109). Unlike many pharmacological agents used in infertility treatment, vitamin D has a mild side effect profile. When taken in physiologic or moderately supraphysiologic doses, adverse effects are rare, and most adults can safely use several thousand IU daily without untoward symptoms. The safety of vitamin D supplementation is further supported by randomized trials in reproductive-age women and ART populations, in which no significant adverse events attributable to supplementation were reported (40, 87, 110, 111).

The primary safety concern with vitamin D is hypervitaminosis D, which leads to hypercalcemia, excess calcium in the blood (112). Symptoms of vitamin D–induced hypercalcemia can include nausea, vomiting, loss of appetite, excessive thirst, frequent urination, kidney stone formation, and in severe cases arrhythmias or confusion (113). However, such toxicity occurs only at very high serum 25(OH)D levels, typically well above the upper physiological range. In practice, reaching these toxic levels usually requires sustained intake of extremely high doses or a massive single overdose (114, 115). In healthy adults, available data suggest that daily vitamin D intakes up to about 10,000 IU may often be tolerated without overt toxicity, although well-defined lowest-observed-adverse-effect levels (LOAEL) remain uncertain and risk of toxicity appears to increase when 25(OH)D concentrations climb into the high end of the spectrum, possibly exceeding ~150 ng/mL, or when very high doses are sustained for extended periods (116, 117). Fertility patients supplementing within recommended ranges (e.g. ≤4000 IU daily for maintenance, or structured high-dose therapy for a short period) are highly unlikely to experience adverse effects (118). Large randomized trials using 4,000 IU daily in pregnant women, for example, found no increase in adverse outcomes compared to standard prenatal doses, reinforcing vitamin D's safety in reproduction (95, 119, 120). Clinicians generally monitor serum calcium and, in high-dose regimens, 25(OH)D, and avoid unnecessary mega-doses of vitamin D to reduce the risk of hypercalcemia. Adequate hydration and, in selected patients, monitoring of urinary calcium excretion are recommended, because vitamin D increases intestinal calcium absorption and can precipitate hypercalcemia in susceptible individuals. Reported side effects of vitamin D toxicity are usually those of hypercalcemia and include gastrointestinal symptoms (nausea, vomiting, constipation) and occasionally headache. In patients with disorders of calcium metabolism such as primary hyperparathyroidism or granulomatous diseases, vitamin D supplementation should be used cautiously with close biochemical monitoring (121–125). Another theoretical concern is that excessive bolus dosing of vitamin D might trigger regulatory mechanisms that blunt its effectiveness. For instance, one analysis suggested that giving a large dose at once can induce the enzyme CYP24A1 (24-hydroxylase), which accelerates vitamin D breakdown, potentially leading to diminishing returns (126, 127). While this is more of an efficacy concern than a safety issue per se, it underscores that more is not always better with vitamin D; dosing regimens should be rational rather than indiscriminately high.

There is no convincing evidence in humans for mutagenic or teratogenic effects of vitamin D, or for suppression of the hypothalamic, pituitary–gonadal axis, and maintaining sufficient vitamin D may support reproductive health.

8.3.3 Combining Vitamin D with Conventional Treatments

Combining vitamin D with conventional infertility treatments has gained increasing attention as a strategy to enhance therapeutic outcomes by addressing metabolic, endocrine, and immunologic pathways that standard treatments may not fully target. In women with PCOS, co-supplementation with vitamin D alongside agents such as metformin and clomiphene has been shown to improve ovulation and clinical pregnancy rates compared with standard therapy alone. Trials demonstrate that vitamin D contributes to greater reductions in insulin resistance, luteinizing hormone, and testosterone levels, and may alleviate symptoms such as oligomenorrhea and acne, suggesting a synergistic role in correcting both reproductive and metabolic disturbances common in PCOS (56, 89, 128).

In ART, vitamin D is increasingly incorporated as part of pretreatment optimization. Several clinical studies show that ensuring vitamin D sufficiency prior to ovarian stimulation can enhance endometrial receptivity and embryo developmental potential (129). A pilot randomized study using a combined nutraceutical regimen, containing vitamin D, reported improved embryo quality even among women with normal baseline vitamin D levels, indicating that vitamin D may provide benefits beyond simple repletion (87). In contrast, a large randomized trial in which women with low vitamin D received a single 600,000 IU bolus of vitamin D3 2–12 weeks before IVF/embryo transfer found no improvement in clinical pregnancy, miscarriage or live birth rates compared with placebo. Based on these findings, the authors suggested that vitamin D may need to be corrected months before IVF to cover the full folliculogenesis window, and observational data now emphasize assessment and treatment of preconception vitamin D deficiency before infertility treatment (32, 130).

Preliminary data suggest that supplementation with vitamin D may modulate endometrial receptivity via upregulation of VDR and decidualization markers, especially in challenging cases such as RIF, but large-scale clinical trials are still lacking (131).

8.4 CHALLENGES AND CONTROVERSIES

8.4.1 Regulatory and Standardization Issues

In infertility care, vitamin D is not regulated or prescribed as a formal medication with standardized therapeutic protocols. It is typically used as an over-the-counter dietary supplement, which provides easy accessibility but also introduces uncertainties regarding product quality, potency, and dosing, given the lack of drug-level regulatory oversight. (1, 132–134). In addition, there are still no standardized, unified guidelines from professional societies specifying who should be tested, when testing should be performed, and for what precise purpose in the context of infertility (1, 135). As a result, clinics and individual physicians often act on the basis of personal interpretation and preference. Even at the laboratory level there are persistent challenges: different methods for measuring 25(OH)D automated immunoassays in routine practice versus LC-MS/MS in research, can produce slightly divergent results, complicating comparison across studies and clinical decision-making (136, 137). Programs such as the Vitamin D Standardization Program aim to reduce these discrepancies so that, for example, a value of 20 ng/mL has a comparable meaning across laboratories and can be used more confidently as a threshold for deficiency and treatment (136, 138). A persistent challenge in the reproductive field is the absence of a unified definition for vitamin D deficiency. Major scientific bodies continue to use different diagnostic thresholds: while Endocrine Society guidelines classify deficiency as <20 ng/mL, insufficiency as 20–30 ng/mL, and sufficiency as >30 ng/mL, the Institute of Medicine endorses a lower cut-off of <20 ng/mL as the primary marker of inadequacy. Comparative analyses show that these discrepancies have created substantial confusion and hinder the development of consistent clinical recommendations (136, 139). Reproductive studies add further variability, with some investigations focusing solely on severe deficiency, whereas others adopt ≥30 ng/mL as an optimal target for reproductive or pregnancy-related outcomes (105, 140). Such heterogeneity complicates evidence synthesis and limits the ability to formulate enforceable infertility-specific guidelines, leaving vitamin D testing and supplementation in infertility largely discretionary (141). Additional sources of variability arise from the supplement market itself, as analyses show that the actual vitamin D content in over-the-counter formulations frequently diverges from the labeled dose (142). Insurance reimbursement for vitamin D testing also varies across health systems, and importantly, no regulatory agency like the U.S. FDA, has approved vitamin D for the specific indication of infertility treatment. Collectively, these factors indicate that until assay methods, deficiency thresholds, and clinical policy frameworks are harmonized, significant differences in practice patterns across clinics and countries will likely persist.

8.4.2 Variability in Patient Responses

A key consideration in the use of vitamin D for infertility is the marked variability in patient response. Individuals with true deficiency, for example <30 ng/mL, typically exhibit the greatest improvement after supplementation, whereas those with sufficient baseline levels gain little additional benefit. Genetic factors including polymorphisms in the vitamin D receptor, vitamin D–binding protein, and metabolic enzymes, can further alter tissue responsiveness and may, in conditions such as endometriosis, increase infertility risk or necessitate higher vitamin D levels to achieve comparable biological effects (69, 143, 144). Beyond genetics, several individual characteristics modulate treatment response, including obesity, infertility etiology, skin pigmentation, and comorbidities such as PCOS or malabsorption syndromes (57). Obesity, for instance, reduces bioavailable vitamin D due to sequestration in adipose tissue, often requiring higher or prolonged dosing (145). Conversely, patients with PCOS may experience more pronounced benefits because of vitamin D's metabolic and anti-inflammatory actions (57). Differences in absorption and dosing response also mean that some individuals benefit more from daily regimens than from intermittent high-dose therapy. Collectively, these factors highlight the need for a personalized approach that considers baseline status, metabolic and genetic background, and the underlying cause of infertility to identify those most likely to respond favorably.

8.4.3 Gaps in Research and Need for Further Studies

Despite the rapid expansion of the literature, important research gaps remain in the study of vitamin D and female infertility (146, 147). Most randomized and cohort studies of vitamin D in infertility have focused on intermediate reproductive outcomes such as ovulation, fertilization, embryo quality, implantation, biochemical pregnancy, or clinical pregnancy, while relatively few trials have been large enough or specifically powered to detect effects on live birth as the primary endpoint (50). Consequently, recent systematic reviews and meta-analyses conclude that, although vitamin D supplementation may improve some intermediate outcomes (especially clinical pregnancy in deficient women), the evidence remains insufficient to make definitive recommendations regarding live birth (69). To address this gap, authors repeatedly call for large, adequately powered, preferably multicenter randomized controlled trials that enroll infertile patients with confirmed vitamin D deficiency, randomize them to supplementation versus placebo, and incorporate stratification by infertility diagnosis together with long-term follow-up to live birth (148). There is also no consensus on the optimal supplementation regimen for infertility care. Meta-analyses show that the apparent benefits of vitamin D depend on baseline 25-hydroxyvitamin D [25(OH)D] status and vary across regimens that differ in total dose, daily dose, duration, and whether vitamin D is given alone or in combination with other agents (69). Likewise, observational and preconception studies in IVF populations highlight that even the appropriate target 25(OH)D level is still debated. It means that some data suggest that correcting deficiency (<20–30 ng/mL) is most important, but it remains unclear whether aiming simply for general sufficiency around ≥30 ng/mL is enough or whether higher ranges (40–50 ng/mL) confer additional benefit for assisted reproduction outcomes (32). Mechanistically, although the presence of VDR in reproductive tissues and plausible roles in immune modulation, hormone regulation, and endometrial receptivity are well recognized, human studies directly interrogating these pathways are still relatively scarce. Detailed investigations using endometrial biopsies, changes in cytokine profiles, follicular fluid composition, or epigenetic effects on sperm are needed. Additional gaps include limited data on male factor infertility and couple-level outcomes, as well as insufficient evidence in special populations such as women with endometriosis, recurrent pregnancy loss, or immune-mediated infertility. Furthermore, long-term outcomes related to pregnancy and offspring health, pre-eclampsia, gestational diabetes, neonatal outcomes, in relation to preconception vitamin D status are incompletely characterized, and the safety profile of very high 25(OH)D levels in the periconceptional period is not fully defined. These gaps represent opportunities for future research to clarify mechanisms, standardize dosing targets, and ultimately define the place of vitamin D within formal infertility guidelines (8, 9, 149–151).

8.5 FUTURE DIRECTIONS AND RESEARCH OPPORTUNITIES

8.5.1 Emerging Trends in Vitamin D for Reproductive Health

In recent years, vitamin D has increasingly become incorporated into routine infertility evaluations, reflecting a shift from its traditional classification as a skeletal health nutrient toward recognition of its broader endocrine, metabolic, and immunomodulatory functions in reproductive physiology. Recent evidence shows vitamin D influences ovarian function, follicular development, endometrial receptivity, and steroid hormone regulation, processes central to fertility. Accordingly, clinics are more likely to measure serum 25-hydroxyvitamin D (25(OH)D) preconceptionally or before assisted reproduction, and to recommend supplementation when deficiency is identified, driven by accumulated data on the high prevalence of vitamin D insufficiency in individuals with reproductive disorders (9). Concurrently, research efforts have expanded toward delineating vitamin D's role in specific reproductive disorders, PCOS, vitamin D is now considered a potentially beneficial adjunct owing to its effects on insulin resistance and chronic inflammation (152); in endometriosis, emerging studies emphasize its anti-proliferative and immunomodulatory actions as a possible mechanism for improving reproductive potential (97). Parallel interest in male factor infertility has further underscored the relevance of adequate vitamin D levels for semen parameters and androgen regulation (97, 153).

8.5.2 New Innovations in Infertility Treatment

A parallel emerging trend is the incorporation of vitamin D into comprehensive preconception care frameworks aimed at optimizing modifiable physiological, nutritional, and metabolic parameters prior to conception. Increasingly, fertility specialists emphasize that repletion of vitamin D, alongside folate, iron, and lifestyle modifications, should occur before pregnancy rather than after its establishment, aligning with a preventive model of reproductive care. While rigorous effectiveness data are still under development, this clinical shift is supported by growing public awareness and patient-driven requests for micronutrient assessment including vitamin D, as part of fertility planning. In addition, interdisciplinary collaborations across endocrinology, immunology, urology, and reproductive medicine, combined with increasing studies using large datasets, advanced biostatistics, and molecular insights into vitamin D's mechanisms, support the positioning of vitamin D as a relevant factor in preconception health optimization (9). At a public health level, recent reviews highlight vitamin D deficiency as a risk factor for reproductive disorders, pregnancy complications, and suboptimal fertility outcomes, suggesting that maintaining adequate vitamin D status in women of reproductive age may warrant broader preventive recommendation (97).

8.5.3 Potential for Personalized Approaches in Fertility Enhancement

Beyond technological advances in reproductive medicine, there is a growing movement to embed supportive biological interventions such as vitamin D optimization into standard infertility care pathways. Some fertility centers now implement structured, holistic protocols in which vitamin D status is assessed and corrected prior to IVF or other ART, recognizing the potential for micronutrient status to influence ovarian response, endometrial receptivity, and implantation success (9, 97). Technological tools, including digital health platforms and fertility-coaching applications, are being developed to help patients monitor adherence to supplementation and optimize their vitamin D status according to sunlight exposure, diet, and other environmental factors, though robust data on effectiveness are still emerging. On the research front, mechanistic studies indicate that vitamin D acts through VDR in reproductive tissues to modulate gene expression related to folliculogenesis, steroidogenesis, immune function, and implantation offering a biologic rationale for its inclusion in fertility treatment protocols (28, 97). Although targeted delivery systems (such as intrauterine gels, local release devices, or vaginal/uterine formulations) remain largely conceptual and under-investigated, the notion of integrating vitamin D (or its analogues) into novel therapeutic delivery frameworks represents a forward-looking direction in fertility medicine (9, 97).

REFERENCES

1. Basile S, Salvati L, Artini PG, Pinelli S. Vitamin D and infertility: A narrative review. *Gynecol Reprod Endocrinol Metable.* 2021;2:15–20.
2. Bhatti AA, Zubair H, Ali S, Jahan S, Siddiqui A, Shahab M. Vitamin D receptor antagonism on mRNA expression of reproductive hormones at hypothalamic and pituitary level of adult male rats. *Rawal Medical Journal.* 2022;47(3):751.
3. van Tienhoven XA, Ruiz de Chávez Gascón J, Cano-Herrera G, Sarkis Nehme JA, Souroujon Torun AA, Bautista Gonzalez MF, et al. Vitamin D in reproductive health disorders: A narrative review focusing on infertility, endometriosis, and polycystic ovarian syndrome. *International Journal of Molecular Sciences.* 2025;26(5):2256.
4. Farhangnia P, Noormohammadi M, Delbandi A-A. Vitamin D and reproductive disorders: A comprehensive review with a focus on endometriosis. *Reproductive Health.* 2024;21(1):61.
5. Morgante G, Darino I, Spanò A, Luisi S, Luddi A, Piomboni P, et al. PCOS physiopathology and vitamin D deficiency: Biological insights and perspectives for treatment. *Journal of Clinical Medicine.* 2022;11(15):4509.
6. Harmon Q, Kissell K, Jukic A, Kim K, Sjaarda L, Perkins N, et al. Vitamin D and reproductive hormones across the menstrual cycle. *Human Reproduction.* 2020;35(2):413–23.
7. Han Y, Cao Q, Qiao X, Huang W. Effect of vitamin D supplementation on hormones and menstrual cycle regularization in polycystic ovary syndrome women: A systemic review and meta-analysis. *Journal of Obstetrics and Gynaecology Research.* 2023;49(9):2232–44.
8. Guo J, Liu S, Wang P, Ren H, Li Y. Characterization of VDR and CYP27B1 expression in the endometrium during the menstrual cycle before embryo transfer: Implications for endometrial receptivity. *Reproductive Biology and Endocrinology.* 2020;18(1):24.
9. van Tienhoven XA, Ruiz de Chávez Gascón J, Cano-Herrera G, Sarkis Nehme JA, Souroujon Torun AA, Bautista Gonzalez MF, et al. Vitamin D in reproductive health disorders: A narrative review focusing on infertility, endometriosis, and polycystic ovarian syndrome. *International Journal of Molecular Sciences.* 2025;26(5):2256.

10. Li M, Hu S, Sun J, Zhang Y. The role of vitamin D3 in follicle development. *Journal of Ovarian Research.* 2024;17(1):148.
11. Bakhshalizadeh S, Amidi F, Shirazi R, Shabani Nashtaei M. Vitamin D3 regulates steroidogenesis in granulosa cells through AMP-activated protein kinase (AMPK) activation in a mouse model of polycystic ovary syndrome. *Cell Biochemistry and Function.* 2018;36(4):183–93.
12. Merhi Z, Doswell A, Krebs K, Cipolla M. Vitamin D alters genes involved in follicular development and steroidogenesis in human cumulus granulosa cells. *Journal of Clinical Endocrinology & Metabolism.* 2014;99(6):E1137–E45.
13. Tóth BE, Takács I, Valkusz Z, Jakab A, Fülöp Z, Kádár K, et al. Effects of vitamin D3 treatment on polycystic ovary symptoms: A prospective double-blind two-phase randomized controlled clinical trial. *Nutrients.* 2025;17(7):1246.
14. Subramanian A, Gernand AD. Vitamin D metabolites across the menstrual cycle: A systematic review. *BMC Women's Health.* 2019;19(1):19.
15. Harmon QE, Kissell K, Jukic AMZ, Kim K, Sjaarda L, Perkins NJ, et al. Vitamin D and reproductive hormones across the menstrual cycle. *Human Reproduction.* 2020;35(2):413–23.
16. Kim G-M, Jeon G-H. Serum vitamin D levels and ovarian reserve markers in secondary amenorrhea patients: Is there a link? *Obstetrics & Gynecology Science.* 2020;63(4):521–8.
17. Heidari H, Abbasi K, Feizi A, Kohan S, Amani R. Effect of vitamin D supplementation on symptoms severity in vitamin D insufficient women with premenstrual syndrome: A randomized controlled trial. *Clinical Nutrition ESPEN.* 2024;59:241–8.
18. Guo D, Ning X, Bai T, Tan L, Zhou Y, Guo Z, et al. Interaction between vitamin D homeostasis, gut microbiota, and central precocious puberty. *Frontiers in Endocrinology.* 2024;15:1449033.
19. Kazeminia M, Rajati F, Rasulehvandi R, Rajati M. The effect of vitamin D on the hormonal profile of women with polycystic ovarian syndrome: A systematic review and meta-analysis. *Middle East Fertility Society Journal.* 2024;29(1):45.
20. Gao B, Zhang C, Wang D, Li B, Shan Z, Teng W, et al. Causal association between low vitamin D and polycystic ovary syndrome: A bidirectional mendelian randomization study. *Journal of Ovarian Research.* 2024;17(1):95.
21. Shahraki SK, Emadi SF, Salarfard M, Chenari Z, Tadayyonfar F, Alikamali M. Effect of vitamin D supplementation on the severity of stress urinary incontinence in premenopausal women with vitamin D insufficiency: A randomized controlled clinical trial. *BMC Womens Health.* 2022;22(1):431.
22. Zinn C, Lenferna De La Motte K-A, Rush A, Johnson R. Assessing the nutrient status of low carbohydrate, high-fat (LCHF) meal plans in children: A hypothetical case study design. *Nutrients.* 2022;14(8):1598.
23. Vo R, Smith M, Patton N. A model of the multidimensional nature of experienced dietitian clinical decision-making in the acute care setting. *Journal of Human Nutrition and Dietetics.* 2020;33(5):614–23.
24. Dastorani M, Aghadavod E, Mirhosseini N, Foroozanfard F, Zadeh Modarres S, Amiri Siavashani M, et al. The effects of vitamin D supplementation on metabolic profiles and gene expression of insulin and lipid metabolism in infertile polycystic ovary syndrome candidates for in vitro fertilization. *Reprod Biol Endocrinol.* 2018;16(1):94.
25. Patel BP, Anderson GH, Vien S, Bellissimo N, McCrindle BW, Hamilton JK. Obesity, sex and pubertal status affect appetite hormone responses to a mixed glucose and whey protein drink in adolescents. *Clinical Endocrinology.* 2014;81(1):63–70.
26. Badihi E, Sharifi P, Moradi A, Kamrani A, Hassanzadeh A, Soltani-Zangbar MS, et al. The effect of vitamin D supplementation and vaginal probiotics on fertility in women with recurrent implantation failure: A randomized clinical trial. *Hum Immunol.* 2025;86(3):111259.
27. Várbíró S, Takács I, Tűű L, Nas K, Sziva RE, Hetthéssy JR, et al. Effects of vitamin D on fertility, pregnancy and polycystic ovary syndrome – A review. *Nutrients.* 2022;14(8):1649.
28. Berry S, Seidler K, Neil J. Vitamin D deficiency and female infertility: A mechanism review examining the role of vitamin D in ovulatory dysfunction as a symptom of polycystic ovary syndrome. *Journal of Reproductive Immunology.* 2022;151:103633.
29. Jennings BS, Hewison M. Vitamin D and endometriosis: Is there a mechanistic link? *Cell Biochemistry and Function.* 2025;43(1):e70037.
30. Kalaitzopoulos DR, Samartzis N, Daniilidis A, Leeners B, Makieva S, Nirgianakis K, et al. Effects of vitamin D supplementation in endometriosis: A systematic review. *Reproductive Biology and Endocrinology.* 2022;20(1):176.
31. Cappello C, Tremolaterra F, Pascariello A, Ciacci C, Iovino P. A randomised clinical trial (RCT) of a symbiotic mixture in patients with irritable bowel syndrome (IBS): Effects on symptoms, colonic transit and quality of life. *International Journal of Colorectal Disease.* 2013;28(3):349–58.
32. Hasan HA, Barber TM, Cheaib S, Coussa A. Preconception vitamin D level and in vitro fertilization: Pregnancy outcome. *Endocrine Practice.* 2023;29(4):235–9.

33. Zhou X, Wu X, Luo X, Shao J, Guo D, Deng B, et al. Effect of vitamin D supplementation on in vitro fertilization outcomes: A trial sequential meta-analysis of 5 randomized controlled trials. *Front Endocrinol (Lausanne)*. 2022;13:852428.
34. Kyozuka H, Murata T, Fukuda T, Imaizumi K, Yamaguchi A, Yasuda S, et al. Preconception vitamin D intake and obstetric outcomes in women using assisted reproductive technology: The Japan Environment and Children's Study. *BMC Pregnancy Childbirth*. 2022;22(1):542.
35. Wojtusik J, Johnson PA. Vitamin D regulates anti-Mullerian hormone expression in granulosa cells of the hen. *Biology of Reproduction*. 2012;86(3):91, 1–7.
36. Grzesiak M, Waszkiewicz E, Wojtas M, Kowalik K, Franczak A. Expression of vitamin D receptor in the porcine uterus and effect of 1, 25 (OH) 2D3 on progesterone and estradiol-17β secretion by uterine tissues in vitro. *Theriogenology*. 2019;125:102–8.
37. Tehrani FR, Behboudi-Gandevani S. *Vitamin D and Human Reproduction. A Critical Evaluation of Vitamin D: Basic Overview*. IntechOpen; 2017.
38. Rudick BJ, Ingles SA, Chung K, Stanczyk FZ, Paulson RJ, Bendikson KA. Influence of vitamin D levels on in vitro fertilization outcomes in donor-recipient cycles. *Fertility and Sterility*. 2014;101(2):447–52.
39. Firouzabadi RD, Rahmani E, Rahsepar M, Firouzabadi MM. Value of follicular fluid vitamin D in predicting the pregnancy rate in an IVF program. *Archives of Gynecology and Obstetrics*. 2014;289(1):201–6.
40. Bezerra Espinola MS, Bilotta G, Aragona C. Positive effect of a new supplementation of vitamin D3 with myo-inositol, folic acid and melatonin on IVF outcomes: A prospective randomized and controlled pilot study. *Gynecological Endocrinology*. 2021;37(3):251–4.
41. Mirzaei M. Effect of auriculotherapy and vitamins on the outcomes of assisted reproductive technologies and mental health in infertile women. *Health Providers*. 2025;5(1):97–108.
42. Maghsoumi-Norouzabad L, Zare Javid A, Mansoori A, Dadfar M, Serajian A. Evaluation of the effect of vitamin D supplementation on spermatogram, seminal and serum levels of oxidative stress indices in asthenospermia infertile men: A study protocol for a triple-blind, randomized controlled trial. *Nutrition Journal*. 2021;20(1):49.
43. Stothers L, Macnab AJ, Bajunirwe F, Mutabazi S, Berkowitz J. Associations between the severity of obstructive lower urinary tract symptoms and care-seeking behavior in rural Africa: A cross-sectional survey from Uganda. *PLoS One*. 2017;12(3):e0173631.
44. Lerchbaum E, Obermayer-Pietsch B. Mechanisms in endocrinology: Vitamin D and fertility: A systematic review. *European Journal of Endocrinology*. 2012;166(5):765–78.
45. Holick MF, Binkley NC, Bischoff-Ferrari HA, Gordon CM, Hanley DA, Heaney RP, et al. Evaluation, treatment, and prevention of vitamin D deficiency: An endocrine society clinical practice guideline. *Journal of Clinical Endocrinology & Metabolism*. 2011;96(7):1911–30.
46. Fernando M, Ellery SJ, Marquina C, Lim S, Naderpoor N, Mousa A. Vitamin D-binding protein in pregnancy and reproductive health. *Nutrients*. 2020;12(5):1489.
47. Dragomir RE, Toader OD, Mutu DEG, Stănculescu RV. The key role of vitamin D in female reproductive health: A narrative review. *Cureus*. 2024;16(7).
48. Chu J, Gallos I, Tobias A, Tan B, Eapen A, Coomarasamy A. Vitamin D and assisted reproductive treatment outcome: A systematic review and meta-analysis. *Human Reproduction*. 2018;33(1):65–80.
49. Cozzolino M, Busnelli A, Pellegrini L, Riviello E, Vitagliano A. How vitamin D level influences in vitro fertilization outcomes: Results of a systematic review and meta-analysis. *Fertility and Sterility*. 2020;114(5):1014–25.
50. Zhou X, Wu X, Luo X, Shao J, Guo D, Deng B, et al. Effect of vitamin D supplementation on in vitro fertilization outcomes: A trial sequential meta-analysis of 5 randomized controlled trials. *Frontiers in Endocrinology*. 2022;13:852428.
51. Polyzos NP, Anckaert E, Guzman L, Schiettecatte J, Van Landuyt L, Camus M, et al. Vitamin D deficiency and pregnancy rates in women undergoing single embryo, blastocyst stage, transfer (SET) for IVF/ICSI. *Human Reproduction*. 2014;29(9):2032–40.
52. Hu K-L, Gan K, Wang R, Li W, Wu Q, Zheng B, et al. Vitamin D supplementation prior to in vitro fertilisation in women with polycystic ovary syndrome: A protocol of a multicentre randomised, double-blind, placebo-controlled clinical trial. *BMJ Open*. 2020;10(12):e041409.
53. Asadi M, Matin N, Frootan M, Mohamadpour J, Qorbani M, Tanha FD. Vitamin D improves endometrial thickness in PCOS women who need intrauterine insemination: A randomized double-blind placebo-controlled trial. *Archives of Gynecology and Obstetrics*. 2014;289(4):865–70.
54. Song G. Vitamin D deficiency and polycystic ovary syndrome: An opinion and positioning article. *Frontiers in Nutrition*. 2025;12:1602472.
55. Yang M, Shen X, Lu D, Peng J, Zhou S, Xu L, et al. Effects of vitamin D supplementation on ovulation and pregnancy in women with polycystic ovary syndrome: A systematic review and meta-analysis. *Frontiers in Endocrinology*. 2023;14:1148556.

56. Zhang B, Yao X, Zhong X, Hu Y, Xu J. Vitamin D supplementation in the treatment of polycystic ovary syndrome: A meta-analysis of randomized controlled trials. *Heliyon*. 2023;9(3):e14291.
57. Cochrane KM, Bone JN, Williams BA, Karakochuk CD. Optimizing vitamin D status in polycystic ovary syndrome: A systematic review and dose–response meta-analysis. *Nutrition Reviews*. 2023;82(9):1176–86.
58. Eller ABP, Ejzenberg D, Monteleone PAA, Soares Jr JM, Baracat EC. Vitamin D and in vitro fertilization: A systematic review. *Journal of Assisted Reproduction and Genetics*. 2023;40(4):735–43.
59. Cozzolino M, Busnelli A, Pellegrini L, Riviello E, Vitagliano A. How vitamin D level influences in vitro fertilization outcomes: Results of a systematic review and meta-analysis. *Fertility and Sterility*. 2020;114(5):1014–25.
60. Hasan HA, Barber TM, Cheaib S, Coussa A. Preconception vitamin D level and in vitro fertilization: Pregnancy outcome. *Endocrine Practice*. 2023;29(4):235–9.
61. Ko JKY, Shi J, Li RHW, Yeung WSB, Ng EHY. 100 Years of vitamin D: Effect of serum vitamin D level before ovarian stimulation on the cumulative live birth rate of women undergoing in vitro fertilization: A retrospective analysis. *Endocrine Connections*. 2022;11(2):e210444.
62. Neysanian GH, Taebi M, Rezaeian A, Nasr-Esfahani MH, Jahangirifar M. The effects of serum and follicular fluid vitamin D levels on assisted reproductive techniques: A prospective cohort study. *Int J Fertil Steril*. 2021;15(4):280–5.
63. Ekanayake DL, Małopolska MM, Schwarz T, Tuz R, Bartlewski PM. The roles and expression of HOXA/Hoxa10 gene: A prospective marker of mammalian female fertility? *Reproductive Biology*. 2022;22(2):100647.
64. Maurya VK, Bashir K, Aggarwal M. Vitamin D microencapsulation and fortification: Trends and technologies. *Journal of Steroid Biochemistry and Molecular Biology*. 2020;196:105489.
65. Wang K, Dong F, Ma S, Bu Z. The association between vitamin D deficiency and clinical pregnancy rate in IVF patients with different age. *Frontiers in Endocrinology*. 2025;15:1485238.
66. Chukhnina EG, Kazachkov EL, Voropaeva EE, Kazachkova EA, Polina ML, Douglas NI. The effect of vitamin D metabolic status and endometrial immune patterns on the outcomes of ART programs. *International Journal of Biomedicine*. 2021;11(2):188–96.
67. Nikbakht R, Moramezi F, Farhadi S, Cheraghian B. Vitamin D deficiency in infertile women with polycystic ovary syndrome: A case-control study. *Int J Pharm Res Allied Sci*. 2016;5(2):144–50.
68. Al-Jaroudi D, Al-Banyan N, Aljohani NJ, Kaddour O, Al-Tannir M. Vitamin D deficiency among subfertile women: Case-control study. *Gynecological Endocrinology*. 2016;32(4):272–5.
69. Meng X, Zhang J, Wan Q, Huang J, Han T, Qu T, et al. Influence of vitamin D supplementation on reproductive outcomes of infertile patients: A systematic review and meta-analysis. *Reprod Biol Endocrinol*. 2023;21(1):17.
70. Iliuta F, Pijoan JI, Lainz L, Exposito A, Matorras R. Women's vitamin D levels and IVF results: A systematic review of the literature and meta-analysis, considering three categories of vitamin status (replete, insufficient and deficient). *Human Fertility*. 2022;25(2):228–46.
71. Bindayel IA. Low vitamin D level in Saudi women with polycystic ovary syndrome. *Frontiers in Nutrition*. 2021;8:611351.
72. Eftekhar M, Mirhashemi ES, Molaei B, Pourmasumi S. Is there any association between vitamin D levels and polycystic ovary syndrome (PCOS) phenotypes? *Archives of Endocrinology and Metabolism*. 2019;64(1):11–6.
73. Moini A, Dashtkoohi M, Haghollahi F, Abiri A, Tajik N. Exploring the relationship between vitamin D levels and body mass index in women with polycystic ovary syndrome. *BMC Nutrition*. 2025;11(1):1–9.
74. Maaherra Armstrong P, Augustin H, Bärebring L, Osmancevic A, Bullarbo M, Thurin-Kjellberg A, et al. Prevalence of vitamin D insufficiency and its determinants among women undergoing in vitro fertilization treatment for infertility in Sweden. *Nutrients*. 2023;15(12):2820.
75. Chu J, Gallos I, Tobias A, Robinson L, Kirkman-Brown J, Dhillon-Smith R, et al. Vitamin D and assisted reproductive treatment outcome: A prospective cohort study. *Reproductive Health*. 2019;16(1):106.
76. Xu C, An X, Tang X, Yang Y, Deng Q, Kong Q, et al. Association between vitamin D level and clinical outcomes of assisted reproductive treatment: A systematic review and dose-response meta-analysis. *Reproductive Sciences*. 2025;32(5):1446–58.
77. Pludowski P, Takacs I, Boyanov M, Belaya Z, Diaconu CC, Mokhort T, et al. Clinical practice in the prevention, diagnosis and treatment of vitamin D deficiency: A Central and Eastern European expert consensus statement. *Nutrients*. 2022;14(7):1483.
78. Kaur J, Khare S, Sizar O, Givler A. *Vitamin D Deficiency*. StatPearls [Internet]: StatPearls Publishing; 2025.
79. Zhang X, Liu Z, Xia L, Gao J, Xu F, Chen H, et al. Clinical features of vitamin D deficiency in children: A retrospective analysis. *Journal of Steroid Biochemistry and Molecular Biology*. 2020;196:105491.
80. Demay MB, Pittas AG, Bikle DD, Diab DL, Kiely ME, Lazaretti-Castro M, et al. Vitamin D for the prevention of disease: An endocrine society clinical practice guideline. *Journal of Clinical Endocrinology & Metabolism*. 2024;109(8):1907–47.

81. Bleizgys A. Vitamin D dosing: Basic principles and a brief algorithm (2021 update). *Nutrients.* 2021;13(12):4415.
82. Obstetricians ACo, Gynecologists. Vitamin D: Screening and supplementation during pregnancy. Committee Opinion No. 495. *Obstet Gynecol.* 2011;118:197–8.
83. Zhang Y, Jukic AMZ, Song H, Zhang L, Yang F, Wu S, et al. Serum vitamin D concentrations, time to pregnancy, and pregnancy outcomes among preconception couples: A cohort study in Shanghai, China. *Nutrients.* 2022;14(15):3058.
84. Luo R, Wang J, Yang Y, Xu C, Yang M, Zhu D, et al. The role of serum vitamin D in patients with normal ovarian reserve undergoing the first IVF/ICSI cycle. *Frontiers in Endocrinology.* 2023;14:1249445.
85. Budani MC, Tiboni GM. Effects of supplementation with natural antioxidants on oocytes and preimplantation embryos. *Antioxidants.* 2020;9(7):612.
86. Xu F, Wolf S, Green Or, Xu J. Vitamin D in follicular development and oocyte maturation. *Reproduction.* 2021;161(6):R129–R37.
87. Baldini GM, Russo M, Proietti S, Forte G, Baldini D, Trojano G. Supplementation with vitamin D improves the embryo quality in in vitro fertilization (IVF) programs, independently of the patients' basal vitamin D status. *Archives of Gynecology and Obstetrics.* 2024;309(6):2881–90.
88. Jiang S, Chen Z, Li L. Assessing vitamin D's impact on pregnancy success: A predictive model for assisted reproductive technology outcomes. *Frontiers in Reproductive Health.* 2025;7:1510484.
89. Zhuang L, Wei C, Jianxiang C, Zhang Y. Efficacy of vitamin D combined with metformin and clomiphene in the treatment of patients with polycystic ovary syndrome combined with infertility. *Iranian Journal of Public Health.* 2019;48(10):1802.
90. Aşır F, Duran SÇ, Afşin M, Duran E, Korak T, Şahin F. Investigation of vitamin D levels in men with suspected infertility. *Life.* 2024;14(2):273.
91. Calagna G, Catinella V, Polito S, Schiattarella A, De Franciscis P, D'Antonio F, et al. Vitamin D and male reproduction: Updated evidence based on literature review. *Nutrients.* 2022;14(16):3278.
92. Westhofen R, Weidinger G, Hoffmann P, Daxecker A, Antonitsch L. Vitamin D: Harmless nutritional supplement or serious medication? *Clinical Case Reports.* 2025;13(4):e70345.
93. Özdemir AA, Gündemir YE, Küçük M, Sarıcı DY, Elgörmüş Y, Çağ Y, et al. Vitamin D deficiency in pregnant women and their infants. *Journal of Clinical Research in Pediatric Endocrinology.* 2018;10(1):44.
94. Marcinowska-Suchowierska E, Kupisz-Urbańska M, Łukaszkiewicz J, Płudowski P, Jones G. Vitamin D toxicity–a clinical perspective. *Frontiers in Endocrinology.* 2018;9:550.
95. Hollis BW, Johnson D, Hulsey TC, Ebeling M, Wagner CL. Vitamin D supplementation during pregnancy: Double-blind, randomized clinical trial of safety and effectiveness. *Journal of Bone and Mineral Research.* 2011;26(10):2341–57.
96. Johnson DD, Wagner CL, Hulsey TC, McNeil RB, Ebeling M, Hollis BW. Vitamin D deficiency and insufficiency is common during pregnancy. *American Journal of Perinatology.* 2011;28(01):007–12.
97. Farhangnia P, Noormohammadi M, Delbandi AA. Vitamin D and reproductive disorders: A comprehensive review with a focus on endometriosis. *Reprod Health.* 2024;21(1):61.
98. Pilz S, Trummer C, Pandis M, Schwetz V, Aberer F, Gruebler M, et al. Vitamin D: Current guidelines and future outlook. *Anticancer Research.* 2018;38(2):1145–51.
99. Skiba MA, Islam RM, Bell RJ, Davis SR. Understanding variation in prevalence estimates of polycystic ovary syndrome: A systematic review and meta-analysis. *Human Reproduction Update.* 2018;24(6):694–709.
100. Mu Y, Cheng D, Yin T-l, Yang J. Vitamin D and polycystic ovary syndrome: A narrative review. *Reproductive Sciences.* 2021;28(8):2110–7.
101. Williams A, Babu JR, Wadsworth DD, Burnett D, Geetha T. The effects of vitamin D on metabolic profiles in women with polycystic ovary syndrome: A systematic review. *Hormone and Metabolic Research.* 2020;52(07):485–91.
102. Tóth EB, Takács I, Szekeres L, Szabó B, Bakos B, Lakatos P. Safety and efficacy of weekly 30,000 IU vitamin D supplementation as a slower loading dose administration compared to a daily maintenance schedule in deficient patients: A randomized, controlled clinical trial. *J Pharmacovigil.* 2017;5(4):233. https://doi.org/10.4172/2329-6887.1000233.
103. Lerchbaum E, Theiler-Schwetz V, Kollmann M, Wölfler M, Pilz S, Obermayer-Pietsch B, et al. Effects of vitamin D supplementation on surrogate markers of fertility in PCOS women: A randomized controlled trial. *Nutrients.* 2021;13(2):547.
104. Pludowski P, Grant WB, Karras SN, Zittermann A, Pilz S. Vitamin D supplementation: A review of the evidence arguing for a daily dose of 2000 international units (50 µg) of vitamin D for adults in the general population. *Nutrients.* 2024;16(3):391.
105. du Fossé NA, van der Hoorn M-LP, van Lith JMM, le Cessie S, Lashley EELO. Advanced paternal age is associated with an increased risk of spontaneous miscarriage: A systematic review and meta-analysis. *Human Reproduction Update.* 2020;26(5):650–69.

106. Manson JE, Bassuk SS, Buring JE. Principal results of the VITamin D and OmegA-3 TriaL (VITAL) and updated meta-analyses of relevant vitamin D trials. *Journal of Steroid Biochemistry and Molecular Biology*. 2020;198:105522.
107. EFSA Panel on Dietetic Products N, Allergies. Dietary reference values for vitamin D. *EFSA Journal*. 2016;14(10):e04547.
108. Cashman KD. Vitamin D deficiency: Defining, prevalence, causes, and strategies of addressing. *Calcified Tissue International*. 2020;106(1):14–29.
109. Fichera M, Török P, Tesarik J, Della Corte L, Rizzo G, Garzon S, et al. Vitamin D, reproductive disorders and assisted reproduction: Evidences and perspectives. *International Journal of Food Sciences and Nutrition*. 2020;71(3):276–85.
110. Abedi S, Taebi M, Nasr Esfahani MH. Effect of vitamin D supplementation on intracytoplasmic sperm injection outcomes: A randomized double-blind placebo-controlled trial. *Int J Fertil Steril*. 2019;13(1):18–23.
111. Doryanizadeh L, Morshed-Behbahani B, Parsanezhad ME, Dabbaghmanesh MH, Jokar A. Calcitriol effect on outcomes of in vitro fertilization in infertile women with vitamin D deficiency: A double-blind randomized clinical trial. *Zeitschrift für Geburtshilfe und Neonatologie*. 2021;225(03):226–31.
112. Fedorov Y, Kovpak A. Vitamin D toxicity and clinical consequences of hypervitaminosis. *SSP Modern Pharmacy and Medicine*. 2025;5(2):1–8.
113. Tonon CR, Silva TAAL, Pereira FWL, Queiroz DAR, Junior ELF, Martins D, et al. A review of current clinical concepts in the pathophysiology, etiology, diagnosis, and management of hypercalcemia. *Medical Science Monitor: International Medical Journal of Experimental and Clinical Research*. 2022;28:e935821–1.
114. Schlingmann KP. Vitamin D–dependent hypercalcemia. *Endocrinology and Metabolism Clinics*. 2021;50(4):729–42.
115. Wimalawansa SJ. Physiological basis for using vitamin D to improve health. *Biomedicines*. 2023;11(6):1542.
116. Lim K, Thadhani R. Vitamin D toxicity. *Brazilian Journal of Nephrology*. 2020;42(2):238–44.
117. Vieth R. Vitamin D supplementation, 25-hydroxyvitamin D concentrations, and safety. *American Journal of Clinical Nutrition*. 1999;69(5):842–56.
118. McGuire T. Fertility: Supporting the fertility treatment journey. *AJP: Australian Journal of Pharmacy*. 2021;102(1207):32–42.
119. Enkhmaa D, Tanz L, Ganmaa D, Enkhtur S, Oyun-Erdene B, Stuart J, et al. Randomized trial of three doses of vitamin D to reduce deficiency in pregnant Mongolian women. *EBioMedicine*. 2019;39:510–9.
120. Bi WG, Nuyt AM, Weiler H, Leduc L, Santamaria C, Wei SQ. Association between vitamin D supplementation during pregnancy and offspring growth, morbidity, and mortality: A systematic review and meta-analysis. *JAMA Pediatrics*. 2018;172(7):635–45.
121. Ozkan B, Hatun S, Bereket A. Vitamin D intoxication. *Turkish Journal of Pediatrics*. 2012;54(2):93–8.
122. Shane E. General management and treatment of acute and chronic hypercalcemia in adults. In *Hypercalcemia: Clinical Diagnosis and Management*. Springer; 2022. p. 75–87.
123. Vitamin D. *Fact Sheet for Health Professionals*. National Institutes of Health Office of Dietary Supplements. https://odsod nih gov/factsheets/VitaminC-HealthProfessional. 2017.
124. Walker MD, Shane E. Hypercalcemia: A review. *JAMA*. 2022;328(16):1624–36.
125. Gordon L, Zipursky R, Cheung CC, Sasidharan Pillai S. Vitamin D intoxication in an adolescent due to over-supplementation: A case report and review of literature. *AACE Endocrinol Diabetes*. 2025;3(4):100247. https://doi.org/10.1016/j.aed.2025.10.008.
126. Mazess RB, Bischoff Ferrari HA, Dawson Hughes B. Vitamin D: Bolus is bogus – A narrative review. *JBMR Plus*. 2021;5(12).
127. Sorrenti V, Buriani A, Davinelli S, Scapagnini G, Fortinguerra S. Vitamin D physiology, deficiency, genetic influence, and the effects of daily vs. bolus doses of vitamin D on overall health: A clinical approach. *Nutraceuticals*. 2023;3(3):403–20.
128. Rasheedy R, Sammour H, Elkholy A, Salim Y. The efficacy of vitamin D combined with clomiphene citrate in ovulation induction in overweight women with polycystic ovary syndrome: A double blind, randomized clinical trial. *Endocrine*. 2020;69(2):393–401.
129. Smits A. *Opportunities for Improvement of Oocyte Quality in Metabolically Compromised Conditions: From Fundamental Discoveries in the Well Until the Development of Preconception Care Strategies in an Obese Mouse Model*. University of Antwerp; 2022.
130. Somigliana E, Sarais V, Reschini M, Ferrari S, Makieva S, Cermisoni GC, et al. Single oral dose of vitamin D3 supplementation prior to in vitro fertilization and embryo transfer in normal weight women: The SUNDRO randomized controlled trial. *American Journal of Obstetrics and Gynecology*. 2021;225(3):283.e1–e10.
131. Kuroshli Z, Novin MG, Nazarian H, Abdollahifar M-A, Zademodarres S, Pirani M, et al. The efficacy of vitamin D supplement in the expression and protein levels of endometrial decidualization factors in women with recurrent implantation failure. *Reproductive Sciences*. 2024;31(3):675–86.

132. Ko EY, Sabanegh Jr ES. The role of over-the-counter supplements for the treatment of male infertility – fact or fiction? *Journal of Andrology*. 2012;33(3):292–308.
133. van Tienhoven XA, Ruiz de Chávez Gascón J, Cano-Herrera G, Sarkis Nehme JA, Souroujon Torun AA, Bautista Gonzalez MF, et al. Vitamin D in reproductive health disorders: A narrative review focusing on infertility, endometriosis, and polycystic ovarian syndrome. *Int J Mol Sci*. 2025;26(5).
134. Cohen PA. The supplement paradox: Negligible benefits, robust consumption. *JAMA*. 2016;316(14):1453–4.
135. Lee IT, Weiss MS, Miranian D, Pattipati S, Rajpal S, Martin CE, et al. Variation in practice patterns surrounding vitamin D testing and supplementation among infertility patients. *Fertility and Sterility*. 2023;120(4):e169.
136. Sempos C, Binkley N. 25-Hydroxyvitamin D assay standardisation and vitamin D guidelines paralysis. *Public Health Nutrition*. 2020;23(7):1153–64.
137. Kader S, Akdağ T, Ecer B, Abuşoğlu S, Unlu A. Comparison between liquid chromatography-tandem mass spectrometry and immunoassay methods for measurement of plasma 25 (OH) vitamin D. *Turkish Journal of Biochemistry*. 2022;47(6):710–8.
138. Control CfD, Prevention. *Vitamin D Standardization Certification Program*. CDC; 2020.
139. Aoun A, Maalouf J, Fahed M, El Jabbour F. When and how to diagnose and treat vitamin D deficiency in adults: A practical and clinical update. *Journal of Dietary Supplements*. 2020;17(3):336–54.
140. Zhang H, Wang S, Tuo L, Zhai Q, Cui J, Chen D, et al. Relationship between maternal vitamin D levels and adverse outcomes. *Nutrients*. 2022;14(20):4230.
141. Irani M, Merhi Z. Role of vitamin D in ovarian physiology and its implication in reproduction: A systematic review. *Fertility and Sterility*. 2014;102(2):460–8. e3.
142. Rombel N, Lim C, Majeed A, Abdul-Jabbar S, McClelland GR, Jones SA. Understanding the impact of vitamin D supplement formulation, quality and provision to older adults in UK residential care homes. *RSC Pharm*. 2025;2:683–90. https://doi.org/10.1039/D5PM00003C.
143. Moradkhani A, Azami M, Assadi S, Ghaderi M, Azarnezhad A, Moradi Y. Association of vitamin D receptor genetic polymorphisms with the risk of infertility: A systematic review and meta-analysis. *BMC Pregnancy Childbirth*. 2024;24(1):398.
144. Kahlon BK, Simon-Collins M, Nylander E, Segars J, Singh B. A systematic review of vitamin D and endometriosis: Role in pathophysiology, diagnosis, treatment, and prevention. *F&S Reviews*. 2023;4(1):1–14.
145. Tobias DK, Luttmann-Gibson H, Mora S, Danik J, Bubes V, Copeland T, et al. Association of body weight with response to vitamin D supplementation and metabolism. *JAMA Network Open*. 2023;6(1):e2250681.
146. Muscogiuri G, Altieri B, de Angelis C, Palomba S, Pivonello R, Colao A, et al. Shedding new light on female fertility: The role of vitamin D. *Reviews in Endocrine and Metabolic Disorders*. 2017;18(3):273–83.
147. Pilz S, Zittermann A, Obeid R, Hahn A, Pludowski P, Trummer C, et al. The role of vitamin D in fertility and during pregnancy and lactation: A review of clinical data. *International Journal of Environmental Research and Public Health*. 2018;15(10):2241.
148. Morshed-Behbahani B, Doryanizadeh L, Shahali S, Shahabi S, Montazeri A. Effect of and the association between vitamin D and outcomes of assisted reproductive techniques among infertile men and women: Protocol for an overview of systematic reviews and meta-analysis. *BMJ Open*. 2023;13(3):e060483.
149. Keane KN, Cruzat VF, Calton EK, Hart PH, Soares MJ, Newsholme P, et al. Molecular actions of vitamin D in reproductive cell biology. *Reproduction*. 2017;153(1):R29–R42.
150. Guo J, Tian X, Liu H, Lu Q, Cao G. P-304 vitamin D promotes endometrial stromal cell decidualization via a VDR-mediated mechanism. *Human Reproduction*. 2025;40(Suppl. 1).
151. Yan T-F, Qi J-J, Li L-X, Li F. The association between serum vitamin D levels and male fertility: A systematic review and meta-analysis. *Andrologia*. 2023;2023(1):9002938.
152. Katyal G, Kaur G, Ashraf H, Bodapati A, Hanif A, Okafor DK, et al. Systematic review of the roles of inositol and vitamin D in improving fertility among patients with polycystic ovary syndrome. *Clinical and Experimental Reproductive Medicine*. 2024;51(3):181.
153. Rinendyaputri R, Nikmah UA, Maria SS. Re: Vitamin D supplementation for improving sperm parameters in infertile men: A systematic review and meta-analysis of randomized clinical trials. *Arab Journal of Urology*. 2023;21(4):213.

9 Folic Acid and Folate

Erfan Zaker, Maryam Azizi-Kutenaei, and Farzaneh Fesahat

9.1 ITS ROLE IN DNA SYNTHESIS AND OOCYTE HEALTH

Folate and folic acid belong to the vitamin B9 family, which plays an essential role in one-carbon metabolism. The body converts folic acid (the synthetic form) into tetrahydrofolate (THF) by way of the enzyme dihydrofolate reductase. THF and its derivatives carry single-carbon units that enter pathways for synthesis of purines and thymidylate. Without sufficient folate supply, the cells cannot build enough adenine, guanine or thymine bases for DNA replication and repair (1). For instance, in pyrimidine synthesis a key step occurs when 5,10-methylene-THF donates a methylene group to deoxyuridine monophosphate (dUMP) which then becomes deoxythymidine monophosphate (dTMP) via the enzyme thymidylate synthase. When folate is deficient, the dUMP/dTMP ratio increases and uracil can be mis-incorporated into DNA, causing strand breaks and genome instability (2). The folate cycle interconnects with the methionine cycle. THF derivatives accept methyl groups from serine or glycine and transfer them to homocysteine, forming methionine. Methionine then becomes S-adenosylmethionine (SAM), the main methyl donor for DNA methylation. DNA methylation regulates gene expression, and altered folate status may disturb epigenetic regulation (1, 3).

In reproductive tissues this biochemistry has special relevance. Oocytes and the surrounding follicular cells undergo rapid growth and division, so they require continuous supply of nucleotides and methylation capacity. Studies show that oocytes accumulate folate and express folate transporter and metabolism genes in follicles and early embryos (4). In animal models, folic acid supplementation of oocyte maturation culture improved blastocyst rates and increased expression of folate-methionine cycle enzymes (e.g., in goats) (5). These features can be observed in Table 9.1.

9.2 CLINICAL APPLICATIONS IN INFERTILITY TREATMENT

Folate status shows a clear link with markers of reproductive potential. Studies in IVF clinics report that follicular fluid acts as a mirror for oocyte needs, and folate sits inside this fluid near the oocyte. Reviews on follicular-fluid metabolomics describe shifts in small molecules that track oocyte competence and embryo viability, so a stable folate supply looks important for this micro-environment (17).

Observational work on women who seek fertility care shows a relation between diet quality, blood folate, and chance of pregnancy after IVF. A cohort from the Food, Lifestyle and Fertility Outcome project found higher red blood cell folate and a higher probability of pregnancy when the diet favored fish, legumes, and vegetables with lower refined carbohydrates. This pattern suggests a role for folate status during treatment (18).

Direct assessments of serum folate in infertility care also show a signal. A systematic review and meta-analysis on women under assisted reproduction examined folate levels and success rates. The authors reported associations between folate status and clinical outcomes across several datasets. Although effect sizes varied, the direction supported a beneficial role for adequate folate (19).

Evidence links homocysteine with poorer IVF metrics, so the folate–homocysteine axis matters. A recent review on homocysteine and fertility summarized data across male and female factors and described worse oocyte competence and embryo quality when homocysteine rose, which usually points to low folate or B12 status. New clinical work also tested homocysteine correction before IVF and reported higher oocyte counts, better embryo grades, and more clinical pregnancies after correction (20).

Data from follicular-fluid studies add biological context. Reviews and original papers describe that the fluid around the oocyte contains metabolites from plasma and granulosa cells; changes in these components track maturation quality. While these papers do not measure folate in every dataset, they support the idea that one-carbon nutrients can affect the niche that supports the oocyte (16).

Folate enters one-carbon metabolism and supplies methyl units for methionine and S-adenosylmethionine. When folate intake stays low, total homocysteine goes up. High

DOI: 10.1201/9781003741541-9

Table 9.1: Biological Roles of Folate in Female Reproduction

Biological Process	Role of Folate/Folic Acid	Reproductive Implication
DNA synthesis	Provides one-carbon units for purine and thymidylate synthesis	Supports oocyte growth and early embryonic cell division (6, 7)
DNA repair	Prevents uracil misincorporation and strand breaks	Maintains genome stability in oocytes (8, 9)
One-carbon metabolism	Regenerates methionine and S-adenosylmethionine (SAM)	Enables DNA and histone methylation (10, 11)
Epigenetic regulation	Supplies methyl groups for DNA methylation	Regulates gene expression during oocyte maturation and implantation (12, 13)
Homocysteine metabolism	Lowers circulating homocysteine	Reduces oxidative stress and vascular dysfunction (14, 15)
Follicular microenvironment	Accumulates in follicular fluid	Supports oocyte competence and embryo viability (14, 16)

homocysteine links with oxidative stress and with weak methyl supply for DNA methylation in endometrium. These two factors can disturb gene regulation during the implantation window. A recent basic study described how methionine availability shapes methylation of immune-tolerance genes in the uterus and how this process influences receptivity. The authors tied methionine status to reduced IL-5 transcription through Eomes control, which suggests a direct route from one-carbon flux to the uterine milieu (11).

Clinical datasets in IVF support the homocysteine signal. A Human Reproduction study on monofollicular fluid connected biomarkers from the homocysteine pathway with embryo quality and pregnancy after IVF, so homocysteine appears close to oocyte–embryo competence and to implantation chance (21). Women who start IVF with higher serum homocysteine often face lower implantation and clinical pregnancy, and this trend looks stronger in the MTHFR C677T TT genotype (21). A recent cohort also reported a positive correlation between homocysteine levels and the count of failed IVF attempts, while authors noted that folic acid, vitamin B12, and vitamin B6 can lower homocysteine in mild cases (22).

Observational work in US fertility clinics adds detail from the endometrial side. Higher total folate intake before treatment associated with higher implantation, higher clinical pregnancy, and higher live birth per initiated cycle. The same cohort reported about 20% higher live birth in women who took more than 800 micrograms per day of supplemental folate, with an intake–response curve that rose until about 1200 micrograms per day. These outcomes need a receptive endometrium in addition to a viable embryo, so the data support better uterine readiness when methyl supply looks rich. Cycle-level indicators point to a role for one-carbon status during stimulation. In a randomized ovarian-stimulation study, estradiol response and follicle counts differed by protocol, and the tables track folate and homocysteine values across time points. The dataset places homocysteine close to gonadotropin response, which affects the quality of the endometrium later in the cycle. Not every study shows a direct gain in pregnancy outcomes after simple folic acid use. A Swedish cohort of women with unexplained infertility showed higher plasma folate and lower homocysteine than fertile controls, but pregnancy and live birth after treatment did not change across folate strata. The same paper still confirmed an inverse relation between plasma folate and homocysteine. Clinicians also discuss preconception homocysteine as a screening factor. A hospital-based study proposed that women with previous IVF/ICSI failure may benefit from correction of high homocysteine before a new cycle. Authors argued for vitamin B support that includes folate, especially when labs show mild hyperhomocysteinemia (23, 24). Reviews from 2025 summarized female data in the same direction and placed endometrial receptivity and implantation on the list of outcomes that connect to the folate–homocysteine axis (20). A summary of the mentioned applications can be seen in Table 9.2.

9.3 CURRENT CLINICAL EVIDENCE SUPPORTING THE USE OF FOLIC ACID AND FOLATE

Infertility is a significant global health issue, affecting an estimated 15–17% of couples worldwide. This high prevalence has spurred scientific interest in modifiable factors that could improve fertility outcomes. One such factor is nutrition, particularly vitamin supplementation, in the

Table 9.2: Clinical Evidence Linking Folate Status to Fertility and ART Outcomes

Clinical Context	Folate-Related Factor	Observed Outcome
IVF/ICSI cycles	Higher serum or RBC folate	Improved oocyte quality and pregnancy rates (25, 26)
ART outcomes	Elevated homocysteine	Lower implantation and clinical pregnancy (14, 22)
Preconception nutrition	High dietary or supplemental folate intake	Higher implantation and live birth rates (27, 28)
PCOS	Folate with myo-inositol	Improved oocyte maturation and embryo quality (29, 30)
Recurrent IVF failure	Homocysteine correction with folate/B vitamins	Reduced miscarriage and improved embryo metrics (20, 31)
MTHFR polymorphisms	Use of 5-methyltetrahydrofolate	Improved uterine and ART outcomes in selected patients (8, 32, 33)

preconception period (34). Among the various nutrients, folate has gained prominence due to its critical role in DNA synthesis, repair, and methylation, processes essential for oocyte development and early embryogenesis (15). Folic acid, the synthetic form of folate, is widely recommended for women attempting to conceive, primarily to prevent neural tube defects in the fetus (35). However, beyond congenital anomaly prevention, there is a strong scientific rationale and growing body of research exploring how adequate folate status and folic acid supplementation may enhance female fertility and assisted reproduction outcomes (24).

The rationale for folate in reproductive medicine rests on basic cell biology and also on clinical outcomes. Folate enters one-carbon metabolism, and this pathway feeds nucleotide biosynthesis and DNA methylation. Gametes and very early embryos show rapid cell division, so a shortage of folate may disturb chromatin structure, meiosis, and genome integrity. Clinicians also face the related question of homocysteine, because low folate usually raises homocysteine, and excess homocysteine may harm the vascular and oxidative balance in the ovaries and endometrium. Recent human data give support to these ideas. Several trials in the last 5 years report better intermediate or final IVF outcomes with folate-containing regimens, while a few neutral trials define limits and help with dose or target group selection (12, 36, 37).

Clinical trials in women who undergo IVF or ICSI provide the most direct view. One double-blind randomized study from Iran tested myo-inositol plus folic acid against folic acid alone in women who planned an IVF cycle. The trial reported a higher number of mature MII oocytes and better embryo metrics in the combination arm after 2 months, with no safety signal (38). Another randomized controlled study in poor ovarian responders compared the same combination with folic acid alone. The investigators found gains in fertilization, embryo quality, and number of oocytes, which suggests that women with weak responses may gain special benefit from folate delivered with inositol support (39). A previous randomized trial in PCOS patients assigned myo-inositol plus melatonin plus folic acid or myo-inositol plus folic acid. The arm with melatonin showed higher oocyte and embryo quality and higher pregnancy rates. The report placed folic acid as a constant background nutrient in both groups, while the total pattern points toward a role for folate-dependent redox and methyl pathways in PCOS oocyte competence (40).

Another randomized study enrolled 120 women who had IVF with blastocyst transfer. All participants took myo-inositol, melatonin, and folic acid through stimulation; then one arm added vitamin D3 during the luteal phase. The vitamin D3 arm showed a higher implantation rate, which supports a multi-nutrient model where folic acid stays as a core element inside the program (41). Trials with mHealth coaching for subfertile couples give another angle. A large multicenter RCT improved folic acid supplement use and serum folate in the intervention arm and kept the design inside IVF settings, even if pregnancy rates were similar between groups. This result supports feasibility and real-world uptake of folate, which matters before any effect on live birth appears (36).

Observational work connects folate status with ART success. A study at a US academic center related higher pretreatment total folate intake to better fertilization and higher numbers of MII oocytes per cycle (12). A meta-analysis that focused on women who underwent ART found that higher folate levels associated with higher pregnancy rates across several cohorts, which supports a dose–response pattern at least for early outcomes (19). A more recent umbrella or methods-focused review across supplements judged the totality of female infertility data and listed folate or folate-containing regimens among the few nutrients with consistent signals in ovarian and implantation endpoints (42). Nutrition studies outside ART also matter. Two large preconception cohorts observed higher fecundability in women who took folic acid–containing supplements relative to non-users, which supports a general fertility effect that may carry into ART (43).

The homocysteine story links folate biology to endpoints that clinics care about. Several IVF cohorts measured serum or red cell folate and homocysteine before stimulation and then tracked pregnancy or implantation. Higher homocysteine was associated with lower clinical pregnancy and lower implantation, and this pattern looked strongest in women with the MTHFR C677T TT genotype (44). Earlier work from a Dutch IVF cohort reported that biomarkers across the homocysteine pathway related to embryo quality and pregnancy rate, which gave one of the first human signals for this mechanism (21). An Italian IVF study measured baseline serum folate, red cell folate, and homocysteine, and the team found that women with high homocysteine had lower cumulative pregnancy after IVF (45). Researchers also described higher homocysteine in women who had several failed embryo transfers, which maintains clinical attention on this target even when the level stays inside a lab's "normal" range (22).

Genetics may modify the expected benefit from folate form or dose. A prospective study in women with the MTHFR 677TT genotype tested 5-methyltetrahydrofolate and assessed IVF outcomes and uterine artery flow. The authors reported better uterine indices and signals for improved outcomes relative to standard care, which suggests that methylfolate may suit some genotypes better than synthetic folic acid (46). An integrative molecular review also mapped folate-pathway SNPs against ART endpoints and proposed that variants in MTHFR, MTRR, and related genes may change the need for folate quantity or form (47).

Male factor trials help with the couple-level picture. A multicenter randomized, double-blind trial in France assigned infertile men who planned IVF-ICSI to 15 mg folic acid per day or placebo for at least 3 months. The folic acid arm showed a higher biochemical pregnancy rate and a trend toward higher clinical pregnancy after fresh transfer; sperm DNA fragmentation decreased in the treatment group (48). A much larger US randomized trial assigned men to 5 mg folic acid plus zinc or placebo for 6 months. The primary results showed no improvement in live birth or semen quality, so the evidence points to a possible benefit in selected settings and not a general rule for all men (49).

Evidence outside strict RCTs also supports folate in reproductive care. A review in Reproductive BioMedicine Online in 2023 surveyed adjuvants in IVF and placed B vitamin complexes and folate strategies among plausible options in specific patient groups. The authors called for standardization of dose and for trials with live birth as the primary outcome, which matches the design of the male trials and the general wish in the field (50). A fresh synthesis on diet and IVF reconfirmed positive links between folate-rich patterns and early ART metrics (51). A 2025 perspective on folic acid fortification and embryo development returned to the cell cycle and methylation logic from a modern viewpoint and argued that periconception folate status likely shapes oocyte maturation and very early embryo progression (52).

9.3.1 Case Studies: Successful Integration of Folic Acid and Folate in Assisted Reproductive Technologies

Scientific interest in folate inside ART grows because folate enters one-carbon pathways which provide methyl groups for DNA and histone methylation (53). These reactions support oocyte competence, early embryo development, and long-term epigenetic health. ART success still stays modest for many couples, and small, safe nutritional steps before and during treatment may shift outcomes in a positive way. Folate sits in one-carbon metabolism, it supports DNA synthesis and methylation, and it controls homocysteine, so it has a direct biochemical logic in oocyte competence and early embryo development (54).

One well-known cohort from the United States tracked women who started IVF with measured serum folate. Women who stood in the highest serum folate quartile had higher chances for clinical pregnancy and for live birth compared with the lowest quartile; the analysis kept age, BMI, and race as covariates. A combined pattern of high folate with high vitamin B12 looked most favorable for live birth in that dataset. This cohort sits inside a population exposed to folic acid fortification, so baseline folate already had a high range, but the gradient still appeared (55).

An Italian prospective study divided 209 IVF or ICSI patients into tertiles by baseline serum and RBC folate. Women who stood in the highest RBC folate tertile, above 329 ng per mL, had higher odds for clinical pregnancy and for live birth per started cycle than women with lower RBC folate; the model used age, BMI, smoking, stimulation protocol, and indication as covariates. Median RBC and serum folate also looked higher in the group that reached pregnancy. This study supports the practical value of a steady, stored folate pool before stimulation (19).

Some centers tried targeted supplementation strategies. A hospital-based program in Japan screened women with past frozen embryo transfer failures. The team gave 800 micrograms per day folic acid for 12 weeks to part of the group and then did FET. Homocysteine levels went down after supplementation, and the miscarriage rate after FET went down as well; the study did not show a rise in clinical pregnancy, but the loss reduction carried clinical value for these patients. This intervention aligns with the biological link between folate status, endothelial health, and placental function (24).

Another clinic compared two supplement paths during ART: folic acid alone versus a vitamin B complex that contained 5-methyltetrahydrofolate and vitamin B12. The B-complex group reached higher clinical pregnancy and higher live birth, with adjusted odds that favored the complex. The difference in oocyte numbers and cleavage also went in the same direction. Genotype for MTHFR did not change these associations inside that study. While the design was retrospective, the result suggests that some patients may benefit when the regimen provides the active folate form together with B12 (56).

9.3.2 Best Practices for Incorporating Folic Acid and Folate into Infertility Treatment Protocols

Beyond preventing neural tube defects in early pregnancy, which is the original rationale for periconceptional folic acid supplementation, there is growing interest in folic acid as a therapeutic adjunct in infertility treatments (57). Many women undergoing IVF or other ART already take prenatal vitamins or folic acid supplements – in one survey over 70% of patients did so (58). However, until recently, clinical guidelines only explicitly recommended folic acid to prevent fetal neural tube defects, not to enhance conception per se (59, 60). This has led to a gap between widespread empirical use and the need for evidence-based guidance on folate in infertility protocols. Over the last few years, multiple international studies and reviews have emerged to address this gap. These studies examine how folic acid/folate supplementation might improve outcomes like oocyte quality, fertilization, embryo development, implantation, and pregnancy maintenance (42).

Determining the optimal timing and duration of folic acid/folate supplementation is crucial for maximizing its benefits in infertility treatment. Current public health recommendations (aimed at preventing neural tube defects) advise that women start taking folic acid before conception – ideally at least 1 month prior – and continue through early pregnancy (61). In the context of infertility care, this preconception window is equally, if not more, important. Gametogenesis and follicular development occur over months before ovulation; thus, ensuring replete folate status during the ~90 days of follicle maturation is thought to improve oocyte quality. There is general consensus that women pursuing IVF or other ART should begin a prenatal or folic acid supplement well in advance of ovarian stimulation, typically 2–3 months before starting treatment (62–64). This allows time to build up tissue folate levels (especially red blood cell folate) that correlate with improved IVF outcomes.

When it comes to duration of supplementation, most protocols continue folic acid throughout the treatment cycle and into the early pregnancy period (if achieved). Folate supplementation is typically maintained during ovarian stimulation, through egg retrieval, and after embryo transfer – essentially treating it as a continuous preconception and postconception support. Continuing folic acid into the luteal phase and beyond makes sense not only for neural tube defect prevention (through the first 12 weeks of gestation) but also because adequate folate may support early embryonic development and implantation processes (5, 50). Some reproductive endocrinologists advise staying on folic acid at least until a pregnancy is confirmed and often through the end of the first trimester (61). In cases where pregnancy is not achieved, the patient simply remains on the supplement as they prepare for any subsequent treatment cycles or attempts.

It is worth noting that evidence from clinical studies, while somewhat limited, supports the importance of starting folate supplementation prior to IVF rather than only during the cycle. A pioneering randomized trial by Boxmeer et al. (14) found that women who took a folic acid supplement in the weeks before and during IVF had a modified follicular fluid environment, trending toward improved embryo quality compared to unsupplemented women.

Integrating folic acid/folate into fertility treatment protocols has become standard practice, with a few important refinements based on emerging evidence. In clinical ART settings, folic acid is essentially treated as a foundational supplement: virtually all patients are advised to be on a folate-containing prenatal vitamin during their infertility journey.

Pretreatment phase: In the months leading up to an IVF (or IUI) cycle, patients are started on folic acid (if not already taking it). The goal in this phase is to build up adequate folate stores and ensure homocysteine is in the optimal range before ovarian stimulation. Many clinics conduct a baseline nutritional workup for patients with recurrent IVF failures or certain risk factors – this may include measuring serum folate, vitamin B12, and homocysteine levels (24, 65).

If any abnormalities are found (e.g., high homocysteine or low folate), they are corrected through intensified supplementation prior to proceeding with treatment. For example, if a woman's homocysteine is elevated, the clinician might prescribe high-dose folic acid (4–5 mg) for 8–12 weeks and then recheck levels, aiming to get homocysteine down (since elevated homocysteine has been linked to lower fertilization rates and higher miscarriage risk (24).

Ovarian stimulation phase: During the controlled ovarian hyperstimulation for IVF, folic acid is continued daily. It is often simply part of the prenatal or supplement regimen the patient is already on. There is no disruption – even on the day of egg retrieval and in the immediate post-retrieval period, folic acid supplementation is maintained (unless the patient is instructed to be NPO for anesthesia, in which case they resume it right after). Some clinics include folic acid in their stimulation checklists and ensure it's listed among medications to take. In clinical trials of fertility supplements, folic acid is so fundamental that it is commonly given to all study participants as a background treatment, even in the placebo group. For instance, in antioxidant trials for female infertility, the "placebo" often contains folic acid (<1 mg) to meet ethical requirements, with only the additional antioxidant being the variable (42, 66). This underscores that folic acid is considered a non-negotiable part of fertility care, integrated by default. During stimulation, having adequate folate may help oocyte maturation (as suggested by higher MII oocyte counts in women on folate-rich supplementation) (67).

Luteal phase and early pregnancy support: After embryo transfer (ET), folic acid remains part of the protocol alongside other medications like progesterone. The early post-ET period is critical for implantation – folate's contribution to cellular division and methylation continues to be relevant as the embryo undergoes rapid cell proliferation and the placenta begins to form. Clinicians advise patients to keep taking folic acid through the "2-week wait" and, if pregnancy is confirmed, throughout the first trimester (and often beyond) (61).

9.4 SAFETY, DOSAGE, AND EFFICACY

Evidence from clinical trials and observational studies supports a favorable safety profile for folic acid within recommended doses, though its direct impact on fertility outcomes remains mixed. In a multicenter prospective study of women with unexplained infertility, administration of 400 µg/day folic acid for 12 weeks resulted in an 80% conception rate without any reported adverse effects (68), illustrating that folic acid is well tolerated and may enhance fecundity in some women. A prospective cohort from the EARTH study reported that women consuming high supplemental folic acid (~800 µg/day) experienced shorter time to pregnancy, lower risk of anovulation and improved menstrual function (69). However, not all data are uniformly positive. A prospective study on IVF outcomes found that higher serum folate levels improved embryo quality only up to a middle tertile; beyond this plateau, additional folate did not further enhance outcomes (70). Another umbrella review concluded that folic acid supplementation is primarily recommended to prevent neural tube defects rather than to improve conception rates and noted that a randomized trial of a vitamin B complex containing 400 µg folic acid showed no significant difference in live birth or clinical pregnancy rates versus placebo (71).

Targeted supplementation may produce specific benefits in subgroups. A Japanese cohort of women with a history of failed frozen embryo transfers received 800 µg/day folic acid for 12 weeks; supplementation significantly reduced serum homocysteine and lowered miscarriage rates, although clinical pregnancy rates were unchanged (31). A randomized trial comparing high-dose (4 mg/day) and standard-dose (0.4 mg/day) folic acid during the periconception period found no difference in congenital malformations but reported fewer spontaneous abortions and preterm births with high-dose supplementation (72). Conversely, a review of randomized interventions for managing anovulation in PCOS reported that when folic acid served as the control, there was no significant difference in ovulation or pregnancy rates compared with inositol combinations (73). International guidelines universally recommend folic acid supplementation for women attempting to conceive. The US Preventive Services Task Force advises that all women planning or capable of pregnancy consume 0.4–0.8 mg of folic acid daily, starting at least one month before conception and continuing through early pregnancy (74). These doses have strong evidence for preventing neural tube defects and form the standard of care. A study recommends 400 µg/day for low-risk women, increasing to 5 mg/day for those with a previous neural tube defect–affected pregnancy or conditions such as diabetes, obesity or anticonvulsant therapy (33). The Canadian Preventive Medicine guidance similarly advises 0.4 mg beginning 3 months before conception and continuing through breastfeeding, and suggests higher doses in complex pregnancies (75). A small case series in women with methylenetetrahydrofolate reductase polymorphisms reported that replacing folic acid with 5 methyltetrahydrofolate (5 MTHF) (median dose 2325 µg/day) led to 11 conceptions and 10 live births, illustrating that bioactive folate forms may be beneficial when genetic variants impair folic acid metabolism. Collectively, these recommendations converge on a baseline of 400 µg/day, with individualized adjustments (e.g., 800 µg to 4 mg) for women with a high risk of neural tube defects, MTHFR variants or elevated homocysteine (76).

At recommended doses, folic acid has an excellent safety profile. The PCOS meta-analysis noted above found no significant difference in serum folate between PCOS and control groups but did identify higher homocysteine, suggesting that folic acid deficiency is not prevalent yet supplementation may correct metabolic imbalances (77). A modified Delphi consensus involving gynecologists and reproductive endocrinologists highlighted folic acid among the few supplements (along with vitamin B12 and myo-inositol) with strong agreement for preconception use; the panel recommended folic acid for reducing neural tube defect risk and regulating homocysteine in PCOS (78). A protocol for a randomized trial on diminished ovarian reserve notes that folic acid participates in one-carbon metabolism, lowers homocysteine and may improve ovarian function, and does not report any adverse events (79).

Guidelines stress caution with very high doses. Though water soluble and readily excreted, excessive folic acid can accumulate as unmetabolized folic acid (UMFA) when intake exceeds metabolic capacity. A retrospective study of multivitamin supplementation in infertility clinics observed that some IVF centers routinely prescribe 5–15 mg/day folic acid; the authors argued that such high doses may lead to UMFA and advocated using 500 µg/day of 5 MTHF instead (80). High folate levels could theoretically mask vitamin B12 deficiency or interfere with cellular signaling, although population studies have not demonstrated significant harm. Conversely, some evidence suggests benefits of higher intake: the randomized trial comparing 4 mg vs. 0.4 mg reported fewer spontaneous abortions and preterm births with the higher dose (72).

Integration of folic acid with other supplements or medications is common in fertility management. Meta-analysis of randomized trials in PCOS found that adding myo-inositol to 400 µg/day folic acid improved oocyte quality, increased the proportion of top grade embryos and clinical pregnancy rates, and reduced the risk of ovarian hyperstimulation syndrome (OHSS) by about 16% (81). These benefits likely derive from synergistic effects on insulin sensitivity and ovarian microcirculation. In addition, co administration of myo-inositol with melatonin and folic acid improved intrafollicular melatonin concentrations, increased the number of mature oocytes and enhanced embryo quality compared with folic acid alone (82). PCOS specific benefits extend beyond oocyte numbers; folic acid supplementation has been shown to reduce body mass index, especially in PCOS patients with elevated homocysteine (30), indicating that it may improve metabolic profiles. These data support incorporating folic acid into broader nutraceutical regimens for PCOS.

Folic acid also interacts beneficially with conventional pharmacologic treatments. Folic acid acts as a substrate for methotrexate antagonism; therefore women taking antifolate drugs or antiepileptics may require higher folic acid doses to maintain adequate levels. Expert consensus states that B complex vitamins, including folic acid, help regulate homocysteine and improve insulin resistance in PCOS (78). Observational reports suggest that co-supplementation with vitamin B complexes and antioxidants may enhance oocyte quality, although rigorous trials are lacking. Notably, in trials where folic acid served as the placebo or control, no adverse interactions with ovulation induction drugs or gonadotropins were observed (28). Finally, metabolic synergy extends beyond vitamins: amino acid homeostasis is crucial for folliculogenesis, and adequate folate facilitates methionine/homocysteine recycling and supports methyl donors for embryo development (83).

9.5 CHALLENGES AND CONTROVERSIES

The aim of supplementation is to reduce the risk of congenital abnormalities and to optimize reproductive health. The book proposal at the center of this study notes that infertility affects 10–15% of couples worldwide and up to 20% in some Middle Eastern countries; oxidative stress, inflammation, and hormonal imbalance are identified as major contributors to fertility problems (84). Folic acid and its natural derivative folate are essential cofactors in one-carbon metabolism and play key roles in DNA synthesis, methylation, and homocysteine remethylation. These functions support gametogenesis, early embryogenesis, and epigenetic regulation, and a deficiency may impair oocyte competence, embryo quality, and implantation. Several observational studies and meta-analyses have indicated that folate intake correlates with higher antral follicle counts, improved menstrual regularity, and reduced the risk of ovulatory infertility (69). Folate supplementation has been shown to decrease plasma homocysteine and improve metabolic profiles, particularly when combined with vitamins B6 and B12. Indeed, high serum homocysteine is associated with diminished ovarian reserve and poor oocyte quality; supplementation with folic acid and vitamins B6 and B12 reduces homocysteine by 25% and improves embryo quality (85). Randomized trials report that women with unexplained infertility treated with 400 μg/day folic acid for 12 weeks achieved an 80% conception rate with no adverse effects (86), and prospective cohorts from the EARTH study observed that women consuming about 800 μg/day supplemental folic acid had shorter time to conception and improved menstrual function (27). Nonetheless, the overall evidence base is mixed, and it remains unclear whether folic acid directly enhances fertility or acts primarily by correcting underlying deficiencies.

Despite its long-standing use, folic acid supplementation remains a subject of controversy in reproductive medicine. Some systematic reviews of nutrient supplementation for infertility stress that preconception health recommendations focus on folic acid primarily to prevent neural tube defects, with few trials evaluating fertility outcomes. Evidence for folate's effect on conception rates is inconsistent; an umbrella review found no significant benefit of a vitamin B complex containing 400 μg folic acid on live birth or clinical pregnancy rates compared with placebo (71). Similarly, in vitro fertilization (IVF) trials show that increased folate intake improves embryo quality only up to a threshold; beyond the middle tertile of serum folate there is no further gain in embryo competence and some studies even report negative associations (70). Other RCTs comparing high-dose (5 mg or 4 mg) and standard-dose (0.4 mg) folic acid found no difference in congenital malformations but did report fewer spontaneous abortions and preterm births at high doses (72). These divergent findings have fueled debates among clinicians and policymakers regarding optimal dosing, appropriate forms of folate, and whether fortification and supplementation policies should be standardized. Moreover, emerging research into genetic polymorphisms, epigenetic effects and potential adverse outcomes such as insulin resistance or twin births has added complexity to what was once considered a straightforward intervention.

The purpose of this section was to critically examine the challenges and controversies surrounding folic acid and folate supplementation for female infertility. The discussion is structured into three thematic areas: regulatory and standardization issues, variability in patient responses, and gaps in research. Over 60 recent (mostly 2019–2025) international publications were reviewed, each cited only once to respect the guidelines. Throughout, reference is made to evidence from randomized trials, observational studies, systematic reviews, and national guidelines, with an emphasis on mechanistic insights and methodological limitations. By synthesizing the current literature, this section aims to provide a balanced appraisal of the benefits and risks of folate supplementation in reproductive medicine and to identify directions for future research and policy development.

9.5.1 Regulatory and Standardization Issues

Public health authorities in many countries mandate folic acid fortification of staple foods and recommend periconceptional supplementation. Nevertheless, guidance on dosing, timing, and the choice between synthetic folic acid and natural or methylated folate varies markedly across jurisdictions. A systematic review of folic acid supplementation in European women of reproductive age found poor adherence to guidelines and highlighted the need to standardize recommendations, particularly for women with obesity. While most European countries advise 0.4 mg/day beginning at least one month before conception and continuing through the first trimester, high-risk women (those with previous neural tube defect-affected pregnancies, diabetes or taking anticonvulsants) are often advised to take 4–5 mg/day (87).

Regulatory bodies must also decide which chemical form of folate to endorse. Folic acid, the synthetic oxidized form of folate, is stable and inexpensive and has been authorized for use in drugs and food fortification by the United States Pharmacopeia and the European Pharmacopoeia. In contrast, 5 methyltetrahydrofolate (5 MTHF), the biologically active form, has greater initial bioavailability but is less stable and more sensitive to light (32). Advocates of 5 MTHF argue that it bypasses enzymatic reduction by dihydrofolate reductase and does not lead to accumulation of unmetabolized folic acid, which has been detected in the circulation of individuals exposed to high intake from fortified foods. An expert opinion from Italy emphasizes that some individuals carry polymorphisms in the MTHFR gene that impair conversion of folic acid to 5 MTHF; for these people, supplementation with 5 MTHF may be more effective and less likely to mask vitamin B12 deficiency (88).

Debate over mandatory fortification further complicates regulatory decisions. A review of contemporary issues in folic acid fortification noted that increased population folate intake may have unforeseen adverse effects, including accumulation of unmetabolized folic acid, masking of vitamin B12 deficiency, potential genotoxicity, increased twin births, insulin resistance, and epigenetic alterations (89). Similar concerns have been raised in more recent analyses: a narrative review on excess folate intake argued that high folic acid exposure may alter DNA methylation and increase the risk of cancer, neurodevelopmental disorders, and metabolic disease (90).

9.5.2 Variability in Patient Responses

Inter-individual variability in response to folic acid or folate supplementation is influenced by genetic polymorphisms, sex, underlying health conditions and lifestyle factors. Among the most studied determinants are polymorphisms in the MTHFR gene, particularly C677T and A1298C. These variants reduce enzyme activity, potentially decreasing the conversion of folic acid to 5 MTHF and raising homocysteine levels. A retrospective cohort study involving IVF patients reported that the MTHFR 677TT genotype was associated with fewer transferable embryos and lower cumulative live birth rate under a short gonadotropin-releasing hormone agonist protocol, though no differences were observed under a long protocol (91). Another retrospective study of 1160 women genotyped for MTHFR combinations noted that previous research had yielded conflicting results because the C677T and A1298C polymorphisms influence enzyme activity jointly rather than independently (92). Meta-analyses have also produced inconsistent findings; some report associations between MTHFR variants and recurrent implantation failure or spontaneous miscarriage, while others find no effect (93). These discrepancies may reflect differences in sample size, supplementation regimens, and confounder adjustment.

Clinical practice has responded to genetic variability by tailoring folate type and dosage. A case series of Australian patients with infertility and MTHFR polymorphisms documented that practitioners commonly stopped folic acid and prescribed high-dose 5 MTHF or folinic acid (~2.3 mg/day); 11 of 12 patients conceived within a year. The study emphasized that such prescriptions depart from national guidelines and called for trials to determine whether adjusting recommendations based on MTHFR genotype improves outcomes. The same report explained that folic acid is reduced to dihydrofolate and then to tetrahydrofolate by dihydrofolate reductase, whereas 5 MTHF enters the folate cycle directly; genetic variants in MTHFR or dihydrofolate reductase genes may therefore alter folate metabolism (94). A cohort study of donor oocyte IVF cycles reported that variants in genes such as ABCB1 and MTR were associated with increased miscarriage risk but not with overall pregnancy outcomes; the authors recommended personalized supplementation only for women with specific genotypes (95). Clearly, patient responses to folate are heterogeneous, and a one-size-fits-all approach may be inadequate.

Sex differences further contribute to variability. In men, folate participates in spermatogenesis by supporting DNA synthesis, methylation and snRNA maturation. A randomized trial among infertile men (FOLFIV study) showed that high-dose folic acid (15 mg/day) increased biochemical pregnancy rates and reduced sperm DNA fragmentation, although standard semen parameters were unchanged (96). A mechanistic review on folic acid and male fertility explained that folate deficiency disrupts RNA splicing and epigenetic programming in sperm, and that supplementation improves snRNA function and semen parameters (97). Paternal exposures to methyl donors, including folic acid, vitamin B12 and methionine, have been shown in animal models to induce epigenetic modifications in offspring (98), suggesting that paternal supplementation could influence reproductive outcomes and long-term health in ways that remain poorly understood.

Underlying health conditions such as polycystic ovary syndrome and obesity modulate folate requirements and responses. PCOS is characterized by insulin resistance, hyperandrogenism, and chronic anovulation and is often accompanied by elevated homocysteine (29). A meta-analysis found that folate and vitamin B12 levels are similar between women with PCOS and controls, but homocysteine levels are significantly higher in PCOS (77). Consequently, co-supplementation with folic acid and other B vitamins may be particularly beneficial in this group. Clinical trials have evaluated combinations of myo-inositol and folic acid, given that inositol improves insulin sensitivity and folic acid supports DNA methylation. In women with PCOS undergoing IVF, 4 g/day myo-inositol plus 400 µg folic acid increased the proportion of mature oocytes and fertilization rate compared with folic acid alone (99). A randomized trial in non-PCOS women found that 2 g/day myo-inositol plus 200 µg folate reduced gonadotropin dose requirements and increased mature oocyte yield relative to 400 µg folate alone (100).

Variability also stems from baseline folate status and dose. A prospective study on IVF outcomes observed that increased serum folate improved embryo quality only up to a middle tertile; additional folate did not further enhance outcomes. A separate prospective study showed that high serum folate and riboflavin improved oocyte competence, but benefit plateaued at mid-range concentrations, and vitamin B12 deficiency negatively impacted embryo quality (70). In a trial examining ovulation induction in PCOS, folic acid served as the control and produced similar ovulation and pregnancy rates as inositol combinations. A case–control study measuring vitamins in follicular fluid during intracytoplasmic sperm injection (ICSI) cycles found that high folic acid levels were associated with a 43.7-fold higher probability of pregnancy, whereas women with poor ovarian reserve had lower follicular folate, vitamin D, B12, and melatonin (101). Together, these studies reveal a complex dose–response curve in which insufficient folate impairs fertility, modest supplementation confers benefits, but excessive intake may offer no additional gain and could potentially have deleterious effects.

9.6 GAPS IN RESEARCH AND NEED FOR FURTHER STUDIES

Although folic acid supplementation is universally recommended for neural tube defect prevention, substantial gaps remain regarding its role in fertility enhancement. Many clinical trials on folate and fertility are small and heterogeneous and lack rigorous control of confounding variables (49, 102). The NICE evidence review emphasized that there is no direct evidence for the commonly prescribed high dose of 5 mg; included trials used 4 mg, and the evidence quality was low (103).

Questions also persist about the optimal form of folate. Clinical practice has increasingly turned to 5 MTHF for individuals with MTHFR polymorphisms; a multivitamin study suggested that (6S) 5 MTHF at 500 µg/day may be preferable to high doses of folic acid (5–15 mg) to avoid accumulation of unmetabolized folic acid and potential epigenetic effects (80). Similarly, health professionals working with recurrent pregnancy loss reported changing from folic acid to active folate forms but noted that guidelines fail to provide advice on dosing or duration (104). These gaps point to a need for comprehensive guidelines that address both maternal and paternal supplementation and consider genetic variability.

Finally, research is needed to evaluate the long-term reproductive and transgenerational effects of folate supplementation. In low- and middle-income countries, evidence for micronutrient supplementation affecting miscarriage or stillbirth remains limited (105), highlighting a need for culturally diverse research. The design of future trials should include adequate sample sizes, consider both maternal and paternal contributions, control for confounders, and evaluate endpoints beyond neural tube defect prevention.

9.6.1 Future Directions and Research Opportunities

Global interest in these vitamins stems from their established role in preventing neural tube defects, yet infertility remains a widespread problem – affecting roughly 10–15% of couples worldwide – and the *Middle East Fertility Society Journal* notes that new technologies are needed alongside micronutrient optimization to address this challenge (106). Many women begin supplementation too late, use the wrong dose or formulation, or cease use during early pregnancy, illustrating the need for better education and regulatory harmonization (6). These inconsistencies and the rapid pace of biomedical innovation provide fertile ground for future research.

At a molecular level, folic acid is a synthetic compound that must be reduced and methylated through dihydrofolate reductase and methylenetetrahydrofolate reductase to form 5 methyltetrahydrofolate, the biologically active circulating form (7). Variations in genes encoding folate metabolizing enzymes, including MTHFR and other components of the one-carbon cycle, can markedly reduce enzymatic activity and impair conversion to 5 MTHF (8). An expert consensus underscores that folic acid is the only supplement universally recommended for women seeking conception, yet emphasizes that scientific evidence for improved IVF outcomes remains limited (78). Guidelines from the US Preventive Services Task Force recommend 400–800 µg/day for all women planning pregnancy (107), while high-dose regimens (5 mg/day) are recommended only for women with risk factors like previous neural tube defects or antiepileptic drug use (33). Taken together, these observations highlight both the centrality of folate in reproduction and the persistent controversies surrounding dosage, formulation, and timing.

Beyond female biology, paternal folate status and microenvironment also affect reproductive outcomes. A systematic review of paternal folate status and sperm quality notes that high and low folate concentrations are both associated with impaired spermatogenesis and that animal studies link paternal folate deficiency with congenital anomalies in offspring. However, human evidence remains sparse, and researchers call for large-scale trials to determine whether optimizing paternal folate improves fertility or reduces miscarriage (108). Complementary studies on the paternal gut microbiome suggest that dysbiosis can perturb hormone homeostasis and impair fertility; modulating the microbiome via diet or probiotics represents a promising future therapy (109). Similarly, epigenetic clocks – biomarkers that quantify biological age – may offer novel insights into reproductive ageing; integrating epigenetic data into fertility assessments could allow clinicians to personalize interventions and develop strategies to reverse "epigenetic ageing" (110). These varied findings illustrate the need to broaden the scope of folate research beyond female supplementation and to incorporate paternal health, multi omics data, and gene–environment interactions.

9.6.2 Emerging Trends in Folic Acid and Folate for Reproductive Health

Folate research is expanding beyond its classical role in preventing neural tube defects into a complex exploration of epigenetics, paternal contributions, nanomedicine and digital health. One striking trend is the investigation of folate's impact on DNA methylation and biological ageing. A controlled trial in healthy adults showed that daily supplementation with 400 or 800 μg folic acid for 8 weeks significantly increased red blood cell folate and accelerated the epigenetic clock, suggesting that folate influences DNA methylation patterns beyond pregnancy (9). These findings raise questions about long-term effects of supplemental folate on epigenetic ageing and underscore the need to determine optimal dosing and timing across the reproductive lifespan (10, 13). This holistic approach will enable clinicians to stratify patients based on genetic and epigenetic profiles and to monitor responses using molecular biomarkers.

Emerging evidence also highlights the interplay between folate and other nutrients. Folate functions within the one-carbon cycle alongside vitamin B12, B6, and methionine. A comprehensive meta-analysis of neural tube defects notes that vitamin B12 deficiency remains prevalent despite folic acid fortification, and genetic polymorphisms such as MTHFR exacerbate risk. The authors advocate for future clinical trials that combine folic acid and vitamin B12 supplementation while monitoring additional biomarkers like methylmalonic acid (111). Another systematic review found that preconception folic acid utilization in sub-Saharan Africa is low and uneven, urging longitudinal studies and culturally tailored interventions to increase supplementation and improve reporting accuracy (112). Emerging digital health strategies may help address such disparities; a study of electronic medical record (EMR) modifications showed that integrating folic acid testing into standard anemia screening increased deficiency detection and underscored the need for scalable digital interventions (113). As digital health technologies evolve, leveraging automated reminders and telehealth could enhance adherence to folate supplementation and support data collection for research.

Nanotechnology represents another frontier in reproductive medicine. Researchers are exploring nanoparticles that co deliver pharmaceuticals and gene silencing molecules to reproductive tissues. For example, lipid nanoparticles have been engineered to carry therapeutic agents and RNA molecules capable of gene editing; these formulations hold translational promise for treating uterine disorders and could eventually deliver gene editing tools to the endometrium or embryo. In pre-eclampsia models, targeted lipid nanoparticles delivering VEGF mRNA to the placenta restored endothelial function and improved fetal outcomes (114). Although these studies remain preclinical, they signal future possibilities for folate-related therapies; as folate is integral to methylation and gene expression, coupling folate metabolism modulators with RNA therapeutics could yield synergistic benefits. Another review notes that, despite advances, nanomedicine for non-malignant endometrial disorders remains underexplored and calls for research on targeted drug delivery, imaging, and gene therapy. Integrating nanotechnology with folate interventions could enhance tissue specificity and reduce systemic exposure.

Taken together, the emerging trends highlight an expansion of folate research into epigenetics, paternal health, nanomedicine, digital health, and metabolic integration. The future of folate in reproductive medicine will rely on interdisciplinary collaboration, multi omics technologies, sex-specific research, and culturally tailored interventions. Translating these discoveries into practice will require robust clinical trials, ethical frameworks, and engagement with policymakers to harmonize guidelines.

9.6.3 New Innovations in Infertility Treatment

Advances in in vitro activation (IVA) of dormant follicles also offer hope for women with diminished ovarian reserve. A pilot study of ovarian cortex fragmentation followed by autologous transplantation reported increased antral follicle counts and pregnancies in 22% of participants. The authors caution that evidence is limited and that supportive therapies – including platelet-rich plasma, mitochondrial transfer, and androgen supplementation – remain experimental (115). Nonetheless, IVA exemplifies how manipulating the ovarian microenvironment can restore fertility and underscores the need to explore combinations of folate supplementation with ovarian activation techniques.

Artificial intelligence is rapidly being integrated into infertility care. Machine learning systems evaluate embryo morphology, predict ploidy, and rank embryos for transfer. A prospective comparison of an AI-driven euploidy ranking model with physician assessments demonstrated that the AI system achieved superior performance across all score categories and improved embryo selection and IVF outcomes (116). However, a diagnostic meta-analysis noted significant heterogeneity among AI models, emphasizing the need for prospective, multicenter, and blinded studies with standardized outcome definitions and diverse data sources to enhance reliability (117). A related review warns that models trained in one clinical environment may not generalize to others, urging establishment of benchmark datasets and protocols to ensure reproducibility (118).

Gene editing and embryo engineering represent transformative innovations. CRISPR–Cas9 technology has been applied in animal models to correct genetic mutations underlying infertility and to study gene function in gametogenesis. A recent interdisciplinary review highlighted the potential of gene therapy and stem cell technologies to treat infertility while emphasizing that ethical considerations and legal frameworks must evolve alongside scientific advances (119).

Nanomedicine has also begun to influence infertility treatment. Lipid nanoparticles carrying gene silencing RNAs or therapeutic mRNAs have been delivered to reproductive tissues in preclinical models, improving placental angiogenesis and fetal growth (114). Incorporating folate molecules onto nanoparticles could facilitate targeted delivery to folate receptor-rich tissues, reducing off-target effects.

Emerging male infertility interventions illustrate the breadth of innovation. The FOLFIV trial found that high-dose folic acid (15 mg/day) improved biochemical pregnancy rates in couples undergoing ICSI and decreased sperm DNA fragmentation, although it did not alter standard semen parameters (96). In another trial, combining folic acid with zinc did not improve sperm DNA methylation or live birth rates (120), underscoring the need to identify which men benefit from supplementation. More broadly, research into paternal folate status, microbiota modulation, and epigenetic therapies holds promise for male fertility. As AI and gene editing technologies progress, combining them with micronutrient optimization may yield synergistic gains.

9.6.4 Potential for Personalized Approaches in Fertility Enhancement

Personalized medicine aims to tailor interventions to individual genetic, epigenetic, metabolic, and environmental profiles. For folate and fertility, this means considering genetic polymorphisms, metabolic status, sex differences, diet, and co-nutrients to optimize dosage and formulation. MTHFR polymorphisms serve as a paradigm: heterozygous or homozygous variants at C677T or A1298C reduce enzyme activity and impair conversion of folic acid to 5 MTHF (8). These findings demonstrate the importance of genotyping women and men before prescribing folate supplementation and support research on 5 MTHF as a more suitable form for individuals with reduced MTHFR activity. Personalization also involves optimizing dosage. High-dose regimens have been proposed for high-risk women, but evidence remains inconclusive. NICE and WHO recommend 4–5 mg/day for women with previous neural tube defects, diabetes, or antiseizure medication use, yet the evidence base is limited and does not address outcomes beyond neural tube defects (103). A study reiterated that routine 400 μg/day is appropriate for most women but that 5 mg/day should be reserved for high-risk groups (121). Personalized medicine will require stratifying patients by genetic variants, metabolic biomarkers, and comorbidities and designing trials to test differential dosing regimens.

REFERENCES

1. Crider KS, Yang TP, Berry RJ, Bailey LB. Folate and DNA methylation: A review of molecular mechanisms and the evidence for folate's role. *Advances in Nutrition*. 2012;3(1):21–38.
2. Mellor C, Larson EA, Wang M. Mechanisms of genome instability from cellular folate stress. *Journal of Cell Biology*. 2025;224(9).
3. Maynard AG, Petrova B, Kanarek N. Notes from the 2022 folate, vitamin B12, and one-carbon metabolism conference. *Metabolites*. 2023;13(4):486.
4. Kwong WY, Adamiak SJ, Gwynn A, Singh R, Sinclair KD. Endogenous folates and single-carbon metabolism in the ovarian follicle, oocyte and pre-implantation embryo. *Reproduction*. 2010;139(4):705–15.
5. Saini S, Sharma V, Ansari S, Kumar A, Thakur A, Malik H, et al. Folate supplementation during oocyte maturation positively impacts the folate-methionine metabolism in pre-implantation embryos. *Theriogenology*. 2022;182:63–70.
6. Gomes S, Lopes C, Pinto E. Folate and folic acid in the periconceptional period: Recommendations from official health organizations in thirty-six countries worldwide and WHO. *Public Health Nutrition*. 2016;19(1):176–89.
7. Paduch-Jakubczyk W, Dubińska M. The role of folic acid and its derivatives in reproductive health. *Actual Gynecology & Obstetrics/Aktuální Gynekologie a Porodnictví*. 2024;16.
8. Carboni L. Active folate versus folic acid: The role of 5-MTHF (methylfolate) in human health. *Integr Med (Encinitas)*. 2022;21(3):36–41.
9. Michels KB, Binder AM. Impact of folic acid supplementation on the epigenetic profile in healthy unfortified individuals – A randomized intervention trial. *Epigenetics*. 2024;19(1):2293410.
10. Kok DE, Dhonukshe-Rutten RA, Lute C, Heil SG, Uitterlinden AG, van der Velde N, et al. The effects of long-term daily folic acid and vitamin B12 supplementation on genome-wide DNA methylation in elderly subjects. *Clinical Epigenetics*. 2015;7(1):121.
11. Cai S, Xue B, Li S, Wang X, Zeng X, Zhu Z, et al. Methionine regulates maternal-fetal immune tolerance and endometrial receptivity by enhancing embryonic IL-5 secretion. *Cell Reports*. 2025;44(2):115291.
12. Jenkins T, Aston K, Carrell D, DeVilbiss E, Sjaarda L, Perkins N, et al. The impact of zinc and folic acid supplementation on sperm DNA methylation: Results from the Folic Acid and Zinc Supplementation Randomized Clinical Trial (FAZST). *Fertility and Sterility*. 2022;117(1):75–85.
13. García-García I, Grisotto G, Heini A, Gibertoni S, Nusslé S, Gonseth Nusslé S, et al. Examining nutrition strategies to influence DNA methylation and epigenetic clocks: A systematic review of clinical trials. *Frontiers in Aging*. 2024;5:1417625.
14. Boxmeer JC, Macklon NS, Lindemans J, Beckers NG, Eijkemans MJ, Laven JS, et al. IVF outcomes are associated with biomarkers of the homocysteine pathway in monofollicular fluid. *Human Reproduction*. 2009;24(5):1059–66.
15. Revelli A, Nuzzo AM, Moretti L, Arduino S, Roero S, Scali R, et al. Effects of homocysteine circulating levels on human spontaneous fertility and in vitro fertilization outcomes: A literature review. *Nutrients*. 2025;17(20):3211.
16. Albeitawi S, Bani-Mousa S-U, Jarrar B, Aloqaily I, Al-Shlool N, Alsheyab G, et al. Associations between follicular fluid biomarkers and IVF/ICSI outcomes in normo-ovulatory women – A systematic review. *Biomolecules*. 2025;15(3):443.
17. Zhang Y, He C, He Y, Zhu Z. Follicular fluid metabolomics: Tool for predicting IVF outcomes of different infertility causes. *Reproductive Sciences*. 2025;32(4):921–34.
18. Silvestris E, Lovero D, Palmirotta R. Nutrition and female fertility: An interdependent correlation. *Frontiers in Endocrinology*. 2019;10.
19. Paffoni A, Reschini M, Noli SA, Viganò P, Parazzini F, Somigliana E. Folate levels and pregnancy rate in women undergoing assisted reproductive techniques: A systematic review and meta-analysis. *Reproductive Sciences*. 2022;29(2):341–56.
20. Revelli A, Nuzzo AM, Moretti L, Arduino S, Roero S, Scali R, et al. Effects of homocysteine circulating levels on human spontaneous fertility and in vitro fertilization outcomes: A literature review. *Nutrients*. 2025;17(20):3211.
21. Boxmeer JC, Macklon NS, Lindemans J, Beckers NGM, Eijkemans MJC, Laven JSE, et al. IVF outcomes are associated with biomarkers of the homocysteine pathway in monofollicular fluid. *Human Reproduction*. 2009;24(5):1059–66.
22. Manzur NF, Gluska H, Feferkorn I, Skvirsky S, Ben-Shlomo I, Wiener-Megnazi Z. Homocysteine serum levels correlate with the number of failed IVF cycles even when within normal range. *Archives of Gynecology and Obstetrics*. 2023;307(6):1975–82.
23. Gaskins AJ, Afeiche MC, Wright DL, Toth TL, Williams PL, Gillman MW, et al. Dietary folate and reproductive success among women undergoing assisted reproduction. *Obstetrics and Gynecology*. 2014;124(4):801–9.

24. Ogawa S, Ota K, Takahashi T, Yoshida H. Impact of homocysteine as a preconceptional screening factor for in vitro fertilization and prevention of miscarriage with folic acid supplementation following frozen-thawed embryo transfer: A hospital-based retrospective cohort study. *Nutrients*. 2023;15(17):3730.
25. Gaskins AJ, Afeiche MC, Wright DL, Toth TL, Williams PL, Gillman MW, et al. Dietary folate and reproductive success among women undergoing assisted reproduction. *Obstet Gynecol*. 2014;124(4):801–9.
26. Murto T, Skoog Svanberg A, Yngve A, Nilsson TK, Altmae S, Wanggren K, et al. Folic acid supplementation and IVF pregnancy outcome in women with unexplained infertility. *Reprod Biomed Online*. 2014;28(6):766–72.
27. Cueto HT, Jacobsen BH, Laursen ASD, Riis AH, Hatch EE, Wise LA, et al. Dietary folate intake and fecundability in two preconception cohorts. *Human Reproduction*. 2022;37(4):828–37.
28. Alesi S, Habibi N, Silva TR, Cheung N, Torkel S, Tay CT, et al. Assessing the influence of preconception diet on female fertility: A systematic scoping review of observational studies. *Hum Reprod Update*. 2023;29(6):811–28.
29. Asemi Z, Karamali M, Esmaillzadeh A. Metabolic response to folate supplementation in overweight women with polycystic ovary syndrome: A randomized double-blind placebo-controlled clinical trial. *Molecular Nutrition & Food Research*. 2014;58(7):1465–73.
30. Han Y, Hou Y, Han Q, Yuan X, Chen L. Dietary supplements in polycystic ovary syndrome–Current evidence. *Front Endocrinol (Lausanne)*. 2024;15:1456571.
31. Ogawa S, Ota K, Takahashi T, Yoshida H. Impact of homocysteine as a preconceptional screening factor for in vitro fertilization and prevention of miscarriage with folic acid supplementation following frozen-thawed embryo transfer: A hospital-based retrospective cohort study. *Nutrients*. 2023;15(17).
32. Samaniego-Vaesken ML, Morais-Moreno C, Carretero-Krug A, Puga AM, Montero-Bravo AM, Partearroyo T, et al. Supplementation with folic acid or 5-methyltetrahydrofolate and prevention of neural tube defects: An evidence-based narrative review. *Nutrients*. 2024;16(18).
33. Dwyer ER, Filion KB, MacFarlane AJ, Platt RW, Mehrabadi A. Who should consume high-dose folic acid supplements before and during early pregnancy for the prevention of neural tube defects? *BMJ*. 2022;377:e067728.
34. Alrashidi AS, Aljaghwani LF, AlMohimeed RS, Alrashidi Jr AS, Almohimeed RS. The effect of nutrient supplementation on female fertility: A systematic review. *Cureus*. 2024;16(8).
35. Penzias A, Azziz R, Bendikson K, Falcone T, Hansen K, Hill M, et al. Optimizing natural fertility: A committee opinion. *Fertility and Sterility*. 2022;117(1):53–63.
36. Oostingh EC, Koster MPH, van Dijk MR, Willemsen SP, Broekmans FJM, Hoek A, et al. First effective mHealth nutrition and lifestyle coaching program for subfertile couples undergoing in vitro fertilization treatment: A single-blinded multicenter randomized controlled trial. *Fertil Steril*. 2020;114(5):945–54. https://doi.org/10.1016/j.fertnstert.2020.04.051.
37. Mathieu d'Argent E, Ravel C, Rousseau A, Morcel K, Massin N, Sussfeld J, et al. High-dose supplementation of folic acid in infertile men improves IVF-ICSI outcomes: A randomized controlled trial (FOLFIV trial). *JCM*. 2021;10(9).
38. Wdowiak A, Bakalczuk S, Filip M, Laganà AS, Unfer V. The clinical use of myo-inositol in IVF-ET: A position statement from the experts group on inositol in basic and clinical research and on PCOS (EGOI-PCOS), the Polish Society of Andrology, and the International Scientific Association for the Support and Development of Medical Technologies. *JCM*. 2025;14(2):558.
39. Mohammadi S, Eini F, Bazarganipour F, Taghavi SA, Kutenaee MA. The effect of Myo-inositol on fertility rates in poor ovarian responder in women undergoing assisted reproductive technique: A randomized clinical trial. *Reproductive Biology and Endocrinology*. 2021;19(1):61.
40. Pacchiarotti A, Carlomagno G, Antonini G, Pacchiarotti A. Effect of myo-inositol and melatonin versus myo-inositol, in a randomized controlled trial, for improving in vitro fertilization of patients with polycystic ovarian syndrome. *Gynecological Endocrinology*. 2016;32(1):69–73.
41. Bezerra Espinola MS, Bilotta G, Aragona C. Positive effect of a new supplementation of vitamin D3 with myo-inositol, folic acid and melatonin on IVF outcomes: A prospective randomized and controlled pilot study. *Gynecological Endocrinology*. 2021;37(3):251–4.
42. Pandey C, Maunder A, Liu J, Vaddiparthi V, Costello MF, Bahri-Khomami M, et al. The role of nutrient supplements in female infertility: An umbrella review and hierarchical evidence synthesis. *Nutrients*. 2025;17(1):57.
43. Cueto HT, Jacobsen BH, Laursen ASD, Riis AH, Hatch EE, Wise LA, et al. Dietary folate intake and fecundability in two preconception cohorts. *Human Reproduction*. 2022;37(4):828–37.
44. Chen L, Chen H, Wang X, Wei B, Wu Z, Chen S, et al. Association of homocysteine with IVF/ICSI outcomes stratified by (MTHFR) C677T polymorphisms: A prospective cohort study. *Reproductive BioMedicine Online*. 2021;43(1):52–61.
45. Paffoni A, Castiglioni M, Ferrari S, La Vecchia I, Ferraris Fusarini C, Bettinardi N, et al. Homocysteine pathway and in vitro fertilization outcome. *Reproductive Toxicology*. 2018;76:12–6.

46. Kim C-H, Moon J-W, Yoo R-m, Moon SY. Effect of 5-methyltetrahydrofolate in infertile patients with methylenetetrahydrofolate reductase (MTHFR) 677TT mutation undergoing IVF. *Fertility and Sterility*. 2021;116(3):e225.
47. Palomares AR, Ruiz-Galdon M, Liu K, Reyes-Engel A, Rodriguez-Wallberg KA. Profiling the influence of gene variants related to folate-mediated one-carbon metabolism on the outcome of in vitro fertilization (IVF) with donor oocytes in recipients receiving folic acid fortification. *International Journal of Molecular Sciences*. 2022;23(19):11298.
48. Mathieu d'Argent E, Ravel C, Rousseau A, Morcel K, Massin N, Sussfeld J, et al. High-dose supplementation of folic acid in infertile men improves IVF-ICSI outcomes: A randomized controlled trial (FOLFIV Trial). *JCM*. 2021;10(9):1876.
49. Schisterman EF, Sjaarda LA, Clemons T, Carrell DT, Perkins NJ, Johnstone E, et al. Effect of folic acid and zinc supplementation in men on semen quality and live birth among couples undergoing infertility treatment: A randomized clinical trial. *JAMA*. 2020;323(1):35–48.
50. Hart RJ. Nutritional supplements and IVF: An evidence-based approach. *Reproductive BioMedicine Online*. 2024;48(3).
51. Gaskins AJ, Nassan FL, Chiu Y-H, Arvizu M, Williams PL, Keller MG, et al. Dietary patterns and outcomes of assisted reproduction. *American Journal of Obstetrics & Gynecology*. 2019;220(6):567.e1–e18.
52. Ménézo Y, Elder K, Clement P, Dattilo M, Patrizio P. Fortification with folic acid and early human embryo development: lessons from assisted reproduction. *J Assist Reprod Genet*. 2025;42(10):2979–89. https://doi.org/10.1007/s10815-025-03613-3.
53. Bailey LB, Gregory JF, III. Folate metabolism and requirements. *Journal of Nutrition*. 1999;129(4):779–82.
54. Menezo Y, Elder K, Clement A, Clement P. Folic acid, folinic acid, 5 methyl tetrahydrofolate supplementation for mutations that affect epigenesis through the folate and one-carbon cycles. *Biomolecules*. 2022;12(2):197.
55. Gaskins AJ, Chiu Y-H, Williams PL, Ford JB, Toth TL, Hauser R, et al. Association between serum folate and vitamin B-12 and outcomes of assisted reproductive technologies1. *American Journal of Clinical Nutrition*. 2015;102(4):943–50.
56. Cirillo M, Fucci R, Rubini S, Coccia ME, Fatini C. 5-Methyltetrahydrofolate and vitamin B12 supplementation is associated with clinical pregnancy and live birth in women undergoing assisted reproductive technology. *International Journal of Environmental Research and Public Health*. 2021;18(23):12280.
57. Helal NA, Eassa HA, Amer AM, Eltokhy MA, Edafiogho I, Nounou MI. Nutraceuticals' novel formulations: The good, the bad, the unknown and patents involved. *Recent Patents on Drug Delivery & Formulation*. 2019;13(2):105–56.
58. Hart RJ. Nutritional supplements and IVF: An evidence-based approach. *Reprod Biomed Online*. 2024;48(3):103770.
59. Cawley S, Mullaney L, McKeating A, Farren M, McCartney D, Turner M. A review of European guidelines on periconceptional folic acid supplementation. *European Journal of Clinical Nutrition*. 2016;70(2):143–54.
60. De-Regil LM, Peña-Rosas JP, Fernández-Gaxiola AC, Rayco-Solon P. Effects and safety of periconceptional oral folate supplementation for preventing birth defects. *Cochrane Database of Systematic Reviews*. 2015(12).
61. Centers for Disease C, Prevention. *Folic Acid: About Folic Acid*. CDC; 2024.
62. Polzikov M, Blinov D, Barakhoeva Z, Vovk L, Fetisova Y, Ovchinnikova M, et al. Association of the serum folate and total calcium and magnesium levels before ovarian stimulation with outcomes of fresh in vitro fertilization cycles in normogonadotropic women. *Frontiers in Endocrinology*. 2022;13.
63. Kadir M, Hood RB, Mínguez-Alarcón L, Maldonado-Cárceles AB, Ford JB, Souter I, et al. Folate intake and ovarian reserve among women attending a fertility center. *Fertility and Sterility*. 2022;117(1):171–80.
64. Murto T, Skoog Svanberg A, Yngve A, Nilsson TK, Altmäe S, Wånggren K, et al. Folic acid supplementation and IVF pregnancy outcome in women with unexplained infertility. *Reproductive BioMedicine Online*. 2014;28(6):766–72.
65. Kovacs G, Norman R, editors. *How to Improve Preconception Health to Maximize IVF Success*. Cambridge (UK): Cambridge University Press; 2018. p. 162.
66. Showell MG, Mackenzie-Proctor R, Jordan V, Hart RJ. Antioxidants for female subfertility. *Cochrane Database Syst Rev*. 2020;(8):CD007807. https://doi.org/10.1002/14651858.CD007807.pub4.
67. Rizzo P, Raffone E, Benedetto V. Effect of the treatment with myo-inositol plus folic acid plus melatonin in comparison with a treatment with myo-inositol plus folic acid on oocyte quality and pregnancy outcome in IVF cycles. A prospective, clinical trial. *Eur Rev Med Pharmacol Sci*. 2010;14(6):555–61.
68. Jadhav SN, Pitale DL. Effectiveness of folic acid in unexplained infertility. *International Journal of Reproduction, Contraception, Obstetrics and Gynecology*. 2020;9(9):3780–3.

69. Kadir M, Hood RB, Mínguez-Alarcón L, Maldonado-Cárceles AB, Ford JB, Souter I, et al. Folate intake and ovarian reserve among women attending a fertility center. *Fertil Steril.* 2022;117(1):171–80.
70. Zhang L, Wu L-m, Xu W-h, Tian Y-q, Liu X-l, Xia C-y, et al. Status of maternal serum B vitamins and pregnancy outcomes: New insights from in vitro fertilization and embryo transfer (IVF-ET) treatment. *Frontiers in Nutrition.* 2022;9.
71. Pandey C, Maunder A, Liu J, Vaddiparthi V, Costello MF, Bahri-Khomami M, et al. The role of nutrient supplements in female infertility: An umbrella review and hierarchical evidence synthesis. *Nutrients.* 2024;17(1).
72. Bortolus R, Filippini F, Cipriani S, Trevisanuto D, Marchetti F, Mastroiacovo P, et al. Randomized controlled trial of 4.0 mg versus 0.4 mg folic acid supplementation: Follow-up of children at 1 year of age. *Eur J Obstet Gynecol Reprod Biol X.* 2025;25:100370.
73. Mahoney A, D'Angelo A. Treatment options for managing anovulation in women with PCOS: An extensive literature review of evidence-based recommendations for future directions. *Life (Basel).* 2025;15(6).
74. Bibbins-Domingo K, Grossman DC, Curry SJ, Davidson KW, Epling JW, García FA, et al. Folic acid supplementation for the prevention of neural tube defects: US Preventive Services Task Force recommendation statement. *JAMA.* 2017;317(2):183–9.
75. Wilson RD, O'Connor DL. Maternal folic acid and multivitamin supplementation: International clinical evidence with considerations for the prevention of folate-sensitive birth defects. *Prev Med Rep.* 2021;24:101617.
76. Ledowsky CJ, Schloss J, Steel A. Variations in folate prescriptions for patients with the MTHFR genetic polymorphisms: A case series study. *Explor Res Clin Soc Pharm.* 2023;10:100277.
77. Ulloque-Badaracco JR, Al-Kassab-Córdova A, Hernández-Bustamante EA, Alarcón-Braga EA, Cabrera-Guzmán JC, Horruitiner-Mendoza AA, et al. Homocysteine, vitamin B12, and folate circulating levels in women with and without polycystic ovary syndrome: A systematic review and meta-analysis. *Womens Health (Lond).* 2024;20:17455057241279039.
78. Soliman MY, Idris OAF, Momtaz M, Kortam MA, MA EL, Saleh HA, et al. Expert consensus on the role of supplementation in obstetrics and gynecology using modified delphi method. *Arch Gynecol Obstet.* 2024;309(2):639–50.
79. Liao K, Wang Y, Zheng L, Lu D, Wu J, Wu B, et al. Effect of folic acid supplementation on diminished ovarian reserve: Study protocol of a single-centre, open-label, randomised, placebo-controlled clinical trial. *BMJ Open.* 2022;12(7):e057689.
80. Gullo G, Zaami S, Streva AV, Burgio S, Billone V, Kotlik Y, et al. Multivitamin supplementation and fertility outcome: A retrospective single-center cohort study and the clinical and medicolegal value of nutritional counseling. *Life.* 2025;15(1):48.
81. Sene AA, Saeedzarandi M, Yazdizadeh M, Ghaffari SR, Amjadi F, Zandieh Z, et al. The effect of myo-inositol on assisted reproductive technology outcomes in women with polycystic ovarian syndrome: A systematic review and meta-analysis of randomized clinical trial studies. *Int J Reprod Biomed.* 2025;23(5):353–76.
82. Chen H, Wang S, Song M, Yang D, Li H. Oocyte and dietary supplements: A mini review. *Front Cell Dev Biol.* 2025;13:1619758.
83. Yu L, Cai W, Wang C, Shen M, Liu M, Che Q, et al. Alteration of the follicular fluid amino acid profile reveals the important roles of several amino acids in embryo quality in patients with polycystic ovary syndrome. *Reprod Biol Endocrinol.* 2025;23(1):123.
84. Mascarenhas MN, Flaxman SR, Boerma T, Vanderpoel S, Stevens GA. National, regional, and global trends in infertility prevalence since 1990: A systematic analysis of 277 health surveys. *PLoS Medicine.* 2012;9(12):e1001356.
85. Revelli A, Nuzzo AM, Moretti L, Arduino S, Roero S, Scali R, et al. Effects of homocysteine circulating levels on human spontaneous fertility and in vitro fertilization outcomes: A literature review. *Nutrients.* 2025;17(20).
86. Jadhav SN, Pitale DL. Effectiveness of folic acid in unexplained infertility. *International Journal of Reproduction, Contraception, Obstetrics and Gynecology.* 2020;9(9):3781.
87. Loperfido F, Sottotetti F, Bianco I, El Masri D, Maccarini B, Ferrara C, et al. Folic acid supplementation in European women of reproductive age and during pregnancy with excessive weight: A systematic review. *Reprod Health.* 2025;22(1):13.
88. Valensise H, Banzi C, Bonin C, Dell'Avanzo M, Di Simone N, Farsetti D, et al. Optimizing pregnancy outcomes: The role of gynecologists in preconceptional care in Italy. *Int J Womens Health.* 2025;17:1897–909.
89. Choi JH, Yates Z, Veysey M, Heo YR, Lucock M. Contemporary issues surrounding folic acid fortification initiatives. *Prev Nutr Food Sci.* 2014;19(4):247–60.

90. Fardous AM, Heydari AR. Uncovering the hidden dangers and molecular mechanisms of excess folate: A narrative review. *Nutrients*. 2023;15(21).
91. Zeng H, Liu Z, Zhang L, Liu N. MTHFR 677TT is associated with decreased number of embryos and cumulative live birth rate in patients undergoing GnRHa short protocol: A retrospective study. *BMC Pregnancy and Childbirth*. 2022;22(1):170.
92. Lu YJ, Li Q, Chen LX, Tian T, Kang J, Hao YX, et al. Association between maternal MTHFR C677T/A1298C combination polymorphisms and IVF/ICSI outcomes: A retrospective cohort study. *Hum Reprod Open*. 2023;2023(1):hoac055.
93. Tan X, Yu Z, Sao J, Chen L, Shen Y, Ding J, et al. Association between in vitro fertilization outcomes and inherited thrombophilias: A meta-analysis. *Journal of Assisted Reproduction and Genetics*. 2016;33(8):1093–8.
94. Ledowsky CJ, Schloss J, Steel A. Variations in folate prescriptions for patients with the MTHFR genetic polymorphisms: A case series study. *Exploratory Research in Clinical and Social Pharmacy*. 2023;10:100277.
95. Palomares AR, Ruiz-Galdon M, Liu K, Reyes-Engel A, Rodriguez-Wallberg KA. Profiling the influence of gene variants related to folate-mediated one-carbon metabolism on the outcome of in vitro fertilization (IVF) with donor oocytes in recipients receiving folic acid fortification. *Int J Mol Sci*. 2022;23(19).
96. Mathieu d'Argent E, Ravel C, Rousseau A, Morcel K, Massin N, Sussfeld J, et al. High-dose supplementation of folic acid in infertile men improves IVF-ICSI outcomes: A randomized controlled trial (FOLFIV trial). *J Clin Med*. 2021;10(9).
97. He Q, Zhang M, Xiao S, Guo Z. Folic acid and sperm quality improvement: Insights from snRNA sequencing and RNA splicing mechanisms. *Front Nutr*. 2025;12:1648307.
98. Dahlen CR, Amat S, Caton JS, Crouse MS, Diniz W, Reynolds LP. Paternal effects on fetal programming. *Anim Reprod*. 2023;20(2):e20230076.
99. Russo M, Forte G, Montanino Oliva M, Laganà AS, Unfer V. Melatonin and myo-inositol: Supporting reproduction from the oocyte to birth. *Int J Mol Sci*. 2021;22(16).
100. Pacchiarotti A, Carlomagno G, Antonini G, Pacchiarotti A. Effect of myo-inositol and melatonin versus myo-inositol, in a randomized controlled trial, for improving in vitro fertilization of patients with polycystic ovarian syndrome. *Gynecol Endocrinol*. 2016;32(1):69–73.
101. Pourghasem S, Bazarganipour F, Taghavi SA, Kutenaee MA. The effectiveness of inositol and metformin on infertile polycystic ovary syndrome women with resistant to letrozole. *Arch Gynecol Obstet*. 2019;299(4):1193–9.
102. Charles DH, Ness AR, Campbell D, Smith GD, Whitley E, Hall MH. Folic acid supplements in pregnancy and birth outcome: Re-analysis of a large randomised controlled trial and update of Cochrane review. *Paediatric and Perinatal Epidemiology*. 2005;19(2):112–24.
103. National Institute for Health and Care Excellence (NICE). *Evidence Reviews for High-Dose Folic Acid Supplementation Before and During the First 12 Weeks of Pregnancy: Maternal and Child Nutrition: Evidence Review A*. London: National Institute for Health and Care Excellence (NICE); 2025 2025/01.
104. Ledowsky C, Scarf V, Steel A. Health professionals require more defined protocols, better funding and patient resources to support couples with recurrent pregnancy loss. *Sci Rep*. 2025;15(1):28965.
105. Wang D, Nguyen CH, Asghari-Kamrani A, Partap U, Shah I, Fawzi WW. Nutrition and reproductive potential of women in low- and middle-income countries: A systematic review and meta-analysis. *BMJ Global Health*. 2025;10(Suppl. 1):e015713.
106. Hussain A, Abbas M, Zain ul A, Mustafa G, Lateef M, Mansoor A, et al. Innovations and challenges in modern infertility treatment: Bridging technology and psychosocial care. *Middle East Fertility Society Journal*. 2025;30(1):44.
107. Barry MJ, Nicholson WK, Silverstein M, Chelmow D, Coker TR, Davis EM, et al. Folic acid supplementation to prevent neural tube defects: US Preventive Services Task Force reaffirmation recommendation statement. *JAMA*. 2023;330(5):454–9.
108. Hoek J, Steegers-Theunissen RPM, Willemsen SP, Schoenmakers S. Paternal folate status and sperm quality, pregnancy outcomes, and epigenetics: A systematic review and meta-analysis. *Mol Nutr Food Res*. 2020;64(9):e1900696.
109. Zambella E, Inversetti A, Salerno S, Müller M, Di Simone N. The father's microbiome: A hidden contributor to fetal and long-term child health. *Biology (Basel)*. 2025;14(8).
110. Li Piani L, Vigano P, Somigliana E. Epigenetic clocks and female fertility timeline: A new approach to an old issue? *Front Cell Dev Biol*. 2023;11:1121231.
111. Nie L, Liu X, Li X, Ren Z, Cheng X, Wu Y, et al. Beyond folate: The emerging role of maternal vitamin B12 in neural tube development. *Nutrients*. 2025;17(12).
112. Aweke MN, Fentie EA, Agimas MC, Baffa LD, Shewarega ES, Belew AK, et al. Folic acid supplementation during preconception period in sub-Saharan African countries: A systematic review and meta-analysis. *PLoS One*. 2025;20(1):e0318422.

113. Litvak D, Merzon E, Shenhar Y, Green I, Vinker S, Israel A, et al. Improving folic acid supplementation through electronic medical record interface modifications–A retrospective study. *J Clin Med.* 2025;14(14).
114. Herrara V, Tarab-Ravski D, Chauhan SC, Narang N, Mirazul Islam M, Peer D, et al. Nanotechnology strategies for endometrium health: Are we on the right track? *Bioact Mater.* 2025;54:423–49.
115. Salehpour S, Kazemi M, Hosseini S, Hajizadeh N, Karimi B, Abbasi H, et al. Drug-free in vitro activation and autologous transplantation in infertile women with diminished ovarian reserve: An experimental pilot study. *Int J Reprod Biomed.* 2024;22(6):425–32.
116. Wang G, Wang K, Gao Y, Chen L, Gao T, Ma Y, et al. A generalized AI system for human embryo selection covering the entire IVF cycle via multi-modal contrastive learning. *Patterns (N Y).* 2024;5(7):100985.
117. Mina A, Younesi M, Doohandeh T, Darzi S, Ardehjani NA, Sheibani S, et al. Predicting pregnancy outcomes in IVF cycles: A systematic review and diagnostic meta- analysis of artificial intelligence in embryo assessment. *Contracept Reprod Med.* 2025;10(1):59.
118. Thirumalaraju P, Kanakasabapathy MK, Kandula H, Kandula T, Reddy Katkuri AV, Cipriano C, et al. Stability and reliability of artificial intelligence models in embryo selection for in vitro fertilization. *Fertil Steril.* 2026;125(2):277–86. https://doi.org/10.1016/j.fertnstert.2025.08.021.
119. Soczyńska J, Gawełczyk W, Papierkowska J, Muzyka A, Majcherczyk K, Obrycka P, et al. The future of embryo engineering and fertility research in interdisciplinary collaboration. *Front Cell Dev Biol.* 2025;13:1619050.
120. Jenkins T, Aston K, Carrell D, DeVilbiss E, Sjaarda L, Perkins N, et al. The impact of zinc and folic acid supplementation on sperm DNA methylation: Results from the folic acid and zinc supplementation randomized clinical trial (FAZST). *Fertil Steril.* 2022;117(1):75–85.
121. Dwyer ER, Filion KB, MacFarlane AJ, Platt RW, Mehrabadi A. Who should consume high-dose folic acid supplements before and during early pregnancy for the prevention of neural tube defects? *BMJ.* 2022;377.

10 The Role of Probiotics in Gynecological Disorders
RCT-Based Evidence

Ali Afrasiabi, Minoo Vahedi Raad, Maryam Azizi-Kutenaei, and Farzaneh Fesahat

10.1 INTRODUCTION

Preterm delivery continues to represent a major global cause of neonatal mortality and long-term morbidity, carrying substantial clinical, developmental, and socioeconomic implications. Emerging evidence identifies vaginal dysbiosis, particularly bacterial vaginosis and recurrent vulvovaginal infections, as a potentially modifiable risk factor for poor obstetric outcomes, including spontaneous preterm labor (1, 2). The genital tract microbiome serves crucial functions in preserving immunological homeostasis, epithelial barrier function, and controlling pathogen proliferation; compositional alterations characterized by diminished Lactobacillus predominance have been linked to heightened inflammatory responses and consequent increased risk of premature delivery (3, 4).

Probiotic supplementation, particularly with *Lactobacillus* species (e.g. *L. crispatus, L. rhamnosus, L. reuteri*) or multi-strain formulations, presents a promising therapeutic and preventive strategy. Evidence from randomized controlled trials (RCTs) suggests potential benefits of such interventions in restoring vaginal microflora, reducing Nugent scores, prolonging remission of BV, and improving related clinical outcomes (1, 3, 5). In the context of polycystic ovary syndrome (PCOS) and metabolic dysfunction – conditions linked to chronic inflammation, oxidative stress, and hormonal imbalance – adjunctive therapies such as probiotics combined with time-restricted eating (TRE) or calorie restriction have demonstrated favorable effects on metabolic, inflammatory, and antioxidant biomarkers (6, 7). Yet, whether these metabolic-immunologic improvements translate into a reduced risk of preterm birth or improved pregnancy-related outcomes remains inadequately elucidated.

Although several RCTs have evaluated the efficacy of probiotics in preventing recurrence of BV, treating vulvovaginal candidiasis (VVC), or supporting fertility treatments (8–10), findings are heterogeneous. Some trials report significant microbiological or symptomatic improvements (11, 12), whereas others find minimal or no added benefit over standard treatments (13, 14). Moreover, differences in probiotic strain composition, dosage, route (oral, vaginal, transvaginal), duration of administration, and the baseline microbiome or metabolic status of participants complicate cross-study comparisons (2, 15).

Therefore, there is a pressing need to synthesize high-quality evidence from RCTs to clarify: (1) which probiotic strains, dosages, and routes are most effective; (2) in which populations (e.g. women with PCOS, overweight vs. non-overweight, history of BV) probiotic supplementation yields clinically meaningful improvements; and (3) whether improvements in microbiologic or metabolic risk factors translate into reduced rates of preterm birth and other adverse pregnancy outcomes.

10.2 CLINICAL MANIFESTATION OF EFFECTS OF PROBIOTICS

10.2.1 Probiotics in Polycystic Ovary Syndrome

Multiple randomized controlled trials have investigated the efficacy of probiotic supplementation, both as monotherapy and as an adjunct to dietary modifications, on metabolic and reproductive outcomes in women diagnosed with polycystic ovary syndrome. In two distinct randomized trials conducted by Talebi et al. (2023, 2025) involving overweight and obese PCOS patients, the effects of time-restricted eating and calorie restriction were evaluated with and without concurrent probiotic supplementation. The findings from both investigations revealed that TRE regimens, whether implemented alone or in combination with probiotics, resulted in statistically significant enhancements in body weight, metabolic profiles, hormonal parameters, and antioxidant biomarkers, alongside notable reductions in systolic blood pressure and C-reactive protein (CRP) levels. The probiotic interventions were consistently reported to be well-tolerated throughout the study periods (7, 16). In a separate clinical investigation, Azizi-Kutenaee et al. (2022) documented that combination therapy utilizing Lactofem – a probiotic formulation containing *Lactobacillus acidophilus,*

DOI: 10.1201/9781003741541-10

Bifidobacterium bifidus, *L. rutri*, and *L. fermentum* – administered concomitantly with letrozole demonstrated superior outcomes in pregnancy rates, sexual function parameters, and body image scores compared to letrozole monotherapy (8). Complementing these findings, Karimi et al. (2018) observed that synbiotic supplementation produced a significant reduction in serum apelin-36 concentrations, though no substantial modifications were detected in HOMA-IR or CRP values, indicating targeted metabolic effects rather than comprehensive endocrine modulation (17). Furthermore, Zafar et al. (2021) established that the concurrent administration of probiotics with metformin significantly decreased prolactin levels in hyperprolactinemic PCOS patients, thereby augmenting the metabolic effectiveness of conventional therapeutic approaches (6).

10.2.2 Probiotics and Assisted Reproductive Technologies

The efficacy of probiotic supplementation has been evaluated across multiple studies involving women undergoing in vitro fertilization or embryo transfer procedures. Thanaboonyawat et al. (2023) reported that intravaginally administered probiotics during the luteal phase did not yield significant differences in implantation, ongoing pregnancy, or live birth rates; however, a notable reduction in miscarriage rates was observed (18). Earlier research by Gilboa et al. (2005) indicated that vaginal probiotic application immediately following oocyte retrieval failed to demonstrate improved pregnancy outcomes (19). Contrasting these findings, Wei et al. (2024) documented that vaginal Lactobacillus supplementation significantly enhanced clinical pregnancy rates among women with a history of unsuccessful frozen embryo transfer cycles (10). In a different approach, Chan et al. (2023) examined a combined myo-inositol, probiotic, and micronutrient formulation in women attempting conception. While overall pregnancy rates remained comparable to standard prenatal supplements, overweight participants exhibited reduced time to conception, suggesting possible metabolic synergism (20).

10.2.3 Probiotics in Bacterial Vaginosis

This clinical domain represents the most extensively researched area in probiotic trials, encompassing both oral and intravaginal administration routes as complementary or alternative approaches to antibiotic therapy.

Pioneering investigations by Anukam et al. (2006) demonstrated that oral administration of *Lactobacillus rhamnosus* GR-1 and *L. reuteri* RC-14 alongside metronidazole resulted in substantially superior cure rates compared to antibiotic monotherapy (88% versus 40%), while intravaginal probiotic installation alone achieved 90% therapeutic success (11, 21). Subsequent research has produced divergent outcomes. Investigations by Mastromarino et al. (2009), Larsson et al. (2008), and Vicariotto et al. (2014) documented significant enhancements in Nugent scores and extended recurrence-free intervals (22–24). In contrast, Bradshaw et al. (2012) and Eriksson et al. (2005) reported no additional therapeutic advantage beyond conventional treatment (25, 26). Large-scale multicenter randomized controlled trials, including Cohen et al. (2020) evaluating Lactin-V, Reznichenko et al. (2020), and Heczko et al. (2015), consistently established that probiotic interventions – particularly those utilizing *L. crispatus* strains – significantly decreased bacterial vaginosis recurrence and sustained clinical remission (1, 5, 27). Contrarily, clinical studies by Zhang et al. (2021), Qi et al. (2023), and van de Wijgert et al. (2020) proposed that oral probiotic supplementation may enhance vaginal microbiota composition without significantly affecting cure rates, potentially attributable to restricted mucosal colonization (2, 14, 28). Supplementary research by Boroumand Rezazadeh et al. (2024) and Wang Ya et al. (2010) demonstrated equivalent effectiveness between oral and vaginal delivery methods and indicated potential for prolonged prevention of recurrent episodes (4, 15). Further safety evaluations by Happel et al. (2020), Pirotta et al. (2004), and Gille et al. (2016) established the favorable safety profile of probiotics during antibiotic therapies and pregnancy, though their capacity to maintain normative microbiota remained constrained (13, 29, 30).

10.2.4 Probiotics in Vulvovaginal Candidiasis

Clinical trials addressing VVC show moderate benefit from probiotics.

Martinez et al. (2009) demonstrated that combining *L. rhamnosus* GR-1 and *L. reuteri* RC-14 with fluconazole significantly reduced vaginal discharge and yeast presence (31).

However, Zahra et al. (2023) and Thekho et al. (2024) reported that while probiotics alleviated acute symptoms comparably to fluconazole, they were less effective in achieving long-term culture negativity, suggesting a role in symptom relief rather than complete eradication (9, 32).

10.2.5 Probiotics in Pregnancy and Preterm Birth Prevention

Several RCTs have explored probiotic safety and potential obstetric benefits during pregnancy.

Husain et al. (2020) and Gille et al. (2016) found that oral administration of *L. rhamnosus* GR-1 and *L. reuteri* RC-14 did not significantly alter vaginal microbiota composition during gestation (29, 33).

Yang (2020) confirmed probiotic safety and tolerance in pregnant women with intermediate Nugent scores but no improvement in vaginal microbiota outcomes (34).

Krauss-Silva et al. (2011) conducted a large-scale trial in women with asymptomatic BV, finding no significant reduction in preterm birth rates, though probiotics were well tolerated with minimal adverse events (35).

10.2.6 Probiotics in Urinary Tract Infections and Aerobic Vaginitis

Czaja et al. (2007) demonstrated the safety of intravaginal *L. crispatus* CTV-05 in women with recurrent urinary tract infections (UTIs), with only mild irritation reported (36).

Heczko et al. (2015) also found that oral probiotics containing multiple *Lactobacillus* strains reduced recurrence rates and improved vaginal pH and microbiota profiles in women with recurrent BV or aerobic vaginitis (5).

10.2.7 Probiotics and Mental Health/Sexual Function

Beyond gynecological outcomes, Nazir et al. (2024) found that co-administration of Lactofem with SSRIs in women with depressive disorder significantly improved sexual function (FSFI domains) and reduced depression severity, highlighting the potential psychosexual benefits of probiotics (37).

10.3 SUMMARY AND INTEGRATION

Overall, RCT evidence indicates that probiotic supplementation in women's reproductive and sexual health is safe and generally well tolerated. While the benefits vary by condition and strain used, the most consistent effects are seen in reducing BV recurrence, improving select metabolic and reproductive outcomes in PCOS, and enhancing quality of life measures such as sexual satisfaction. However, several large trials report no significant differences compared to placebo or standard therapy, underscoring the need for strain-specific, route-specific, and population-specific protocols in future research (Table 10.1).

10.4 SYNERGISM

Multiple randomized controlled trials have examined the complementary role of probiotic supplementation alongside conventional therapeutic approaches in managing reproductive and gynecological disorders. Clinical evidence indicates that combining probiotics with time-restricted eating regimens yields enhanced clinical outcomes in polycystic ovary syndrome patients. One RCT documented significant improvements in systolic blood pressure, C-reactive protein levels, and total antioxidant capacity following combined probiotic and TRE intervention, though intergroup differences in specific oxidative stress parameters failed to reach statistical significance (16). A subsequent investigation by the same research group demonstrated that both TRE monotherapy and TRE-probiotic combination therapy resulted in substantial weight reduction and significant enhancements across metabolic, hormonal, inflammatory, and antioxidant parameters in overweight and obese PCOS patients when compared to traditional calorie restriction approaches (7).

In pharmacological contexts, synergistic benefits have also been observed. The adjunctive administration of Lactofem with letrozole demonstrated superior outcomes relative to letrozole monotherapy in women with PCOS, evidenced by increased chemical and clinical pregnancy rates, enhanced scores across multiple domains of sexual function, and improved body image perception, indicating a potential synergistic role for probiotics in optimizing ovulation induction regimens (8). Likewise, in women with hyperprolactinemia and PCOS, probiotics combined with metformin significantly reduced serum prolactin levels after 12 weeks compared to metformin monotherapy, highlighting potential synergistic effects in endocrine modulation (6).

In infectious disease contexts, the addition of probiotics to standard antifungal therapy (fluconazole) for vulvovaginal candidiasis showed comparable efficacy in alleviating clinical symptoms but was less effective in preventing recurrence compared to fluconazole alone (32). However, another RCT demonstrated that probiotic supplementation enhanced fluconazole

Table 10.1: Results of RCTs Based on Drug Combinations and Their Results

Author	Year of Publication	Study Design	Number of Enrollments	Kinds of Probiotic and Dosage	Key Findings
Talebi et al.	2025	RCT	90	TRE + probiotic vs. TRE + placebo vs. DCR + placebo; duration 8 weeks	TRE, with or without probiotics, improved SBP, CRP, TAC; probiotics well tolerated
Thekho et al.	2024	RCT	60	Fluconazole ± probiotics (*L. crispatus* 1×10^9, *L. rhamnosus* 1×10^9, *L. gasseri* 0.3×10^9, *L. jensenii* 0.2×10^9)	Symptoms improved in both groups; no significant differences; safe
Thanaboonyawat et al.	2023	RCT	316	Intravaginal Lactobacilli tablets + progesterone vs. progesterone only	No significant differences in pregnancy outcomes; miscarriage rate lower in probiotic group
Azizi-Kutenaee et al.	2022	RCT	40	Lactofem (*L. acidophilus, B. bifidus, L. rutri, L. fermentum*); Myo-inositol + probiotics + micronutrients vs. standard prenatal supplements	Improved chemical/clinical pregnancy, FSFI, and body image scores
Talebi et al.	2023	RCT	90	14:10 TRE + probiotic vs. TRE + placebo vs. DCR + placebo; 8 weeks	Weight loss and improved metabolic, hormonal, inflammatory, antioxidant markers
Chan et al.	2023	RCT	-	Myo-inositol + probiotics + micronutrients vs. standard prenatal supplements	Similar conception rates overall; overweight women benefited
Zafar et al.	2021	RCT	102	Metformin probiotics (180 mg daily)	Probiotics reduced serum prolactin more than metformin alone
Happel et al.	2020	RCT	30	Metronidazole ± commercial oral/vaginal probiotic	No additional benefit from probiotics; both groups improved
Karimi et al.	2018	RCT	88	Synbiotic supplement vs. placebo (12 weeks)	Decreased apelin-36; no improvement in HOMA-IR or CRP
Nazir et al.	2024	RCT	112	SSRI – Lactofem (*L. acidophilus, B. bifidus, L. rutri, L. fermentum*; 2×10^9 CFU each)	Improved sexual satisfaction, FSFI, and depressive symptoms
Zahra et al.	2023	RCT	80	Fluconazole vs. probiotic (*L. acidophilus*)	Fluconazole more effective at preventing recurrence; both controlled acute symptoms

(Continued)

Table 10.1: Results of RCTs Based on Drug Combinations and Their Results (Continued)

Author	Year of Publication	Study Design	Number of Enrollments	Kinds of Probiotic and Dosage	Key Findings
Tomusiak et al.	2015	RCT	160	inVag (*L. fermentum* 57A, *L. plantarum* 57B, *L. gasseri* 57C)	Reduced pH and Nugent score; colonization confirmed
van de Wijgert et al.	2020	RCT	68	Behavioral counseling, metronidazole, Ecologic Femi + Gynophilus LP	BV incidence reduced in metronidazole and Ecologic Femi+ groups
S. Yang	2020	RCT	66	*L. rhamnosus* RC-14 + GR-1 vs. placebo 12 weeks)	Safe; no differences in vaginal microbiota
Qi et al.	2023	RCT	67	MET ± oral probiotics (*L. gasseri* TM13, *L. crispatus* LG55)	No cure rate improvement; restored vaginal health post-cure
Boroumand Rezazadeh et al.	2024	RCT	55	Vaginal vs. oral probiotics	Both improved BV outcomes; no difference between oral vs. vaginal
Zhang et al.	2021	RCT	126	MET ± oral probiotics (*L. rhamnosus* GR-1, *L. reuteri* RC-14; 30 days)	No cure rate improvement; safe
Reznichenko et al.	2020	RCT	166	Oral probiotic (*L. crispatus*, *L. brevis*, *L. acidophilus*) vs. placebo	Reduced recurrence and prolonged remission
Gille et al.	2016	RCT	320	Oral *L. rhamnosus* GR-1 + *L. reuteri* RC-14 vs. placebo (8 weeks)	No effect on vaginal health; safe
Gilboa et al.	2005	RCT	117	Intravaginal probiotics vs. control (IVF)	No improvement in pregnancy outcomes
Wei et al.	2024	RCT	379 (60 supplemented)	Transvaginal Lactobacillus supplementation in FET patients	Improved clinical pregnancy rates in women with prior failed cycles
Husain et al.	2020	RCT	238	Oral *L. rhamnosus* GR-1 + *L. reuteri* RC-14 vs. placebo until delivery	No differences in BV rates or microbiota
Cohen et al.	2020	RCT	228	*L. crispatus* CTV-05 (Lactin-V) vs. placebo (11 weeks)	Reduced BV recurrence; well tolerated
Larsson et al.	2008	RCT	100	Vaginal clindamycin ± Lactobacilli capsules	Probiotics prolonged time to relapse; no effect on initial cure
Mastromarino et al.	2009	RCT	39	Vaginal Lactobacillus tablet vs. placebo (7 days)	All probiotic group BV-free; flora restored
Bradshaw et al.	2012	RCT	–	Oral metronidazole + vaginal probiotic vs. controls	No differences in BV recurrence
Eriksson et al.	2005	RCT	–	Lactobacilli-loaded tampons vs. placebo	No additional benefit
Czaja et al.	2007	RCT	30	*L. crispatus* CTV-05 vs. placebo (5 days)	Safe; some mild side effects

(Continued)

Table 10.1: (Continued)

Author	Year of Publication	Study Design	Number of Enrollments	Kinds of Probiotic and Dosage	Key Findings
Pirotta et al.	2004	RCT	278	Oral or vaginal Lactobacilli vs. placebo (during antibiotics)	No reduction in vulvovaginitis
Laue et al.	2018	RCT	34	Probiotic yogurt (*L. crispatus*, *L. gasseri*, *L. jensenii*, *L. rhamnosus*)	BV prevalence lower; improved symptoms
Heczko et al.	2015	RCT	241	prOVag + antibiotics vs. placebo	Delayed BV/AV relapse; improved microbiological outcomes
Anukam et al.	2006a	RCT	40	Vaginal *L. rhamnosus* GR-1 + *L. reuteri* RC-14 vs. metronidazol	90% cure rate; effective in restoring microbiota
Anukam et al.	2006b	RCT	125	Oral metronidazole ± oral probiotics (*L. rhamnosus* GR-1, *L. reuteri* RC-14)	Higher cure and Lactobacillus recovery with probiotics
Martinez et al.	2009	RCT	55	Fluconazole ± probiotics (*L. rhamnosus* GR-1, *L. reuteri* RC-14)	Reduced yeast presence and vaginal discharge
Vicariotto et al.	2014	RCT	34	Vaginal *L. fermentum* LF15 + *L. plantarum* LP01 tablets	Reduced Nugent scores; restored microbiota
Wang Ya et al.	2010	RCT	120	Vaginal probiotics (*L. rhamnosus*, *L. acidophilus*, *S. thermophilus*)	Reduced BV recurrence; long-term benefit
Krauss-Silva et al.	2011	RCT	644	Oral probiotics vs. placebo (<20 weeks pregnant women with BV)	No significant reduction in preterm birth; safe

therapy by significantly reducing vaginal discharge, yeast culture positivity, and symptomatic persistence in VVC (31). These findings suggest variable synergism depending on strain composition and trial design.

In bacterial vaginosis, probiotic adjuncts to metronidazole or clindamycin have shown mixed results. Some studies indicated that oral probiotic adjunctive treatment did not increase the cure rate compared to metronidazole alone (14), whereas others demonstrated reduced recurrence rates and prolonged remission when probiotics were combined with standard-of-care antibiotics (1, 5). Probiotic supplementation has also been shown to restore vaginal Lactobacillus abundance and reduce Nugent scores after antibiotic cure, supporting a role in long-term microbiota stabilization (24).

Nutritional synergism has also been explored. A multicenter RCT tested myo-inositol, probiotics, and micronutrients as a combined supplement in women attempting natural conception. Although overall time-to-pregnancy and clinical pregnancy rates were similar to control, overweight women receiving the combination supplement showed shorter time-to-conception, comparable to non-overweight women, suggesting a potential synergistic metabolic benefit in this subgroup (20).

Taken together, these findings indicate that while probiotics alone may not consistently outperform standard therapies, their integration with pharmacological agents, dietary regimens, or micronutrient supplementation demonstrates potential synergistic benefits. Such effects appear particularly relevant in PCOS-related endocrine modulation, fertility enhancement, and recurrence prevention in infectious diseases.

10.5 SAFETY PROFILES AND POTENTIAL SIDE EFFECTS

Safety evaluation of probiotic supplementation has been a central component of randomized controlled trials across gynecological, obstetric, and metabolic disorders. Overall, the majority of RCTs consistently report that probiotics are well tolerated, with few, if any, serious adverse events.

10.5.1 Pregnancy-Related Safety

Several large-scale RCTs have investigated oral probiotic supplementation during pregnancy. In a triple-blind trial including 320 women <12 weeks of gestation, oral *Lactobacillus rhamnosus* GR-1 and *L. reuteri* RC-14 were administered for 8 weeks, showing no significant adverse events or detrimental effects on maternal or neonatal outcomes (29). Similarly, oral probiotic use during early pregnancy did not modify the vaginal microbiota but was well tolerated without increased risk of complications (33). In a Brazilian cohort, probiotics administered to women with asymptomatic BV or intermediate infections were also deemed safe, with only minor nonspecific events reported (35). Collectively, these findings suggest that probiotic use during pregnancy is safe, even though efficacy in modifying vaginal microbiota or preventing preterm delivery remains inconclusive.

10.5.2 Gynecological Infections

RCTs on bacterial vaginosis and vulvovaginal candidiasis largely confirm probiotic safety. In Chinese BV patients, oral probiotic adjunctive treatment did not increase cure rates compared to metronidazole but no serious adverse effects occurred (14). Vaginal probiotic tablets significantly reduced symptoms and Nugent scores without safety concerns (23), while intravaginal *Lactobacillus* supplementation was well tolerated in recurrent BV, with no difference in adverse event rates compared to placebo (27). For VVC, probiotic supplementation alongside fluconazole reduced symptom severity and recurrence, with no notable side effects (9, 31). Mild, self-limiting events such as vaginal discharge or irritation were reported in some cases (36), but these were comparable between probiotic and placebo groups.

10.5.3 PCOS and Metabolic Disorders

Multiple RCTs in women with polycystic ovary syndrome have confirmed the tolerability of probiotics. Time-restricted eating with or without probiotics improved metabolic and hormonal markers, and all interventions were well tolerated (7, 16). Synbiotic supplementation selectively improved metabolic parameters without adverse effects (17). In women with hyperprolactinemia and PCOS, probiotics combined with metformin reduced prolactin levels without additional safety concerns compared to metformin alone (6).

10.5.4 General Safety Considerations

Across trials in diverse populations, probiotics have been consistently safe. Studies in women undergoing IVF reported that intravaginal probiotic administration did not influence pregnancy outcomes and was not associated with adverse events (10, 19). Probiotic-containing yogurt improved BV recovery with no safety issues (12). Even in long-term interventions for recurrent BV, both oral and vaginal probiotics demonstrated high tolerability, with adverse events comparable to placebo (1, 5).

10.6 SEXUAL BEHAVIOR

Randomized controlled trials indicate that probiotic supplementation may enhance sexual behavior and sexual function in women with polycystic ovary syndrome and those with treatment-emergent sexual dysfunction associated with psychotropic medications.

In a clinical trial by Azizi-Kutenaee et al. (2022) ($N = 40$) involving PCOS patients, participants were randomized to receive either letrozole monotherapy or letrozole combined with Lactofem capsules containing multiple probiotic strains (*Lactobacillus acidophilus, Bifidobacterium bifidus, L. rutri,* and *L. fermentum*, 2×10^9 CFU each) administered as 500 mg daily. The probiotic regimen involved one month of probiotic pretreatment followed by one month of combined therapy. The combination group showed significantly improved chemical and clinical pregnancy rates (10% versus 0%), enhanced scores across all Female Sexual Function Index (FSFI) domains, increased total FSFI scores, and improved body image perceptions compared to letrozole alone (8).

Complementing these findings, Nazir et al. (2024) ($N = 112$) examined women with depressive disorders experiencing SSRI-associated sexual dysfunction. Participants were randomized to receive either SSRIs with adjunctive Lactofem probiotics (containing the same probiotic strains at identical concentrations) or SSRIs alone for 8 weeks. The probiotic-augmented group demonstrated significantly better outcomes across all FSFI domains, including sexual satisfaction, along with greater reduction in depressive symptom severity compared to the control group (37).

Collectively, current evidence from randomized trials suggests that probiotic supplementation, particularly when combined with pharmacological agents such as letrozole or SSRIs, may yield meaningful improvements in sexual function, reproductive outcomes, and psychological well-being in women with PCOS and mood disorders.

10.7 SYNBIOTICS

Randomized double-blind placebo-controlled trials have increasingly investigated synbiotic formulations – combining probiotics with prebiotics – as a therapeutic strategy for improving reproductive and metabolic health in women.

One such trial evaluated the impact of synbiotic supplementation on metabolic parameters and apelin levels in patients with polycystic ovary syndrome. The study enrolled 88 women with PCOS, aged 19–37 years, who were randomly assigned to receive either a synbiotic supplement ($n = 44$) or a placebo ($n = 44$) over a 12-week period. Results demonstrated a significant reduction in serum apelin-36 levels in the synbiotic group compared to the placebo group (adjusted mean difference: –4.05; 95% CI: –7.15, –0.96; $p = 0.004$). In contrast, no significant changes were observed in insulin resistance, as measured by HOMA-IR, or in the inflammatory marker CRP. These findings suggest that while synbiotic supplementation may selectively modulate certain metabolic biomarkers such as apelin, its effects on broader endocrine and inflammatory pathways in PCOS appear limited (17).

Synbiotic interventions have been studied for their potential effects on fertility outcomes in addition to metabolic parameters. A multicenter, randomized, double-blind, controlled trial investigated a nutritional supplement containing myo-inositol, probiotics, and selected micronutrients in women attempting natural conception (20). Participants between 18 and 38 years of age were randomly assigned to either a standard prenatal supplement (including folic acid, iron, calcium, iodine, and β-carotene) or an experimental formulation enhanced with myo-inositol, probiotics, B vitamins, vitamin D, and zinc. The analysis revealed no statistically significant differences between groups in time-to-conception or clinical pregnancy rates in the overall study population. However, a prespecified subgroup analysis of overweight women demonstrated a statistically significant reduction in time-to-conception in the intervention group compared to controls. This observation suggests that synbiotic-micronutrient supplementation may attenuate obesity-related subfertility (20).

Current evidence from randomized controlled trials indicates that synbiotic regimens are well-tolerated and may provide specific therapeutic advantages, including modulation of metabolic biomarkers such as apelin in PCOS and potentially improved conception timing in overweight women with reduced fertility. Nevertheless, comprehensive clinical benefits across diverse reproductive and endocrine outcomes require further substantiation through larger, methodologically robust clinical trials.

10.8 CHALLENGES AND CONTROVERSIES

Despite the growing interest in probiotics and synbiotics as adjunctive therapies in gynecology, obstetrics, and reproductive medicine, several challenges and controversies remain.

10.8.1 Inconsistent Clinical Efficacy

A significant area of debate centers on the variable clinical outcomes observed across randomized controlled trials. For instance, adjunctive oral probiotic therapy failed to enhance bacterial vaginosis cure rates relative to metronidazole monotherapy in a Chinese patient cohort (14, 38). Parallel findings emerged from obstetric research, where probiotic supplementation administered to pregnant women with elevated preterm delivery risk did not significantly decrease spontaneous birth incidence before either 34 or 37 weeks' gestation (35). Furthermore, in populations undergoing in vitro fertilization, intravaginal probiotic instillation following oocyte retrieval demonstrated no improvement in pregnancy rates or modification of vaginal colonization patterns

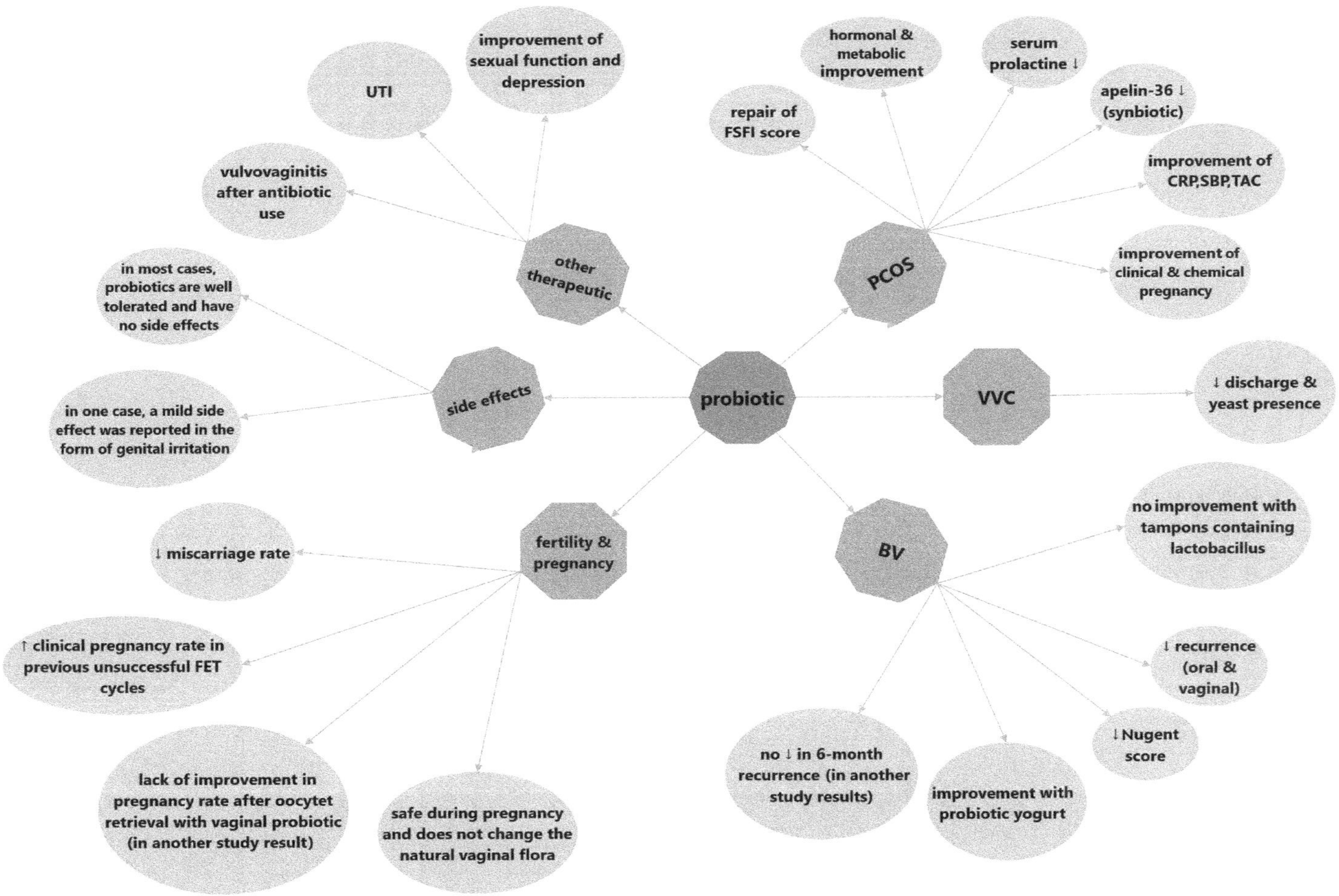

Figure 10.1 A mind map of effects of probiotics on women's infertility. (From the Authors.)

(19). These collective observations underscore that despite compelling biological rationale, the therapeutic efficacy of probiotic interventions remains inconsistently demonstrated across clinical settings.

10.8.2 Strain-Specific and Formulation Variability

Another challenge is the heterogeneity of probiotic strains and formulations used across trials. Some studies demonstrated significant benefits, such as the combination of *Lactofem* with letrozole in PCOS patients, which improved sexual function and pregnancy outcomes (8), while others reported no differences between probiotic and placebo groups, as seen in trials assessing oral lactobacilli in pregnancy (33, 34). This variability complicates the interpretation and generalization of findings, suggesting that therapeutic benefits may be strain-dependent and context-specific.

10.8.3 Duration of Effect and Recurrence Issues

Even when probiotics are initially effective, their benefits may diminish after cessation. In BV, while probiotics combined with antibiotics reduced recurrence in some studies (1, 5), others showed no long-term advantage once supplementation stopped, with high inter-individual variability in microbiota response (2). This raises concerns about sustainability of probiotic effects and the need for maintenance regimens.

10.8.4 Population-Specific Outcomes

Controversies also arise from subgroup analyses. For instance, combined myo-inositol, probiotics, and micronutrient supplementation did not improve conception rates overall, but overweight women appeared to benefit through shorter time-to-conception (20). Similarly, synbiotic supplementation in PCOS patients significantly reduced apelin levels but failed to improve insulin resistance or CRP (17). These findings suggest probiotics and synbiotics may be beneficial only in specific populations or metabolic phenotypes, rather than universally.

10.8.5 Methodological Limitations

Many RCTs have relatively small sample sizes, short follow-up durations, and lack standardized outcome measures, contributing to conflicting results. For example, small pilot studies using intravaginal probiotics in BV showed positive outcomes (24), whereas larger trials with stricter endpoints failed to replicate these results (27). Additionally, high dropout rates in pregnancy-related trials limit statistical power and may underestimate potential effects (35).

10.9 DISCLAIMER

In the preparation of this manuscript, artificial intelligence tools were utilized to enhance language accuracy and clarity. The integration of AI-assisted writing technology supported the efficient refinement of scientific content, ensuring precision in terminology and improved coherence. The author acknowledges that AI served as an aid in the writing process, but all intellectual input, data interpretation, and final content decisions were made independently by the author.

REFERENCES

1. Reznichenko H, Henyk N, Maliuk V, Khyzhnyak T, Tynna Y, Filipiuk I, et al. Oral intake of Lactobacilli can be helpful in symptomatic bacterial vaginosis: A randomized clinical study. *J Low Genit Tract Dis.* 2020;24(3):284–9.
2. van de Wijgert JHHM, Verwijs MC, Agaba SK, Bronowski C, Mwambarangwe L, Uwineza M, et al. Intermittent Lactobacilli-containing vaginal probiotic or metronidazole use to prevent bacterial vaginosis recurrence: A pilot study incorporating microscopy and sequencing. *Scientific Reports.* 2020;10(1):3884.
3. Tomusiak A, Strus M, Heczko PB, Adamski P, Stefański G, Mikołajczyk-Cichońska A, et al. Efficacy and safety of a vaginal medicinal product containing three strains of probiotic bacteria: A multicenter, randomized, double-blind, and placebo-controlled trial. *Drug Des Devel Ther.* 2015;9:5345–54.
4. Ya W, Reifer C, Miller LE. Efficacy of vaginal probiotic capsules for recurrent bacterial vaginosis: A double-blind, randomized, placebo-controlled study. *Am J Obstet Gynecol.* 2010;203(2):120–6.
5. Heczko PB, Tomusiak A, Adamski P, Jakimiuk AJ, Stefański G, Mikołajczyk-Cichońska A, et al. Supplementation of standard antibiotic therapy with oral probiotics for bacterial vaginosis and aerobic vaginitis: A randomised, double-blind, placebo-controlled trial. *BMC Women's Health.* 2015;15(1):115.

6. Urooj Zafar, Syeda Amber Zaidi, Hafiz Syed Muhammad Osama Jafri, Sana Imran, Afreen Bhatty and Fizza Abidi. Effectiveness of metformin and its combination with probiotic in polycystic ovarian disease with hyperprolactinemia: A randomized clinical trial. *J Pharm Res Int (Internet).* 2021 Oct. 26 (cited 2025 Sep. 23);33(47A):268–74.
7. Talebi S, Shab-Bidar S, Mohammadi H, Moini A, Djafarian K. The effects of intermittent fasting diet alone or in combination with probiotic supplementation in comparison with calorie-restricted diet on metabolic and hormonal profile in patients with polycystic ovary syndrome: Study protocol for a randomized clinical trial. *Trials.* 2023;24(1):690.
8. Azizi-Kutenaee M, Heidari S, Taghavi SA, Bazarganipour F. Probiotic effects on sexual function in women with polycystic ovary syndrome: A double blinded randomized controlled trial. *BMC Womens Health.* 2022;22(1):373.
9. Thekho AJ, Mendiratta V, Garg T, Kaur R, Yadav V. Role of probiotic in vulvovaginal candidiasis: A randomised controlled non-blinded trial from India. *Indian J Dermatol.* 2024;69(5):422.
10. Wei Q, Chen H, Zou H, Zhang H, Liu S, Zheng J, et al. Impact of vaginal microecological differences on pregnancy outcomes and endometrial microbiota in frozen embryo transfer cycles. *J Assist Reprod Genet.* 2024;41(4):929–38.
11. Anukam K, Osazuwa E, Ahonkhai I, Ngwu M, Osemene G, Bruce AW, et al. Augmentation of antimicrobial metronidazole therapy of bacterial vaginosis with oral probiotic *Lactobacillus rhamnosus* GR-1 and *Lactobacillus reuteri* RC-14: Randomized, double-blind, placebo controlled trial. *Microbes and Infection.* 2006;8(6):1450–4.
12. Laue C, Papazova E, Liesegang A, Pannenbeckers A, Arendarski P, Linnerth B, et al. Effect of a yoghurt drink containing Lactobacillus strains on bacterial vaginosis in women – A double-blind, randomised, controlled clinical pilot trial. *Benef Microbes.* 2018;9(1):35–50.
13. Happel AU, Singh R, Mitchev N, Mlisana K, Jaspan HB, Barnabas SL, et al. Testing the regulatory framework in South Africa – A single-blind randomized pilot trial of commercial probiotic supplementation to standard therapy in women with bacterial vaginosis. *BMC Infect Dis.* 2020;20(1):491.
14. Zhang Y, Lyu J, Ge L, Huang L, Peng Z, Liang Y, et al. Probiotic Lacticaseibacillus rhamnosus GR-1 and *Limosilactobacillus reuteri* RC-14 as an adjunctive treatment for bacterial vaginosis do not increase the cure rate in a Chinese Cohort: A prospective, parallel-group, randomized, controlled study. *Front Cell Infect Microbiol.* 2021;11:669901.
15. Rezazadeh MB, Zanganeh M, Jarahi L, Fatehi Z. Comparative efficacy of oral and vaginal probiotics in reducing the recurrence of bacterial vaginosis: A double-blind clinical trial. *BMC Womens Health.* 2024;24(1):575.
16. Talebi S, Shab-Bidar S, Askari G, Mohammadi H, Moini A, Djafarian K. Comparison of the impact of intermittent fasting diet alone or in conjunction with probiotic supplementation versus calorie-restricted diet on inflammatory, oxidative stress, and antioxidant capacity biomarkers in women with polycystic ovary syndrome: A randomized placebo-controlled trial. *J Res Med Sci.* 2025;30:5.
17. Karimi E, Moini A, Yaseri M, Shirzad N, Sepidarkish M, Hossein-Boroujerdi M, et al. Effects of synbiotic supplementation on metabolic parameters and apelin in women with polycystic ovary syndrome: A randomised double-blind placebo-controlled trial. *British Journal of Nutrition.* 2018;119(4):398–406. https://doi.org/10.1017/S0007114517003920
18. Thanaboonyawat I, Pothisan S, Petyim S, Laokirkkiat P. Pregnancy outcomes after vaginal probiotic supplementation before frozen embryo transfer: A randomized controlled study. *Sci Rep.* 2023;13(1):11892.
19. Gilboa Y, Bar-Hava I, Fisch B, Ashkenazi J, Voliovitch I, Borkowski T, et al. Does intravaginal probiotic supplementation increase the pregnancy rate in IVF-embryo transfer cycles? *Reprod Biomed Online.* 2005;11(1):71–5.
20. Chan SY, Barton SJ, Loy SL, Chang HF, Titcombe P, Wong JT, et al. Time-to-conception and clinical pregnancy rate with a myo-inositol, probiotics, and micronutrient supplement: Secondary outcomes of the NiPPeR randomized trial. *Fertil Steril.* 2023;119(6):1031–42.
21. Anukam KC, Osazuwa E, Osemene GI, Ehigiagbe F, Bruce AW, Reid G. Clinical study comparing probiotic Lactobacillus GR-1 and RC-14 with metronidazole vaginal gel to treat symptomatic bacterial vaginosis. *Microbes Infect.* 2006;8(12–13):2772–6.
22. Larsson PG, Stray-Pedersen B, Ryttig KR, Larsen S. Human lactobacilli as supplementation of clindamycin to patients with bacterial vaginosis reduce the recurrence rate; a 6-month, double-blind, randomized, placebo-controlled study. *BMC Womens Health.* 2008;8:3.
23. Mastromarino P, Macchia S, Meggiorini L, Trinchieri V, Mosca L, Perluigi M, et al. Effectiveness of Lactobacillus-containing vaginal tablets in the treatment of symptomatic bacterial vaginosis. *Clin Microbiol Infect.* 2009;15(1):67–74.

24. Vicariotto F, Mogna L, Del Piano M. Effectiveness of the two microorganisms *Lactobacillus fermentum* LF15 and *Lactobacillus plantarum* LP01, formulated in slow-release vaginal tablets, in women affected by bacterial vaginosis: A pilot study. *J Clin Gastroenterol.* 2014;48(Suppl. 1):S106–12.
25. Bradshaw CS, Pirotta M, De Guingand D, Hocking JS, Morton AN, Garland SM, et al. Efficacy of oral metronidazole with vaginal clindamycin or vaginal probiotic for bacterial vaginosis: Randomised placebo-controlled double-blind trial. *PLoS One.* 2012;7(4):e34540.
26. Eriksson K, Carlsson B, Forsum U, Larsson PG. A double-blind treatment study of bacterial vaginosis with normal vaginal lactobacilli after an open treatment with vaginal clindamycin ovules. *Acta Derm Venereol.* 2005;85(1):42–6.
27. Cohen CR, Wierzbicki MR, French AL, Morris S, Newmann S, Reno H, et al. Randomized trial of lactin-V to prevent recurrence of bacterial vaginosis. *N Engl J Med.* 2020;382(20):1906–15.
28. Qi F, Fan S, Fang C, Ge L, Lyu J, Huang Z, et al. Orally administrated *Lactobacillus gasseri* TM13 and *Lactobacillus crispatus* LG55 can restore the vaginal health of patients recovering from bacterial vaginosis. *Front Immunol.* 2023;14:1125239.
29. Gille C, Böer B, Marschal M, Urschitz MS, Heinecke V, Hund V, et al. Effect of probiotics on vaginal health in pregnancy. EFFPRO, a randomized controlled trial. *Am J Obstet Gynecol.* 2016;215(5):608. e1–e7.
30. Pirotta M, Gunn J, Chondros P, Grover S, O'Malley P, Hurley S, et al. Effect of lactobacillus in preventing post-antibiotic vulvovaginal candidiasis: A randomised controlled trial. *BMJ.* 2004;329(7465):548.
31. Martinez RC, Franceschini SA, Patta MC, Quintana SM, Candido RC, Ferreira JC, et al. Improved treatment of vulvovaginal candidiasis with fluconazole plus probiotic *Lactobacillus rhamnosus* GR-1 and *Lactobacillus reuteri* RC–14. *Lett Appl Microbiol.* 2009;48(3):269–74.
32. Mollazadeh-Narestan Z, Yavarikia P, Homayouni-Rad A, Samadi Kafil H, Mohammad-Alizadeh-Charandabi S, Gholizadeh P, et al. Comparing the effect of probiotic and fluconazole on treatment and recurrence of vulvovaginal candidiasis: A triple-blinded randomized controlled trial. *Probiotics Antimicrob Proteins.* 2023;15(5):1436–46.
33. Husain S, Allotey J, Drymoussi Z, Wilks M, Fernandez-Felix BM, Whiley A, et al. Effects of oral probiotic supplements on vaginal microbiota during pregnancy: A randomised, double-blind, placebo-controlled trial with microbiome analysis. *BJOG.* 2020;127(2):275–84.
34. Yang S, Reid G, Challis JRG, Gloor GB, Asztalos E, Money D, et al. Effect of oral probiotic *Lactobacillus rhamnosus* GR-1 and *Lactobacillus reuteri* RC-14 on the vaginal microbiota, cytokines and chemokines in pregnant women. *Nutrients.* 2020;12(2).
35. Krauss-Silva L, Moreira ME, Alves MB, Braga A, Camacho KG, Batista MR, et al. A randomised controlled trial of probiotics for the prevention of spontaneous preterm delivery associated with bacterial vaginosis: Preliminary results. *Trials.* 2011;12:239.
36. Czaja CA, Stapleton AE, Yarova-Yarovaya Y, Stamm WE. Phase I trial of a *Lactobacillus crispatus* vaginal suppository for prevention of recurrent urinary tract infection in women. *Infect Dis Obstet Gynecol.* 2007;2007:35387.
37. Hashemi-Mohammadabad N, Taghavi SA, Lambert N, Moshtaghi R, Bazarganipour F, Sharifi M. Adjuvant administration of probiotic effects on sexual function in depressant women undergoing SSRIs treatment: A double-blinded randomized controlled trial. *BMC Psychiatry.* 2024;24(1):44.
38. Rapisarda AMC, Pino A, Grimaldi RL, Caggia C, Randazzo CL, Cianci A. *Lacticaseibacillus rhamnosus* CA15 (DSM 33960) strain as a new driver in restoring the normal vaginal microbiota: A randomized, double-blind, placebo-controlled clinical trial. *Front Surg.* 2022;9:1075612.

11 Conclusion

Amir Masoud Firouzabadi, Samaneh Harimi, Maryam Azizi-Kutenaei, and Farzaneh Fesahat

11.1 INTEGRATED SUMMARY OF MECHANISTIC EVIDENCE

Female infertility represents a multifaceted clinical challenge, accounting for approximately 40% to 50% of all infertility cases globally. This condition emerges from a complex interplay of hormonal imbalances, genetic predispositions, metabolic dysregulation, and environmental stressors. Within this landscape, the quality and quantity of the oocyte stand as the primary determinants of both natural conception and the success of assisted reproductive technologies (ART). Advanced maternal age remains the most significant irreversible factor, as it is inextricably linked to increased meiotic errors, a higher incidence of aneuploidy, and a progressive decline in mitochondrial function. Furthermore, the modern reproductive environment is complicated by metabolic disorders such as polycystic ovary syndrome (PCOS), obesity, and diabetes, which disrupt oocyte maturation through systemic inflammation and insulin resistance.

Central to the pathophysiology of oocyte degradation is the phenomenon of oxidative stress. An imbalance between the production of reactive oxygen species (ROS) and the body's antioxidant defenses leads to catastrophic damage to oocyte DNA, lipids, and proteins. This cellular damage is often exacerbated by lifestyle factors, including chronic stress and poor nutrition, as well as exposure to endocrine-disrupting chemicals like bisphenol A (BPA) and heavy metals. As the field of reproductive medicine evolves beyond the mere pursuit of high oocyte yields, contemporary research has pivoted toward enhancing the "competence" of the oocyte. This shift has brought nutraceuticals to the forefront, as these compounds offer a mechanism-based approach to mitigating oxidative damage, restoring mitochondrial bioenergetics, and optimizing the follicular microenvironment.

11.1.1 Inositol: Restoring Metabolic and Ovarian Harmony

The therapeutic application of inositols has revolutionized the management of ovulatory dysfunction, particularly in the context of PCOS. Myo-inositol (MI) acts as a pivotal second messenger in the FSH signaling pathway, playing a direct role in calcium-mediated oocyte maturation and cytoplasmic integrity. Clinical data robustly support the administration of 4 grams of MI daily to improve insulin sensitivity, lower circulating androgens, and restore the LH/FSH ratio. While D-chiro-inositol (DCI) contributes to metabolic regulation, its overabundance within the ovary can be detrimental to oocyte quality. Therefore, maintaining the physiological MI/DCI ratio of 40:1 is essential for achieving superior clinical outcomes, including increased rates of mature MII oocytes and improved live birth markers in IVF and ICSI cycles.

11.1.2 Alpha-Lipoic Acid: A Universal Shield against Cellular Aging

Alpha-lipoic acid (ALA) serves as a potent, universal antioxidant that safeguards the oocyte and its mitochondrial genome against oxidative damage, a key factor in preserving developmental competence. By scavenging reactive oxygen species and regenerating endogenous antioxidants – including glutathione, vitamin C, vitamin E, and coenzyme Q10 – ALA protects DNA, lipids, and critical cellular structures like the meiotic spindle from oxidative insults. In clinical settings, particularly among women with PCOS or chronic inflammation, ALA supplementation has been shown to reduce systemic inflammatory markers and enhance oocyte quality, maturation, and morphology. Moreover, adding ALA to IVF embryo culture media can buffer developing embryos from oxidative stress in vitro, improving blastocyst development and embryo viability. These effects are especially notable in older women or those with diminished ovarian reserve, highlighting ALA as a multi-level protector against cellular aging in reproductive medicine.

11.1.3 Coenzyme Q10: Reinvigorating Mitochondrial Bioenergetics

Coenzyme Q10 (CoQ10) is a vital component of the mitochondrial electron transport chain, playing a central role in oocyte bioenergetics. The process of oocyte maturation, meiotic division, and early embryonic cleavage is highly energy-intensive, necessitating robust ATP production. CoQ10 facilitates this energy generation while simultaneously acting as a lipid-soluble antioxidant,

DOI: 10.1201/9781003741541-11

neutralizing reactive oxygen species within the mitochondria. This dual action preserves mitochondrial integrity and reduces oxidative damage, which is a major contributor to age-related decline in oocyte quality. Supplementation with CoQ10 has shown particular benefit in women with diminished ovarian reserve (DOR) and those of advanced reproductive age, where mitochondrial efficiency is often compromised. Clinical evidence indicates that CoQ10 therapy is associated with higher fertilization rates, improved embryo morphology, and enhanced developmental competence, effectively addressing one of the most significant hurdles in geriatric reproductive medicine. Moreover, CoQ10 may synergize with other antioxidants in the follicular environment, further supporting oocyte viability and competence.

11.1.4 Melatonin: Safeguarding the Follicular Microenvironment

Melatonin exerts its influence far beyond the regulation of circadian rhythms; it acts as a high-affinity scavenger of free radicals within the follicular fluid. By stimulating essential antioxidant enzymes such as superoxide dismutase (SOD) and glutathione peroxidase (GPx), melatonin creates a protective shield for the developing follicle. When integrated into ART protocols – often in synergy with myo-inositol and folic acid – melatonin has been shown to enhance the clinical pregnancy rate by fostering an environment conducive to successful oocyte maturation and subsequent embryo implantation.

11.1.5 Folates: The Foundations of Genomic Integrity

Folate and its synthetic form, folic acid, are essential nutrients in reproductive health, serving as critical cofactors in one-carbon metabolism, DNA synthesis, and epigenetic programming. Adequate folate levels support the synthesis of purines and thymidylate, maintain genomic stability, and enable proper DNA methylation – processes crucial for oocyte maturation and follicular development. Research consistently demonstrates that optimal serum and red blood cell folate concentrations correlate with improved oocyte quality, higher fertilization rates, and increased live birth outcomes in IVF cycles. Moreover, folate supplementation helps regulate homocysteine levels, reducing oxidative stress and improving the uterine environment. In PCOS patients, combination therapies of folate with inositol derivatives have proven particularly effective in increasing the yield of mature oocytes and enhancing embryo competence.

11.1.6 Micronutrient Synergy: The Critical Role of Selenium and Zinc

Selenium (Se) and Zinc (Zn) act as essential trace elements and cofactors for multiple antioxidant systems that protect oocytes, support ovulation, and facilitate early embryogenesis. Zinc is crucial for processes like "zinc sparks" during fertilization and for proper DNA synthesis in dividing cells, whereas selenium is a key component of selenoproteins, including glutathione peroxidase, which guard oocytes and embryos against oxidative damage and DNA fragmentation. Clinical evidence, including randomized trials, cohort studies, and case reports, indicates that targeted supplementation with Se and Zn can improve oocyte yield, embryo quality, and pregnancy outcomes, particularly in women with oxidative stress-related infertility conditions such as PCOS, endometriosis, premature ovarian insufficiency (POI), and recurrent pregnancy loss. These minerals also play complementary roles in thyroid function and insulin metabolism, further supporting reproductive success in affected patients.

11.1.7 Vitamin D: Endocrine Modulation and Ovarian Response

Vitamin D functions more as a pro-hormone than a simple vitamin, exerting significant influence over the hypothalamic–pituitary–ovarian (HPO) axis. It modulates the expression of genes involved in estrogen synthesis and improves insulin sensitivity, which is crucial for maintaining regular ovulatory cycles. Clinical studies indicate that correcting vitamin D deficiency is a low-cost, high-impact intervention that yields improved reproductive outcomes, particularly in women undergoing ART, by optimizing the endometrial environment and supporting ovarian response.

11.1.7.1 Probiotics: The Emerging Frontier of the Reproductive Microbiome

The reproductive microbiome is an emerging field highlighting the role of probiotics, particularly Lactobacillus strains, in supporting fertility. Clinical trials in women with PCOS have demonstrated that probiotic supplementation, alone or in combination with interventions such as time-restricted eating (TRE) or pharmacological agents like letrozole and metformin, can improve metabolic, hormonal, inflammatory, and antioxidant profiles while enhancing reproductive outcomes and sexual function. In the context of assisted reproductive technologies, while evidence is mixed, some studies indicate that vaginal or transvaginal Lactobacillus supplementation may reduce miscarriage rates and improve clinical pregnancy rates in women with prior unsuccessful embryo transfers. Probiotics also help prevent dysbiosis-related complications such as bacterial vaginosis (BV) and vulvovaginal candidiasis (VVC), which are associated with poor fertility outcomes. Although direct correlations with live birth rates remain to be confirmed in large-scale trials, probiotics are generally safe and well-tolerated, even during pregnancy, and provide a valuable adjunct in a holistic infertility management strategy (Figure 11.1).

11.2 TRANSLATIONAL AND CLINICAL RECOMMENDATIONS

The integration of nutraceuticals into clinical practice offers a low-risk, evidence-based supportive strategy to enhance oocyte quality and optimize the success of ART. To achieve maximal therapeutic efficacy, clinicians should consider the following structured recommendations regarding dosage, duration, and patient-specific applications.

11.2.1 Precision Dosing of Inositol: Restoring the Ovarian Ratio

For patients presenting with PCOS, the administration of MI in combination with DCI is highly recommended. The clinical gold standard is a daily dose of 4 grams of MI and 100 mg of DCI, maintaining the physiological 40:1 ratio. To ensure optimal oocyte maturation and metabolic stabilization, treatment should ideally commence 3 to 6 months prior to the initiation of an IVF or ICSI cycle. Clinicians must be cautious with high-dose DCI monotherapy, as excessive levels can paradoxically impair oocyte quality; maintaining the 40:1 ratio is key to enhancing insulin sensitivity and increasing the yield of mature MII oocytes.

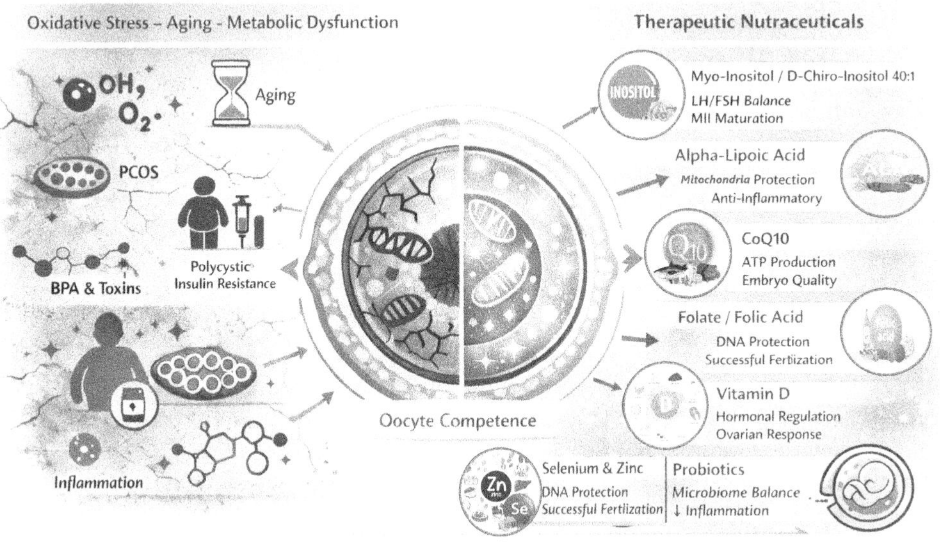

Figure 11.1 The interplay between pathological stressors and therapeutic nutraceuticals. This diagram illustrates the dual landscape of oocyte competence, contrasting systemic degradative factors with targeted nutritional interventions. The left panel depicts how oxidative stress, advanced maternal aging, and metabolic dysregulation (such as PCOS and insulin resistance) trigger cellular damage and systemic inflammation. Conversely, the right panel showcases the protective role of therapeutic nutraceuticals, including inositol, CoQ10, and alpha-lipoic acid, which aim to restore mitochondrial function, protect DNA integrity, and optimize the hormonal environment for successful fertilization and embryo quality. (From the Authors.)

11.2.2 Alpha-Lipoic Acid: Timing the Antioxidant Defense

The clinical efficacy of ALA is highly dependent on timing, dosage, and co-administration strategies. Studies indicate that 200–600 mg/day of ALA for 6–12 weeks prior to ART cycles optimizes oocyte competence, mitochondrial function, and embryo quality. Co-supplementation with myo-inositol or other antioxidants has demonstrated synergistic benefits, particularly in patients with insulin resistance or inflammation-driven infertility.

Practical considerations include the route of administration and formulation: oral ALA is widely studied but bioavailability can be affected by food, whereas vaginal ALA has shown localized benefits in conditions such as subchorionic hematoma and cervical shortening. Future research should focus on large, well-designed RCTs with live birth as the primary endpoint, as well as optimized formulations and studies in challenging patient populations like poor responders and women with recurrent pregnancy loss. Appropriately timed ALA supplementation represents a promising strategy to strengthen antioxidant defense, enhance oocyte and embryo quality, and improve overall reproductive outcomes.

11.2.3 Bioenergetic Support with Coenzyme Q10: A Strategy for Advanced Age

In the management of DOR and women over 35 years, CoQ10 provides critical support for mitochondrial function and overall oocyte quality. Recommended oral supplementation ranges from 120 to 300 mg per day, aimed at enhancing ATP production and reducing ROS-induced mitochondrial and cellular damage. Because mitochondrial CoQ10 pools are gradually replenished, pretreatment should ideally begin at least 2 to 3 months prior to follicular stimulation in ART cycles. Duration and consistency of supplementation are key, as clinical outcomes – including fertilization rates, embryo morphology, and the number of high-quality embryos – have been shown to correlate with the length of CoQ10 pretreatment. Beyond direct mitochondrial support, CoQ10 may also improve the follicular microenvironment, preserving antioxidant capacity and reducing oxidative stress that could otherwise compromise oocyte competence. Taken together, these effects highlight CoQ10 as a valuable intervention for enhancing reproductive potential in women experiencing age-related or reserve-related fertility challenges.

11.2.4 Melatonin: Optimizing the Circadian Follicular Microenvironment

To shield the developing follicle from oxidative insults, a nightly dose of 3–5 mg of melatonin is recommended. Supplementation should start at least one month before the IVF cycle and continue until the day of oocyte retrieval. Beyond its role in sleep, melatonin acts synergistically with other antioxidants like MI and folic acid to improve embryo viability. Due to its sedative properties, it should be strictly administered before bedtime to align with natural circadian rhythms.

11.2.5 Folate and Folic Acid: Foundations of Early Embryogenesis

As a cornerstone of preconception and infertility care, folate (or folic acid) should be administered at 400–800 µg daily, ideally starting at least 3 months before conception or as ART cycles. This timing ensures adequate folate stores throughout the ~90-day period of follicle maturation, which is critical for oocyte quality and epigenetic stability in early embryos. Clinical studies indicate that combining folate with inositols significantly increases the proportion of mature oocytes, improves fertilization and embryo quality, and may reduce the risk of early developmental errors. Bioactive forms of folate, such as 5-methyltetrahydrofolate, should be prioritized in patients with MTHFR or other methylation-related polymorphisms to optimize DNA methylation and one-carbon metabolism. Maintaining adequate folate intake through the ovarian stimulation, luteal phase, and early pregnancy supports both implantation and early embryonic development, complementing standard ART protocols.

11.2.6 Micronutrient Optimization: Selenium and Zinc Synergy

Optimizing Se (55–200 µg/day) and Zn (10–30 mg/day) intake strengthens antioxidant enzyme systems, supports follicular development, and improves ART outcomes. Best practices recommend initiating supplementation 8–12 weeks prior to ART cycles, reflecting the duration of oocyte maturation. While supplementation is generally safe within established therapeutic windows, clinicians should monitor serum levels and oxidative stress markers to avoid potential toxicity. Personalized approaches – considering baseline nutritional status, genetic polymorphisms affecting mineral metabolism, and underlying infertility etiology – maximize efficacy. In conditions like POI, PCOS, and endometriosis, supplementation should be integrated with conventional fertility treatments and, when appropriate, combined with other antioxidants such as vitamins C and E or CoQ10 for synergistic benefits. Ongoing monitoring of ovarian response, hormonal profiles, and pregnancy outcomes ensures the intervention remains both effective and safe.

11.2.7 Vitamin D: Endocrine Calibration and Systemic Health

Given its role in HPO axis regulation and insulin modulation, vitamin D supplementation should be tailored to the patient's baseline serum levels, typically ranging from 1,000 to 4,000 IU daily. A minimum of 8 to 12 weeks is required to achieve stable physiological levels before beginning ovarian stimulation. Correction of vitamin D deficiency is particularly crucial for PCOS and ART patients, as it optimizes the endometrial receptivity and reduces hyperandrogenism.

11.2.8 Probiotics: Cultivating the Reproductive Environment

To optimize the reproductive environment and prevent metabolic and microbiota dysregulation, daily supplementation with 10^9–10^{10} CFU of Lactobacillus strains is recommended. Clinical evidence suggests that probiotics should ideally be introduced 4–6 weeks prior to an ART cycle and maintained throughout treatment to support vaginal health, reduce infections, and modulate systemic inflammation.

Table 11.1: Summary of Key Nutraceuticals, Mechanisms of Action, and Clinical Benefits in Female Infertility

Nutraceutical	Primary Mechanism of Action	Target Population/ Condition	Key Clinical Benefits
Myo-Inositol (MI) & D-Chiro-Inositol (DCI)	Regulation of insulin signaling, restoration of LH/FSH ratio, enhancement of calcium-mediated oocyte maturation	PCOS, insulin resistance	Improved ovulation, increased MII oocytes, enhanced IVF/ICSI outcomes
Alpha-Lipoic Acid (ALA)	Potent antioxidant, mitochondrial protection, reduction of systemic inflammation	PCOS, obesity, inflammatory infertility	Improved oocyte morphology, reduced oxidative stress, enhanced embryo viability
Coenzyme Q10 (CoQ10)	Enhancement of mitochondrial ATP production, ROS scavenging	Advanced maternal age, DOR	Improved fertilization rate, better embryo quality, restored mitochondrial efficiency
Melatonin	Free radical scavenging, stimulation of antioxidant enzymes (SOD, GPx)	ART patients, oxidative stress–related infertility	Improved oocyte maturation, higher clinical pregnancy rates
Folate/Folic Acid	One-carbon metabolism, DNA synthesis, epigenetic regulation	Preconception care, PCOS, ART	Enhanced oocyte quality, reduced developmental errors, improved live birth rates
Selenium (Se)	Selenoprotein-mediated antioxidant defense, DNA protection	PCOS, POI, endometriosis	Reduced DNA fragmentation, improved oocyte yield
Zinc (Zn)	Regulation of meiotic progression, fertilization-associated zinc sparks	Ovulatory disorders, oxidative stress	Improved fertilization potential, early embryo development
Vitamin D	Modulation of HPO axis, insulin sensitivity, gene regulation	PCOS, ART candidates, Vitamin D deficiency	Improved ovarian response, enhanced endometrial receptivity
Probiotics (*Lactobacillus* spp.)	Regulation of reproductive microbiome, reduction of inflammation	PCOS, dysbiosis-related infertility	Improved metabolic balance, reduced infection-related ART failure

Probiotic supplementation has demonstrated synergistic effects in combination with:

- **Dietary interventions**: TRE plus probiotics enhanced metabolic and inflammatory markers in overweight and obese PCOS patients.
- **Pharmacological therapy**: Lactofem combined with letrozole improved chemical and clinical pregnancy rates, sexual function, and body image in PCOS; probiotics with metformin reduced prolactin in hyperprolactinemic patients.
- **Antimicrobial therapy**: Adjunctive probiotics in BV or VVC reduced recurrence rates, improved Nugent scores, and restored Lactobacillus dominance after antibiotic cure.

While the impact on live birth rates requires further validation, probiotics provide a safe, well-tolerated, and complementary approach to improving reproductive outcomes, particularly in populations with PCOS, recurrent infections, or metabolic risk factors. Incorporating probiotics into fertility care may help create a stable, anti-inflammatory, and microbiota-friendly reproductive environment, supporting both natural conception and ART success.

11.3 FINAL THOUGHTS ON THE FUTURE OF NUTRACEUTICALS IN WOMEN'S HEALTH

11.3.1 Toward a New Paradigm in Reproductive Medicine

The evidence synthesized in this work underscores a transformative shift in the management of female infertility. Targeted nutraceuticals – including myo-inositol, alpha-lipoic acid, coenzyme Q10, melatonin, vitamin D, and essential trace elements – have moved from the periphery of "alternative options" to the center of evidence-based supportive therapy. By directly addressing the biochemical hallmarks of infertility, such as oxidative stress, mitochondrial decay, and systemic inflammation, these compounds provide a biological foundation upon which the success of assisted reproductive technologies can be built. The transition from merely increasing oocyte quantity to actively enhancing oocyte "competence" represents the next major milestone in reproductive endocrinology.

11.3.2 Precision Nutraceuticals: The Dawn of Personalized Fertility Care

One of the most compelling trends for the future is the transition toward personalized supplementation. Rather than a "one-size-fits-all" approach, the future of women's health lies in tailoring nutraceutical interventions to the individual's unique metabolic profile, PCOS phenotype, ovarian reserve, and genetic background. By integrating nutritional science with omics technologies – such as nutrigenomics and epigenetics – clinicians will soon be able to prescribe specific synergistic combinations (e.g., MI with melatonin or ALA) that maximize oocyte quality while minimizing unnecessary costs or side effects. This mechanism-based precision will ensure that each patient receives the right molecule at the right dose for their specific reproductive stage.

11.3.3 Synergy of Lifestyle and Bioactive Compounds

The future of nutraceuticals is inextricably linked to a holistic view of the patient. Bioactive compounds do not act in isolation; their efficacy is profoundly influenced by the systemic environment. Integrating these supplements with structured lifestyle modifications – including anti-inflammatory diets, regular physical activity, and psychological stress management – will likely yield the most significant improvements in metabolic and reproductive health. This integrative approach not only treats existing infertility but also serves as a preventive strategy, safeguarding the reproductive potential of women long before they enter the IVF laboratory.

11.3.4 Navigating the Challenges: From Bench to Bedside

Despite the promising data, the path to full clinical standardization requires addressing several critical gaps. The field necessitates large-scale, multicenter randomized controlled trials (RCTs) to define the definitive "therapeutic windows" for various patient populations. Furthermore, as we look toward the next generation, evaluating the long-term safety and potential transgenerational epigenetic effects of high-dose supplementation remains a priority. Additionally, while this work focuses on maternal health, the emerging role of paternal nutraceuticals and their impact on embryo quality is a burgeoning field that warrants intensive investigation to achieve a comprehensive understanding of couple-based fertility.

Index

For Product Safety Concerns and Information please contact our EU
representative GPSR@taylorandfrancis.com
Taylor & Francis Verlag GmbH, Kaufingerstraße 24, 80331 München, Germany

www.ingramcontent.com/pod-product-compliance
Lightning Source LLC
LaVergne TN
LVHW080118031026
849429LV00030B/375
* 9 7 8 1 0 4 1 2 3 5 5 2 1 *